ADVANCES IN NEUROLOGY

Volume 95

ADVANCES IN NEUROLOGY

Volume 95

Myoclonic Epilepsies

Editors

Antonio V. Delgado-Escueta, M.D.
Professor of Neurology and Director of Comprehensive Epilepsy Program
David Geffen School of Medicine at UCLA and
Epilepsy Center of Excellence at VA GLAHS, Los Angeles, CA, USA

Renzo Guerrini, M.D.
Professor of Pediatric Neurology
Head—Epilepsy, Neurophysiology, Neurogenetics Unit
Department of Developmental Neurosciences
University of Pisa and Institute for Clinical Research IRCCS Stella
Maris Foundation, Pisa, Italy

Marco T. Medina, M.D.
Professor of Neurology and Director of
Neurology Training Program
National Autonomous University of Honduras
Tegucigalpa, Honduras

Pierre Genton, M.D.
Neurologist
Centre Saint-Paul-Hôpital Henri Gastaut, Marseille, France

Michelle Bureau, M.D.
Former Head of EEG Department
Centre Saint-Paul-Hôpital Henri Gastaut, Marseille, France

Charlotte Dravet, M.D.
Centre Saint-Paul-Hôpital Henri Gastaut, Marseille, France
Childhood Epilepsy Consultant, INPE-IRCCS Stella Maris Foundation
Pisa, Italy and Catholic University, Roma, Italy

Editorial Assistants

Katerina Tanya Perez-Gosiengfiao, M.D.
Iris E. Martínez-Juárez, M.D.
Reyna M. Durón, M.D.
Comprehensive Epilepsy Program & VA GLAHS Epilepsy Center of Excellence
David Geffen School of Medicine at UCLA, Los Angeles, California

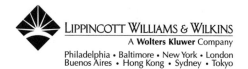

LIPPINCOTT WILLIAMS & WILKINS
A **Wolters Kluwer** Company
Philadelphia • Baltimore • New York • London
Buenos Aires • Hong Kong • Sydney • Tokyo

Library
University of Texas
at San Antonio

Acquisitions Editor: Anne M. Sydor
Developmental Editor: Scott Scheidt
Production Manager: David Murphy
Manufacturing Manager: Benjamin Rivera
Compositor: TechBooks
Printer: Maple Press

© 2005 by LIPPINCOTT WILLIAMS & WILKINS
530 Walnut Street
Philadelphia, PA 19106 USA
LWW.com

Printed in the USA

Library of Congress Cataloging-in-Publication Data

ISBN: 0-7817-5248-5
ISSN: 0091-3952

Care has been taken to confirm the accuracy of the information presented and to describe generally accepted practices. However, the authors, editors, and publisher are not responsible for errors or omissions or for any consequences from application of the information in this book and make no warranty, expressed or implied, with respect to the currency, completeness, or accuracy of the contents of the publication. Application of this information in a particular situation remains the professional responsibility of the practitioner.

The authors, editors, and publisher have exerted every effort to ensure that drug selection and dosage set forth in this text are in accordance with current recommendations and practice at the time of publication. However, in view of ongoing research, changes in government regulations, and the constant flow of information relating to drug therapy and drug reactions, the reader is urged to check the package insert for each drug for any change in indications and dosage and for added warnings and precautions. This is particularly important when the recommended agent is a new or infrequently employed drug.

Some drugs and medical devices presented in this publication have Food and Drug Administration (FDA) clearance for limited use in restricted research settings. It is the responsibility of the health-care provider to ascertain the FDA status of each drug or device planned for use in their clinical practice.

10 9 8 7 6 5 4 3 2 1

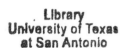

Advances in Neurology Series

Dedication

Charlotte Dravet

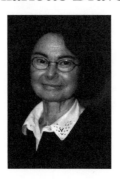

Charlotte Dravet graduated from Marseilles University as a psychiatrist with a primary interest in pediatrics. Henri Gastaut offered her a position as the resident physician at the then newly created Centre Saint Paul, Marseille, where she remained for the rest of her career, although her travels brought her to many places around the globe. She worked as a clinical epileptologist in Marseille under Henri Gastaut and Joseph Roger, in close collaboration with her friend Michelle Bureau as the resident electroencephalographer, and with many epileptologists who spread the teachings of the Marseille School, among whom are Carlo-Alberto Tassinari, Bernardo Dalla Bernardina, Renzo Guerrini, Marco T. Medina and Pierre Genton, to mention only a few. Charlotte Dravet served as President of the French Chapter of the International League Against Epilepsy, and received in 2004 the European Epilepsy Prize.

Her MD thesis was devoted to the delineation of the "Petit Mal variant" or childhood encephalopathy with diffuse slow spike-and-waves and was represented in the seminal paper "Childhood epileptic encephalopathy with diffuse slow spike waves (otherwise known as "petit mal variant") or Lennox Syndrome (Gastaut H, et al., *Epilepsia,* 1966; 139–179). This work led to international recognition of the Lennox-Gastaut syndrome. She also studied the evolution of West syndrome (Dravet C, Got AM, Coquery C, Munari C, Roger J, Soulayrol R and Tassinari *CA. Electroencephalogr Clin Neurophysiol.* 1971;30:372). She was further interested in childhood absence epilepsies ("A study of the distribution of petit mal absences in the child in relation to his activities" with Bureau M, Guey J, and Roger J, in *Electroencephalogr Clin Neurophysiol.* 1968;25:513 and "A study of the rhythm of petit mal absences in children in relation to prevailing situations. The use of EEG telemetry during psychological examinations, school exercises and periods of inactivity" with Guey J, Bureau M, Dravet C, Roger J, in *Epilepsia,* 1969;10:441–451). Her interest also included partial epilepsies in infancy (*Epilepsia* 1989;30:807–812) and myoclonus in degenerative disorders. However, she devoted much creative energy to the delineation of myoclonic epilepsies in childhood, and described both "benign myoclonic epilepsy of infancy" (Dravet C, Bureau M, *Rev Electroencephalogr Neurophysiol Clin.* 1981;11:438–444, and "severe myoclonic epilepsy of infancy" (Les épilepsies graves de l'enfant. Vie Med 1978;8:543–548). In 2001, the Commission on Classification of the International League Against Epilepsy justly decided that severe myoclonic epilepsy of infancy should now be called "the Dravet syndrome." Her life was and still is dedicated to the care of patients with epilepsy and she advocates for their causes.

Contents

Section 1: Introduction to Concepts and Classifications

Section 2: Myoclonic Epilepsies of Infancy and Childhood

Section 3: Myoclonic Epilepsies of Adolescence and Adulthood

Contributing Authors

María Elisa Alonso, MD
Neurogenetics and Molecular Biology
Instituto Nacional de Neurología y Neurocirugía
Tlalpan, Mexico
Genetic Epilepsy Studies (GENESS) International
*   Consortium*

Claudia Amador, MD
Neurology Service Hospital Escuela and Neurology
*   Training Program*
National Autonomous University of Honduras
Tegucigalpa, Honduras

Danielle M. Andrade
Program in Genetics and Genomic Biology
The Hospital for Sick Children
Toronto, Canada

Yutaka Awaya, MD
Department of Pediatrics
Seibo International Catholic Hospital
Tokyo, Japan

Dongsheng Bai, MD
California Comprehensive Epilepsy Program
David Geffen School of Medicine at UCLA
Los Angeles, California
Genetic Epilepsy Studies (GENESS) International
*   Consortium*

Julia N. Bailey, PhD
California Comprehensive Epilepsy Program
David Geffen School of Medicine
Neuropsychiatric Institute
University of California at
Los Angeles, California
Genetic Epilepsy Studies (GENESS) International
*   Consortium*

Michel Baulac, MD
Neurology/Epilepsy Department
Paris VI University
Hôpital Pitie-Salpetriere
Paris, France

Stephanie Baulac, PhD
Neurology/Epilepsy Department
Paris VI University
Hôpital Pitie-Salpetriere
Paris, France

Paolo Bonanni, MD
Epilepsy, Neurophysiology, and Neurogenetics Unit
Department of Child Neurology and Psychiatry
University of Pisa and Research Institute 'Stella
*   Maris' Foundation*
Pisa, Italy

Paola Brovedani, MD
Epilepsy, Neurophysiology and Neurogentics Unit
Department of Child Neurology and Psychiatry
University of Pisa and Research Institute 'Stella
*   Maris' Foundation*
Pisa, Italy

Michelle Bureau, MD
Centre Saint-Paul-Hôpital Henri Gastaut
Marseille, France

Roberto Caraballo, MD
Department of Neurology
Hospital de Pediatria Juan P. Garrahan
Buenos Aires, Argentina

Ignacio Pascual Castroviejo, MD
Pediatric Neurology Department
University Hospital La Paz
Madrid, Spain
Genetic Epilepsy Studies (GENESS) International
*   Consortium*

Ricardo Cersosimo, MD
Department of Neurology
Hospital de Pediatria Juan P. Garrahan
Buenos Aires, Argentina

Elayne M. Chan

Program in Genetics and Genomic Biology
The Hospital for Sick Children
Toronto, Canada

Franz Chaves-Sell, MD

Universidad de Ciencias Médicas and Academia
* Nacional de Medicina de Costa Rica*
Hospital Clinica Biblica
Genetic Epilepsy Studies (GENESS) International
* Consortium*

Ozlem Cokar, MD

Department of Neurology
Haseki Research and Educational Hospital
Fatih-Istanbul, Turkey

Sergio Cordova, MD

National Institute of Neurology and
* Neurosurgery*
Mexico City, Mexico
Genetic Epilepsy Studies (GENESS)
* International Consortium*

Patrick Cossette, MD, MSc, FRCPC

Centre for Research in Neuroscience
McGill University Health Center
* Research Institute*
Service de Neurologie
Centre Hospitalier de l'Université de
* Montréal-Hôpital Notre-Dame*
Montréal, Québec, Canada

Athanasios Covanis, MD

Neurology Department
The Childrens Hospital "Agia Sophia" Goudi
Athens, Greece

Bernardo Dalla Bernardina, MD

Servizio Neuropsichiatria Infantile
Policlinico G.B. Rossi
Universita degli Studi di Verona
Verona, Italy

Francesca Darra, MD

Servizio di Neuropsichiatria Infantile
Policlinico G.B. Rossi
Universita degli Studi di Verona
Verona, Italy

Fabrizio A. De Falco, MD

Department of Neurology
Loreto Nuovo Hospital
Napoli, Italy

Antonio V. Delgado-Escueta, MD

Department of Neurology
David Geffen School of Medicine
* at UCLA*
Los Angeles, California
and Comprehensive Epilepsy Program
Epilepsy Center of Excellence at VA GLAHS
Genetic Epilepsy Studies (GENESS)
* International Consortium*

Hermann Doose, MD

Norddeutsches Epilepsie-Zentrum
Raisdorf, Germany

Charlotte Dravet, MD

Centre Saint-Paul-Hôpital Henri Gastaut
Marseille, France

Martina Durner, MD

Division of Statistical Genetics
Department of Biostatistics
Mailman School of Public Health
Columbia University
New York, New York

Reyna M. Durón, MD

National Autonomous University of Honduras
* Tegucigalpa, Honduras*
California Comprehensive Epilepsy
* Program*
David Geffen School of Medicine at UCLA
Los Angeles, California
Genetic Epilepsy Studies (GENESS)
* International Consortium*

Natalio Fejerman, MD

Department of Neurology
Hospital de Pediatria Juan P. Garrahan
Buenos Aires, Argentina

Elena Fontana, MD

Servizio di Neuropsichiatria Infantile
Policlinico G.B. Rossi
Universita degli Studi di Verona
Verona, Italy

Silvana Franceschetti, MD

Department of Clinical Neurophysiology
Instituto Nazionale
* Neurologico Carlo Besta*
Milan, Italy

Ying-Hui Fu, PhD
Department of Neurology
University of California San Francisco
San Francisco, California

Goryu Fukuma, MD
Department of Pediatrics
School of Medicine
Fukuoka University
Fukuoka, Japan

Yukio Fukuyama, MD
Child Neurology Institute
Tokyo, Japan

Makoto Funatsuka
Department of Pediatrics
Tokyo Women's Medical University
Tokyo, Japan

Pierre Genton, MD
Centre Saint-Paul-Hôpital Henri Gastaut
Marseille, France

Isabelle Gourfinkel-An, MD, PhD
Neurology/Epilepsy Department
Paris VI University
INSERM U289
Hôpital Pitie-Salpetriere
Paris, France

David Greenberg, PhD
Mailman School of Public Health
and New York State Psychiatric Institute
Columbia Genome Center
Columbia-Presbyterian Medical Center
New York, New York

M. Grothe, MD
Department of Neuropediatrics
Klinik für Neuropädiatrie der Universität
Kiel, Germany

Renzo Guerrini, MD
Epilepsy, Neurophysiology, and Neurogenetics Unit
Department of Child Neurology and Psychiatry
University of Pisa and Research Institute 'Stella
* Maris' Foundation*
Pisa, Italy

A. Hahn, MD
Department of Neuropediatrics
Zentrum Kinderheilkunde und Jugendmedizin
University of Giessen
Giessen, Germany

Mark Hallett
Chief, Human Motor Control Section
National Institute of Neurological Disorders
* and Stroke*
National Institutes of Health
Bethesda, Maryland

Kitami Hayashi, MD
Department of Pediatrics
Tokyo Women's Medical University
Tokyo, Japan

Armin Heils, MD
Clinic of Epileptology
Institute of Human Genetics
University of Bonn
Bonn, Germany

Shinichi Hirose, MD
Department of Pediatrics
School of Medicine
Fukuoka University
Fukuoka, Japan

Kaoru Imai
Department of Pediatrics
Tokyo Women's Medical University
Tokyo, Japan

Aurelio Jara-Prado
Neurogenetics and Molecular Biology
Instituto Nacional de Neurología y Neurocirugía
Tlalpan, Mexico
Genetic Epilepsy Studies (GENESS) International
* Consortium*

Sunao Kaneko, MD
Department of Neuropsychiatry
School of Medicine
Hirosaki University
Aomori, Japan

Sonia Khan, MD
Neurosciences Department
Riyadh Armed Forces Hospital
Saudi Arabia
Genetic Epilepsy Studies (GENESS)
* International Consortium*

G. Kurlemann, MD
Department of Neuropediatrics
University of Münster
Münster, Germany

Eric Leguern, MD, PhD
Département de Génétique, Cytogénétique et
Embryologie
INSERM U289
Hôpital Pitie-Salpetriere
Paris, France

Lourdes León, MD
Angel Leaños Hospital
Guadalajara, Mexico
Genetic Epilepsy Studies (GENESS) International
*   Consortium*

Minerva López-Ruiz, MD
Unidad de Neurología y Neurocirugía
Hospital General de Mexico
Mexico City, México

Anne Lortie, MD
Service de Neurologie
Centre Hospitalier de
*   l'Université de Montréal-Hôpital Notre-Dame*
Montréal, Québec, Canada

Jesús Machado-Salas, MD, PhD
Neuroanatomy and Neurosciences CUT
David Geffen School of Medicine at UCLA
Los Angeles, California and Comprehensive
*   Epilepsy Program*
Epilepsy Center of Excellence at VA GLAHS
Genetic Epilepsy Studies (GENESS) International
*   Consortium*

Carla Marini, MD
Epilepsy, Neurophysiology and
*   Neurogentics Unit*
Department of Child Neurology and Psychiatry
University of Pisa and Research Institute 'Stella
*   Maris' Foundation*
Pisa, Italy

Iris E. Martínez-Juárez, MD
California Comprehensive Epilepsy
*   Program*
David Geffen School of Medicine at UCLA
Los Angeles, California
National Institute of Neurology and Neurosurgery
*   Mexico City, Mexico,*
Genetic Epilepsy Studies (GENESS) International
*   Consortium*

Marco T. Medina, MD
Neurology Training Program
Postgraduate Studies Direction
National Autonomous University of Honduras
Tegucigalpa, Honduras
California Comprehensive Epilepy Program
David Geffen School of Medicine at UCLA
Epilepsy Center of Excellence at VA GLAHS
Genetic Epilepsy Studies (GENESS) International
*   Consortium*

Lizardo Mija, MD
Neurological Sciences Institute
Lima, Peru

Berge Minassian, MD
Division of Neurology
The Hospital for Sick Children
Toronto, Canada

Akihisa Mitsudome, MD
Department of Pediatrics
School of Medicine
Fukuoka University
Fukuoka, Japan

Ryoji Morita, PhD
Laboratory for Neurogenetics
RIKEN Brain Science Institute
Saitama, Japan
Genetic Epilepsy Studies (GENESS) International
*   Consortium*

Bernard A. Neubauer, MD
Department of Neuropediatrics
Zentrum Kinderheilkunde und Jugendmedizin
University of Giessen
Giessen, Germany

Adriana Ochoa-Morales
Neurogenetics and Molecular Biology
Instituto Nacional de Neurología y Neurocirugía
Tlalpan, Mexico
Genetic Epilepsy Studies (GENESS) International
*   Consortium*

Hirokazu Oguni, MD, PhD
Department of Pediatrics
Tokyo Women's Medical University
Tokyo, Japan

Makiko Osawa, MD
Department of Pediatrics
Tokyo Women's Medical University
Tokyo, Japan

Deb Pal, PhD
Division of Statistical Genetics
Department of Biostatistics,
Mailman School of Public Health,
and Columbia Genome Center, Columbia
University and Clinical and Genetic
Epidemiology Unit
New York State Psychiatric Institute
New York, New York

Lucio Parmeggiani, MD
Epilepsy, Neurophysiology, Neurogenetics Unit
Department of Child Neurology
University of Pisa and Research Psychiatry
Institute 'Stella Maris' Foundation
Pisa, Italy

Katerina Tanya Perez-Gosiengfiao, MD
California Comprehensive Epilepsy Program
David Geffen School of Medicine at UCLA
Los Angeles, California
Genetic Epilepsy Studies (GENESS) International
Consortium

Gregorio Pineda, MD
Department of Neurology and Pediatrics
David Geffen School of Medicine at UCLA
Los Angeles, California
Genetic Epilepsy Studies (GENESS) International
Consortium

Lucio Portilla, MD
Department of Epilepsy
Institute of Neurological Sciences
Lima, Peru

Louis J. Ptácek, MD
Department of Neurology
University of California, San Francisco
San Francisco, California
Howard Hughes Medical Institute

Jaime Ramos-Peek, MD
National Institute of Neurobiology and Neurosurgery
Mexico City, Mexico
Genetic Epilepsy Studies (GENESS) International
Consortium

Ricardo Ramos-Ramírez, MD
Unidad de Neurología y Neurocirugía
Hospital General de Mexico
Mexico City, México

Astrid Rasmussen-Almarez, MD
Neurogenetics and Molecular Biology
Instituto Nacional de Neurología y
Neurocirugía
Tlalpan, Mexico

Joseph Roger, MD
Centre Saint-Paul-Hôpital Henri Gastant
Marseille, France

Guy A. Rouleau, MD
Centre for Research in Neuroscience
McGill University Health Center
Research Institute
Montreal, Québec, Canada

Francisco Rubio-Donnadieu, MD
National Institute of Neurology and
Neurosurgery
Mexico City, Mexico
Genetic Epilepsy Studies (GENESS) International
Consortium

Jean-Marc Saint-Hilaire, MD
Service de Neurologie
Centre Hospitalier de l'Université de
Montréal-Hôpital Notre-Dame
Montréal, Québec Canada
Center for Research in Neuroscience, McGill
University Health Center Research Institute

Masako Sakauchi
Department of Pediatrics
Tokyo Women's Medical University
Tokyo, Japan

T. Sander, MD
Gene Mapping Center (GMC)
Max-Delbrück-Centrum
Berlin, Germany

Raman Sankar, MD, PhD
Departments of Neurology and Pediatrics
David Geffen School of Medicine at UCLA
Los Angeles, California and
Mattel Children's Hospital at UCLA

Harvey B. Sarnat, MD, F.R.C.P.C.
Departments of Pediatrics, Pathology
(Neuropathology) and Clinical Neurosciences
University of Calgary Faculty of Medicine and
Alberta Children's Hospital
Calgary, Alberta, Canada

Seigo Shirakawa
Department of Pediatrics
Tokyo Women's Medical University
Tokyo, Japan

René Silva, MD
Nuestra Señora de La Paz Hospital
San Miguel, El Salvador
Genetic Epilepsy Studies (GENESS) International
*   Consortium*

Ulrich Stephani, MD
Clinics for Neuropediatrics
Christian-Albrechts-University Germany
Kiel, Germany

Miyabi Tanaka, MD
California Comprehensive Epilepsy Program
David Geffen School of Medicine at UCLA
Los Angeles, California
Genetic Epilepsy Studies (GENESS)
*   International Consortium*

Carlo Alberto Tassinari, MD
Ospedale Bellaria, Bologna, Italy

I. Tuxhorn, MD
Epilepsy Center Bethel
Klinik Mara
Bielefeld, Germany

Eiichiro Uyama, MD
Department of Neurology
Kumamoto University School of Medicine
Kumamoto, Japan

Michel Vanasse
Centre for Research in Neuroscience
McGill University Health Center
*   Research Institute*
Montréal, Quebec, Canada

Karen Weissbecker, PhD
Hayward Genetics Center
Human Genetics Program
Tulane University School of Medicine
New Orleans, Louisiana
Genetic Epilepsy Studies (GENESS) International
*   Consortium*

Bronwyn Westling, MD
Hayward Genetics Center
Human Genetics Program
Tulane University School of Medicine
New Orleans, Louisiana
Genetic Epilepsy Studies (GENESS) International
*   Consortium*

St. Waltz, MD
Department of Neuropediatrics
Klinik für Neuropädiatrie der Universität
Kiel, Germany

James W. Wheless, MD
Departments of Neurology and Pediatrics
University of Texas School of Medicine
Houston, Texas

Federico Zara, MD
Laboratory of Neurogenetics
Department of Neuroscience and Rehabilitation
Institute G. Gaslini
Genova, Italy

Preface

The first mission of this volume is to convert the epilepsy community to the concept that cures of epilepsies will not be found until we accept the epilepsies as diseases. The definition of molecular etiologies of specific epilepsy syndromes speaks eloquently to this concept.

The second mission of this volume is to educate general practitioners, pediatricians, child neurologists and adult neurologists, as well as students and researchers in the neurosciences, about the myoclonic epilepsies and their importance in the totality of the epilepsies. Myoclonic epilepsies account for at least six percent to as much as twenty-five percent (conservative estimate) of all epilepsies. Myoclonic epilepsies are frequently misdiagnosed, underdiagnosed, misunderstood and, hence, *mistreated* (using the wrong antiepileptic drugs).

The book is designed to help the practitioner understand the phenotypes and subvarieties of myoclonic epilepsies and their molecular defects. It should introduce the practitioners to the present advances in molecular genetics that are unraveling the etiologies of myoclonic epilepsies. At the same time, it should prepare him/her to the coming advances in molecular genetics that should further break down the causes of myoclonic epilepsies. While this book incorporates molecular advances, it remains a practical treatise with a strong clinical basis.

To aid the practitioner, the editors (see photo) use their combined experience to provide a table in Chapter one that summarizes the diagnostic characteristics useful in identifying myoclonic epilepsies of infancy and early childhood which are often mistakenly placed under the rubric of Lennox-Gastaut syndrome. A table listing the clinical features of childhood absences mixed with myoclonias that differentiate them from classic juvenile myoclonic epilepsy is also provided in Chapter one. In two separate treatment chapters, one for myoclonic epilepsies of infancy and childhood and another for myoclonic epilepsies of childhood and adolescence, there are two separate treatment algorithms representing the combined experience of the editors and contributing chapter authors. These two algorithms take the practitioner step by step in the decision process involved in choosing the first options for treatment. The algorithms then deal with specific co-morbidities and clinical issues or settings that prompt the addition of a second antiepileptic drug or induce major changes in direction and the use of another antiepileptic drug option. Because double blind randomized studies of antiepileptic drugs are not available in these specific myoclonic epilepsies, the editors consider these algorithms as aids for the practitioner in making decisions in treatment.

The third mission of this book is to stimulate further collaboration and cross-fertilization between investigators within and across continents and the fusion of clinical and molecular studies of the epilepsies. Until now there has been little effort to validate and classify the subvarieties of myoclonic epilepsies except by a few epilepsy units. Collaborations should accelerate further clarification of the phenotypes and subvarieties of the myoclonic epilepsies, which, in turn, should lead to the definition of their specific molecular lesions.

The fourth mission of this book is the most pleasant—to honor the work of Charlotte Dravet and the "school of epileptology" in Marseilles that crystallized in the Centre Saint Paul, which was created by Henri Gastaut in 1960 and was later led by Joseph Roger. It is true that the part of the flowering of epileptology can be traced to a great extent to the schooling received by the international students from Charlotte Dravet and her teachers, Michelle Bureau and their many colleagues. The *raison d'être* behind this volume are the international students of Charlotte Dravet. They gathered informally in 2000 during the American Epilepsy Society annual meeting in Los Angeles and talked about their dream of having a symposium-workshop and a book to honor the life work of Charlotte Dravet. Over the next several months in 2001, Charlotte's colleagues (see photo) joined her students in support for this endeavor. Raul Harris-Collazo, Ph.D., Ortho-McNeil Neuroscience Scientific Liaison, worked closely with the students and colleagues of Dr. Dravet to obtain an educational grant from Ortho-McNeil. Many of Charlotte's students and colleagues participated as chairs, speakers, and attendees at what was a truly international symposium-workshop, "Myoclonic Epilepsies of Infancy, Childhood, Adolescence and Adulthood." This meeting to honor Dr. Charlotte Dravet was held in Seattle on December 5–6, 2002. We are grateful to the many students and colleagues of Dr. Dravet who have contributed to this volume as editors and chapter authors.

As the first and only collation of all that is known about idiopathic myoclonic epilepsies of infancy, childhood, adolescence, and adulthood; this book should be an indispensable resource for teaching students, house officers, and fellows, as well as practitioners of pediatrics, internal medicine, neurology, and neurosurgery.

Antonio V. Delgado-Escueta, MD
Renzo Guerrini, MD
Marco T. Medina, MD
Pierre Genton, MD
Michelle Bureau, MD
March 2004

Editors

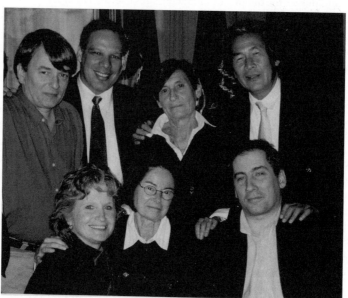

From left to right, top: Pierre Genton, Marco T. Medina, Michelle Bureau, Antonio V. Delgado Escueta. Botton: Susan Pietsch-Escueta, Charlotte Dravet and Renzo Guerrini.

Foreword

Myoclonic epilepsies include a variety of clinical forms that are defined in terms of age of expression, natural history, etiology, pathophysiology, and prognosis. Over the last ten years, important new genetic and pathophysiological data have been produced that make it necessary to reconsider the criteria used to define idiopathic epilepsy. This book comes at the right time to update readers concerning the latest information and will contribute to the ongoing revision of the classification of epilepsies and epileptic syndromes.

The book is partly based on an International Workshop organized in honor of Charlotte Dravet, which saw the participation of the most important specialists in the field. After a first conceptual section, the different types of myoclonic epilepsies of infancy, childhood, adolescence and adulthood, identified on the basis of their clinical pictures and/or etiopathogenesis, are reviewed in great detail by authors who have contributed most to our knowledge of each syndrome. It is enough here to cite the names of two "eponymous founders," Dieter Janz for juvenile myoclonic epilepsy (JME) and Charlotte Dravet for severe myoclonic epilepsy in infancy (SMEI), and that of Antonio Delgado-Escueta himself, who pioneered the molecular genetic investigations into epilepsies that led to collaborative studies of JME and progressive myoclonic epilepsy (PME). The result is a comprehensive overview of the state of the art that whoever is interested in epilepsy as a clinician or basic scientist will find particularly valuable.

It is now clear that the myoclonic jerks associated with EEG polyspike-waves may occur as a *primary* genetically-determined dysfunction of the excitable mechanisms (as in the case of JME) or as part of the clinical picture of genetic encephalopathies such as PME. The clear-cut differences in electroclinical semeiology between the myoclonic symptoms of JME and PME are probably related to pathogenetic differences that are still only partially understood. However, a number of neurophysiological protocols based on combinations of stimulation and recording techniques using sophisticated signal analysis procedures have now been developed and can be expected to extend our knowledge in the near future.

What seems to me to be one of the main merits of the book is that it provides a precise and complete repertoire of the syndromes with myoclonic epilepsy that have been characterized in different age ranges. How far this clinically-based nosography fits the genetic information is not an easy question to answer: the correspondance is very close in cases such as PME, but not in others such as myoclonic astatic epilepsy, which does not seem to correlate with a definite genotype, or those that may include different sub-syndromes associated with different mutations, as has been suggested for JME. The main problems arise from the fact that similar channel gene mutations may have a wide range of clinical expressions in terms of their clinical picture and prognosis. One typical case is that of *SCNAI* mutations, which have been found to be associated with generalised epilepsies with febrile seizures, as well as (GEFS$^+$) syndrome and SMEI. GEFS$^+$ covers a wide spectrum of clinical forms that, at one extreme, fit the definition of idiopathic epilepsy but, at the other, share some characteristics with SMEI, a very severe form of epilepsy whose association with neurological and cognitive impairment makes it incompatible with the criteria for defining idiopathic epilepsy. Whether this variability depends on the type of *SCNAI* mutation, or on the concomitant effect of other gene mutations in accordance with a multigenic model of inheritance, is still an open question. However, it is certainly true that the information being drawn from myoclonic epilepsies is challenging the current concept of idiopathic epilepsy as the result of a gene mutation that directly affects neuronal excitability and leads to "pure" epileptic symptomatology unassociated with any other neurological signs or symptoms.

I am sure that the book will be as successful as it deserves. I enthusiastically accepted the invitation to introduce it to the epileptological community for a number of reasons: its scientific quality, the fact that it will stimulate readers with its new information and ideas, and last but not least because it is dedicated to Charlotte Dravet, whose scientific endowments, patient dedication and teaching skill I learned to appreciate during many years of warm personal friendship.

Giuliano Avanzini, M.D.
ILAE President 2002
Chief, Neurophysiopathology Instituto
Neurologico Carlo Besta
Milan, Italy

Acknowledgments

The editors gratefully acknowledge the restricted educational grant from Ortho-McNeil Pharmaceutical which provided the primary support for the International Symposium-Workshop on "Myoclonic Epilepsies of Infancy, Childhood, Adolescence and Adulthood" in Seattle in December 2002.

We especially appreciate Raul Harris-Collazo, Ph.D., Ortho-McNeil Neuroscience Scientific Liaison, who advocated for this project from concept to completion and participated in various meetings of the editors.

We acknowledge the assistance of the Office of Continuing Medical Education, UCLA School of Medicine, and particularly Ms. Sheryl Crowley, who helped organize the Symposium-Workshop in Seattle.

The editors are grateful to Joan Spellman who organized their working meeting in Malibu, California, in January 2004. During and after this working meeting, Dr. Katerina Tanya Perez-Gosiengfiao, Dr. Reyna M. Durón-Martinez, and Dr. Iris E. Martínez-Juárez assisted the editors by editing chapters, retyping text, formatting figures, tables, and preparing final versions of the chapters for submission to the publisher.

We are especially grateful for the support and assistance of Anne M. Sydor at Lippincott Williams & Wilkins. We also acknowledge the efforts of Scott Scheidt.

1

History and Classification of "Myoclonic" Epilepsies: From Seizures to Syndromes to Diseases

Pierre Genton,* Joseph Roger,* Renzo Guerrini,† Marco T. Medina,‡
Michelle Bureau,* Charlotte Dravet,* and Antonio V. Delgado-Escueta§

*Centre Saint-Paul, Hôpital Henri Gastaut, Marseille, France; †Department of Child Neurology and Psychiatry, University of Pisa and Research Institute 'Stella Maris' Foundation, Pisa, Italy; ‡Neurology Training Program, Postgraduate Direction, National Autonomous University of Honduras, Tegucigalpa, Honduras; §Comprehensive Epilepsy Program, David Geffen School of Medicine at UCLA and Epilepsy Center of Excellence at VA GLAHS, Los Angeles, CA.

INTRODUCTION

The word "paramyoklonus multiplex" was first introduced by Professor Nikolaus Friedreich (1) in Heidelberg, and the shorter term "myoclonus" was used thereafter in various clinical settings. All through the years of the 19th and 20th centuries, clinicians had to cope with a concept of "myoclonic epilepsies," which covered mostly cases that were difficult to classify and even more difficult to treat.

This volume contains detailed descriptions and discussions of a large number of rare and common epilepsies associated with myoclonias. Our aim in this chapter is to review the evolution of attitudes and concepts in this large domain of epileptology and their molecular genetics. We feel that they can be summarized into three separate and successive (but overlapping) stages:

- The first stage, which stretches over more than 2 centuries, corresponds to the description of different forms of epilepsy characterized by a specific seizure type that included a myoclonic component: The seizure type was synonymous with the epilepsy type, which was named accordingly.

- The second stage, which began a few decades ago, saw the introduction of a syndromic approach to the problem of myoclonic epilepsies, with a new importance given to the electroencephalogram (EEG), and to elements of etiology and prognosis; for example, using qualifications like "*benign*" or "*severe*," the definition of epilepsy types along such lines was sometimes complex and could not be summarized in a brief denomination. Therefore, eponymic designations, which pay tribute to the major contributor(s) of the original description of such syndromes, were often (and are still) used.

- The third and present stage is a continuation of the second but is now also based on other findings, especially on molecular genetics. The aim, currently, is to define forms of epilepsy by their seizure-causing molecular mechanisms, that is, to speak about epilepsies as diseases. The potential inclusion, among diagnostic criteria, of descriptive genetics, on the one hand, for example, epilepsy phenotypes, mode of inheritance, and chromosomal locus, versus their molecular lesions, on the other hand have challenged the syndromic concepts. Indeed, recent data have pointed to the complexities of the relationship between phenotype and genotype and the complexities of epilepsy inheritance. Unraveling these complexities will undoubtedly lead to novel and curative treatments.

WHEN A SEIZURE TYPE DEFINES AN EPILEPSY TYPE

The first use of the word "myoclonus" to describe an epileptic entity can be ascribed to Unverricht, who published, in 1891, a monography entitled *"Die Myoklonie"* (2). This constituted the first comprehensive description and discussion of a familial epilepsy disease. In 1903, H. Lundborg described 10 families and wrote a review of "Die progressive Myoklonus–Epilepsie." Since then, this rare, but spectacular and recognizable inherited neurological disease with seizures and myoclonus has been called Unverricht–Lundborg disease. In 1911, Lafora and Glueck described a separate and more rapidly progressive and fatal dementing myoclonus epilepsy with periodic acid Schiff's procedure (PAS)-positive "amyloid bodies" distributed throughout the central nervous system at autopsy. In 1921, Ramsay Hunt described six cases of action myoclonus and cerebellar ataxia, four of whom also had epilepsy. Ramsay Hunt coined the term "dyssynergia cerebellaris myoclonica." These descriptions of myoclonus epilepsies in the early 20th century produced the concept of progressive myoclonus epilepsies, (refer to Chapter 4).

There were, however, much more common epilepsy forms that presented with myoclonic jerks as their most prominent symptom. Already fairly well characterized by its epileptic "secousses" or "impulsions" by Herpin in 1857, and later by its "myoclonie épileptique" by Rabot in 1899, (3) (Fig. 1–1) a form of epilepsy that has a high prevalence worldwide was formally described nearly simultaneously from two sources in the middle of the 20th century. In Germany, Janz, as a clinician, and Christian, as the electroencephalographer, reported a series of patients with "Impulsiv Petit Mal." The denomination was chosen because of the characteristic occur-

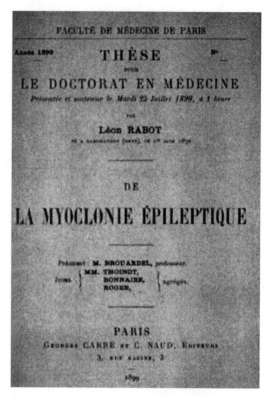

FIG. 1–1. Facsimile of the cover of Dr. Rabot's doctoral thesis on "The Epileptic Myoclonia," Paris, 1899.

rence of minor seizures (hence, "Petit Mal") in the form of brief, forward directed jerks (4,5). From Uruguay came the description, in exactly the same vein, of a "bilateral myoclonic and conscious epilepsy" that had the same general features (6). In France, the condition was thought to be very uncommon and was characterized as "massive bilateral myoclonic jerks of adolescence" (7,8).

In contrast to this nonfatal form of epilepsy with onset in adolescence less common, but much more severe cases, characterized by very debilitating drop attacks with frequent injuries, affecting young children were observed. From Germany came the description based on the spectacular falls that were its trademark. Doose (9) called them "myoclonic-astatic" epilepsy. The falls, which were due to a combination of a massive jerk and a brutal atonia, were the only seizure type, at least initially, in many cases. The context of this epilepsy was highly variable: Most of these children had previously developed normally, many had a family history of epilepsy, and, although the ictal EEG correlates were fairly homogenous, the interictal findings were variable. This description met with little success outside of the German-speaking world, mostly because this entity was not associated with a clear prognosis: Some cases did, indeed remit, without sequel after a short period, whereas others evolved into a severe epilepsy with multiple seizure types, dramatic EEG changes, and mental deterioration. Although a "core" of such patients may have a typical "myoclonic-astatic" epilepsy, most had a condition that clearly went beyond this single seizure type. The definition by Doose of an epilepsy by a seizure type was thus judged to be insufficient: However, by a sort of twist of history, a more comprehensive approach, based on a syndromic diagnosis of severe epilepsies, finally led to the recognition of a genetic form of myoclonic astatic epilepsy.

Among cases with childhood absence epilepsy (CAE), a subgroup with absence seizures that were very typical on the EEG, with regular, 3-Hz spike-and-wave discharges, had particular clinical correlates in the form of both increased axial muscular tone and rhythmic jerks, especially apparent in the upper limbs. The first identification of "epilepsy with myoclonic absences"(10) was justified by this particular neurophysiology, but the identification of this seizure type as a distinct epilepsy syndrome emerged by reason of a particularly poor prognosis, with drug resistance and mental deterioration, setting it clearly apart from typical CAE (11). Here again, a very specific seizure type apparently sufficed to qualify for a distinct epilepsy syndrome.

There were other forms of absence epilepsies that were tentatively individualized on the basis of associated myoclonic features that seemed to define another form of epilepsy [review in Capovilla et al. (12)]. The syndrome of eyelid myoclonias with absences, first mentioned by Jeavons in 1977 (13), has been recognized by many as an uncommon, yet easily identifiable entity. The syndrome of absences with perioral myoclonias was first reported by Panayiotopou-

los et al. in 1994 (14). This entity has not been accepted by all as an independent and distinct disorder, as it is not necessarily associated with a prognosis that sets it apart in general, from CAE. Recent studies have also stressed the fact that typical absences with very early onset, before age 3, may be associated with ictal myoclonic manifestations (15). Such cases are highly heterogenous and cannot be gathered into one single entity or grouped on the basis of myoclonic features.

The description of an epilepsy by a single seizure type has thus met with some limited success. Currently, only few epilepsy syndromes retain a denomination that is based only and mainly on the seizure type: Epilepsy with myoclonic absences and epilepsy with myoclonic-astatic seizures have both been officially sanctioned by the International League Against Epilepsy (ILAE), whereas the syndrome of "eyelid myoclonias with absences" has not.

BEYOND THE SEIZURE TYPE: THE SYNDROMIC APPROACH

By the 1970s, the evolution of concepts and classifications in epilepsy, with better use of the EEG and video-EEG, together with more concerns about prognosis, drug efficacy, and overall impairment, led to a different approach of diagnosis and classification of epilepsies, in general, and myoclonic epilepsies, in particular. Although the broad concept of "myoclonic epilepsies" was still used, usually in circumstances where there was no deep awareness of the plurality and complexity of the field, diversification occurred with a need for more informative and practical knowledge. A seizure type was no longer judged sufficient to define a form of myoclonic epilepsy and to distinguish it from the others.

A good example can be drawn from the history of "Impulsiv Petit Mal," the early stages of which have been reported previously. This condition was first christened as "juvenile myoclonic epilepsy" in Denmark, where, under the influence of the German school, it was already well recognized and where studies were done on its social and psychological consequences (16). The latter denomination was very successful and was used when this "new" disease was rediscovered in North America and thus internationally acknowledged (17) and rightly ascribed as "the Janz syndrome." The change of denomination is significant. Whereas the first denominations stressed the seizure type ("impulsion" or "bilateral and conscious myoclonia"), the latter introduced the age of appearance of symptoms, and, for some authors, the notion of benign prognosis, which was later dropped. It is also of significance that the most comprehensive and successful denomination was produced by those who were actually interested in the social consequences of epilepsy. The social outcome is, indeed, part of the syndromic approach.

Another significant example of the same process occurred in the case of more severe epilepsies of childhood, which are often characterized by drop attacks and mental deterioration. The EEG marker was, in many cases, a slow variant of the 3-Hz generalized spike-and-wave discharge of petit mal, and a "Petit Mal variant" of the severe type was thus reported (18) and accepted by some as the "Lennox syndrome." However, the description remained partial. Various denominations focusing on the seizure type and on the EEG terminology were used in various parts of the world. Some focused on possibly myoclonic features, for example, childhood epileptic encephalopathy with slow spike-waves (19), or severe myokinetic epilepsy of early childhood (20). Some light was shed on this by the epochal work of Drs. Gastaut and Dravet (21,22), who defined the restrictive diagnostic criteria of what was later finally called the Lennox–Gastaut syndrome (LGS). These criteria include the coexistence of several seizure types with typical EEG features and cognitive deterioration. The modern, restrictive definition of the LGS (23,24) has stressed that myoclonias are not major features of this syndrome. There was clearly an overlap (and there were, indeed, many lively discussions) between the LGS and the aforementioned entity described by Doose as "myoclonic-astatic epilepsy" (9). Only in recent years have these syndromes been more accurately separated, as discussed elsewhere in this volume, with emphasis on the "symptomatic" and acquired nature of LGS and on the "idiopathic" and genetically determined nature of myoclonic-astatic epilepsy. Recent neurophysiological data have stressed their differences showing, in particular, bilateral synchrony in the former versus truly generalized changes in the latter (see Chapter 3).

In the 1970s, infants with various seizure types and, especially, a large spectrum of outcomes led Dravet and Bureau (26) to establish new electroclinical correlations that differentiated two groups of infants who presented with myoclonic seizures and did not fulfill the criteria for the LGS. Some had febrile seizures, long clonic seizures during sleep, and later myoclonus, a variety of other seizure types and mental deterioration leading to severe retardation. They did not have tonic seizures and the prominent sleep-related EEG changes so characteristic of LGS. They had a "severe" myoclonic epilepsy in infancy (25). Other infants had isolated myoclonic jerks and a good prognosis and were thus logically described as having a "benign" myoclonic epilepsy in infancy (26). These descriptions thus included age of onset and overall prognosis and were also typical of the syndromic approach to hitherto difficult-to-define epileptic entities.

PRESENT DEVELOPMENTS: TOWARD EPILEPSY DISEASES

The 1989 classification of epilepsies (27) listed epilepsies with myoclonic components among various categories, within the generalized, focal, and undetermined categories, and also into various etiological subgroups (Table 1–1). Positive and negative myoclonias can occur in a variety of epilepsies—focal and generalized; however, the conditions that this volume focuses on are mostly in the categories of idiopathic generalized epilepsies (IGE). A notable exception is represented by severe myoclonic epilepsy in infancy, which was considered to have both generalized and focal features.

A new diagnostic scheme was recently proposed (28) that introduced the possibility of classifying epilepsies according to different axes. Syndromes are simply listed according to age at onset. The changes from the 1989 classification

TABLE 1–1. *Myoclonic epilepsies: Recent changes in ILAE classification*

International classification (27)	Proposed diagnostic scheme (Task Force, 2001: Table IV) (28)

Idiopathic focal epilepsies
  Benign rolandic epilepsies (negative myoclonus)
  Primary reading epilepsy
Symptomatic focal epilepsies
  Epilepsia partialis continua (type I and II)
Idiopathic generalized epilepsies (IGE)
  Benign myoclonic epilepsy in infancy
  Juvenile myoclonic epilepsy
  Other syndromes (including IGE with photosensitivity)
Symptomatic or cryptogenic generalized epilepsies
  Myoclonic-astatic epilepsy (Doose syndrome)
  Lennox–Gastaut syndrome (myoclonic form)
  Epilepsy with myoclonic absences
Symptomatic generalized epilepsies
  Progressive myoclonus epilepsies
Epilepsies undetermined whether generalized or focal
  Severe myoclonic epilepsy in infancy
	List of syndromes
	  Benign myoclonic epilepsy in infancy
	  Dravet's syndrome (severe myoclonic epilepsy in infancy)
	  Epilepsy with myoclonic absences
	  Epilepsy with myoclonic-astatic seizures
	  Lennox–Gastaut syndrome
	  Progressive myoclonus epilepsies
	  IGE with variable phenotypes, including juvenile myoclonic epilepsy
	  Reflex epilepsies, including primary reading epilepsy
	
	Syndromes in development
	  Myoclonic status in nonprogressive encephalopathies
	  Generalized epilepsies with febrile seizures plus

are minimal concerning the myoclonic epilepsies, and mostly cosmetic:

- Given the larger than initially expected range of clinical presentations in severe myoclonic epilepsy, with many patients failing to exhibit prominent myoclonic features, it was suggested to rename this syndrome "Dravet syndrome."
- Other syndromes not included in the 1989 classification (27) were admitted, or admitted pending confirmation.
- Due to the possible overlap among the phenotypes of juvenile myoclonic epilepsy, juvenile absence epilepsy, and epilepsy with grand mal seizures on awakening, it was decided to gather all three syndromes as idiopathic generalized epilepsy (IGE) with variable phenotypes.
- A concept of "epileptic encephalopathies" was introduced that may gather various epilepsy types associated with severe and progressive cognitive and neurological decline. Dravet syndrome and some cases with myoclonic-astatic epilepsy may fit into this new category as well.

However, the recently proposed 2001 diagnostic scheme and classification lags far behind the rapid advances in molecular genetics of the epilepsies. A transformation of our global understanding of the nosology of "idiopathic" epilepsies will need to consider their defined molecular lesions and their acceptance as epilepsy diseases. Recent data, which have emerged from genetic work, have shown the importance of a disease-based approach to epilepsies. Almost 10 years have passed since Steinlein et al. (29) showed the $\alpha4$ subunit of the nicotinic acetylcholine receptor (nACH) as the epilepsy mutation in autosomal dominant nocturnal frontal lobe epilepsy in chromosome 20q13, and 7 years have passed since the identification of potassium (*KCNQ2*, *KCNQ3*) ion channels as epilepsy-causing genes in benign familial neonatal convulsions in chromosomes 20q13 and 8q24 (30,31). These reports clearly showed that mutations in receptors or ion channels can cause epilepsies (32,33). They have led to discoveries of other receptoropathies and channelopathies, such as *SCN1A* (34), *SCN1B* (35), and *SCN2A* (36), in generalized epilepsy with febrile seizures plus (GEFS+; chromosomes 19q13 and 2q21), and the $\alpha1$ and $\gamma2$ subunits of the GABA-A receptor (37–39) in autosomal dominant juvenile myoclonic epilepsy (JME) and (GEFS+) (chromosome 5q34). More recently, a novel glial membrane gene has been associated with autosomal dominant temporal lobe epilepsy with auditory symptoms (40). Thus, there has been ample time for the ILAE commission on classification to incorporate genetic advances in their classification schema.

The genetic complexities that underlie the common myoclonic epilepsies are definitely starting to unravel. Traditionally, it had been argued that because there are ~50,000 to 80,000 functional genes in humans and that mutations may exist in any of them, one can imagine the myriad of genes interacting in a nonadditive fashion (epistasis or epistatic variance components) to produce the genetically complex common idiopathic epilepsies. Thus, the popular concept is that genetically complex myoclonic epilepsies are probably the result of interacting genes in epistasis. The problem is that such modest epilepsy alleles underlying common myoclonic epilepsies would most likely not have a sufficiently large genetic displacement to be detected by linkage analyses.

There are other common diseases, detected by linkage, whose meiotic process of recombinations segregated with the disease in families. Examples include presenilin 1 and 2 in early onset Alzheimer's disease (41,42) and apolipoprotein E3,4 in late-onset Alzheimer's disease (43), calpain 10 in type 2 diabetes mellitus (44), and *BRCA1* and *BRCA2* in breast cancer (45). Most had conjectured that the numerous myoclonic epilepsy genes of modest or small effects, which do not produce a structural change in their gene product, produce only a small or modest functional change in their gene product and would not be detected by linkage analyses. They had not anticipated that a different genetic architecture than those known for Mendelian or non-Mendelian diseases could be present in common myoclonic epilepsies (Fig. 1–2).

An oligogenic model is perhaps the best fit for JME families of European descent residing in New York City. Pal et al. (2002) observed the association of single nucleotide polymorphisms

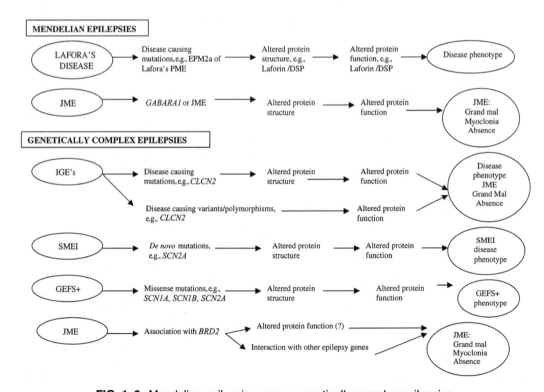

FIG. 1–2. Mendelian epilepsies versus genetically complex epilepsies.

haplotype that stretched to the boundary of *BRD2* in 20 JME probands whose families are genetically linked to and genetically associated with the HLA locus in chromosome 6p. In spite of the absence of mutations, they argued that *BRD2* is a susceptibility gene for JME, consistent with their oligogenic model of interacting loci in chromosome 8 for grand mal, chromosome 6 for JME, and chromosome 5 for petit mal absence epilepsy. This oligogenic model contrasts with the clear-cut Mendelian Ala322Asp mutation in *GABRA1* that cosegregated with eight affected members of one large JME family from Quebec (39). Because these rare *GABRA1* epilepsy alleles followed Mendelian autosomal dominant inheritance, they had high genetic displacement and the chromosome 5q34 locus was detected by linkage analyses.

The recent observations of *CLCN2* mutations in individuals with IGE and JME provide a novel genetic architecture for IGE and JME families (49,50). Actual data in the case of the *CLCN2* mutations and variants show that missense mutations in the same gene (i.e., *CLCN2*) were sufficient to produce the entire JME, CAE, and IGE phenotypes in three families. Variants (nucleotide changes) in the same *CLCN2* gene provided a wide range of susceptibility for the epilepsy phenotypes when tested in still a larger number of other families (i.e., 115 families) (49,50). Thus, the same *CLCN2* gene acts as (a) an epilepsy gene fully responsible for seizure phenotypes through its mutations in some families and (b) as a susceptibility gene that needs to interact with other genes to produce the seizure phenotype in an even larger number of families. These observations may be unique to common myoclonic epilepsies because the conjecture had been that common epilepsies, like other common diseases, would be explained by relatively simple allelic spectra (i.e., a very large number of loci, with each having a low frequency of epilepsy-producing alleles or allelic heterogeneity).

Developments in severe myoclonic epilepsy in infants (SMEI) recently added a new twist and provided an explanation for a sporadic form of epilepsy. *De novo* somatic mutations in the same *SCN1A* gene known to cause the syndrome of GEFS+ were reported to cause a majority of severe myoclonic epilepsy of Dravet (46). In contrast to missense mutations in GEFS+, stop frame shift and nonsense mutations were found in most cases of sporadic severe myoclonic epilepsy of Dravet in Belgium and in 40% to 80% of cases in Japan. In addition, in some families from Japan, Italy, and France, even *de novo* mutations in index cases were associated with additional seizures in nonnuclear members, implying the presence of modifying gene or genes (47,48).

Thus, the success in defining myoclonic epilepsy mutations is not restricted to simple Mendelian epilepsies. *BRD2* as part of an oligogenic model, *CLCN2* with dual genetic effects, and *de novo* mutations of *SCN1A* have all been shown to affect the seizure phenotypes of JME and SMEI.

Thus, genetic data should now be included in the diagnosis and classification of myoclonic epilepsies. Such data should help explain clinical observations of phenotypes and inheritance in these families. Indeed, in large and medium-size pedigrees with multiply affected members, several types of epilepsy phenotypes are usually represented, for example, GEFS+ and JME families from the United Kingdom, Sweden, and New York. Alternatively, in large pedigrees from Belize and Mexico, probands and affected family members can all have the same epilepsy phenotypes. This has led us to understand the fundamental genetic concepts of pleomorphisms (one genotype leading to multiple phenotypes) and locus heterogeneity (multiple genotypes causing a single phenotype) in myoclonic epilepsies (51).

A further example may be given by the GEFS+ syndrome (52). In this clinically and genetically heterogenous familial form of epilepsy, most patients have febrile seizures only, but a significant proportion of patients may have a form of epilepsy not unlike myoclonic-astatic epilepsy. Severe myoclonic epilepsy has also been diagnosed in this context, albeit less frequently. The correlations between genetic anomaly and clinical phenotype are discussed in other chapters, but we must stress here that this is a clear indicator of things to come. A disease, as defined by a precise biological marker or genetic defect, may express itself by a phenotype of epilepsy that hugely

(text continues on page 12)

TABLE 1–2. *Juvenile myoclonic epilepsy: Reports on its frequency*

Juvenile myoclonic epilepsy (JME) Authors	Ref. no.	Year	Location and sample	Type of study	Cases/ population	Prevalence × 1,000 (all epilepsies)	Percentage of JME among all epilepsies
Janz D	(55)	1969	Berlin, Germany	Hospital based	280/6,500	—	4.3
Tsuboi and Christian	(56)	1977	Heidelberg, Germany	Hospital based	399/7,400	—	5.4
Asconapé et al.	(57)	1984	Winston-Salem, North Carolina	Hospital based. Intensive treatment team for epilepsy at the North Carolina Baptist Hospital	12/275		4
Gooses	(58)	1984	Berlin	Video-EEGs in neurology clinics	126/1,069	—	11.9
Kramer et al.	(59)	1998	Tel Aviv, Israel	Pediatric neurology outpatient clinic of an urban hospital, 20-yr cohort	4/440		0.9
Kun et al.	(60)	1999	Singapore, Republic of Singapore	Military service survey (all male citizens age 18)	5/89 JME	4.9/1,000 males	5.6
Manonmani et al.	(63)	1999	Malaysia	University Hospital Kuala Lumpur	9/165	—	5.5
Murthy et al.	(64)	1998	Hyderabad, India	Hospital based	124/2,531	—	4.9
Panayiotopoulos et al.	(65)	1994	Saudi Arabia	Hospital based	66/672	—	10.2
Manford et al.	(66)	1992	Buckinghamshire, England	Hospital and community based	9/594	—	1.5
Figueredo et al.	(67)	1999	Santa Catarina, Brazil	Hospital based. Epilepsy clinic	26/939	—	2.8
Reutens and Berkovic	(68)	1995	Melbourne, Australia	Hospital based. Austin Hospital, Melbourne, Australia	21/101	—	21
Jha et al.	(69)	2002	Hyderabad, India	Hospital based	84/1,026	—	8.1
Fong et al.	(61)	2003	Hong Kong west region	Hospital based, Epilepsy Clinic at Queen Mary Hospital	5/636	1.5/1000	0.68
Jain et al.	(62)	2003	New Delhi, India	Hospital based. Neurosciences Center, All India Institute of Medical Sciences (AIIMS)	500/5,509	—	9.1
Nicoletti et al.	(74)	1999	Cordillera Province, Bolivia	Door to door survey	3/9955	3/1000	2.4

TABLE 1–3. *Myoclonic astatic epilepsy and others: Reports on its frequency*

Myoclonic astatic epilepsy (MAE)	Authors	Ref. no.	Year	Location and sample	Type of study	Cases/population	Prevalence of all epilepsies per 1,000	Percentage of MAE among all epilepsies studied
	Pazzaglia et al.	(70)	1978	Italy	Hospital based	—	—	1.4
	Doose and Sitepu	(71)	1983	Germany	Hospital based	—	—	1–2
	Kramer et al.	(59)	1998	Tel Aviv, Israel	Pediatric neurology outpatient clinic of an urban hospital, 20-yr cohort	1/440		0.2
	Oguni et al.	(72)	2002	Tokyo, Japan	Hospital based, epilepsy clinic	81/3,600	—	2.25
	Medina et al.	(73)	2004	Salama, rural Honduras	Door-to-door survey	1/6473	0.15	1/90 = 1.1
All myoclonic epilepsies including progressive	Ferrer-Vidal	(53)	1999	Review of bibliographic data	Published series on generalized epilepsies	408/6,450	—	6.3

9

TABLE 1–4. *Myoclonic seizures in infancy and early childhood*

	Myoclonic seizures in infancy and early childhood			
Seizure types, onset and evolution	*Subvariety #1:* Febrile & afebrile convulsive seizures at onset, followed by myoclonic, tonic-clonic, partial unilateral seizures and atypical absence. *Subvariety #2:* Same as subvariety #1, but myoclonic seizures are rare and not prominent. Clinical seizures triggered by sunlight and contrasting patterns.	Myoclonic seizures. Rare simple febrile seizures. No other seizure types except tonic-clonic later in late childhood and adolescence.	The most distinct & main complaints are myoclonic and absence seizures. Myoclonic seizures with astatic drop seizures are almost always present, but may occur infrequently. Rare generalized clonic seizures or tonic-clonic seizures, especially at onset. No tonic seizures.	Onset with generalized tonic-clonic seizures in most. Myoclonic and myoclonic-astatic (atonic by polygraphy) seizures in all. 60% with absences. Frequent nonconvulsive status. Isolated axial tonic seizures may occur at night. In some patients, simple febrile seizures may precede other seizure types.
EEG	Diffuse spike- & polyspike-waves; multifocal & focal abnormalities &/or parietal theta. About 1/3 have spikes–polyspike-waves triggered by light patterns.	Generalized spike- & polyspike-waves; normal background. Few with photosensitivity.	Generalized 3- to 6-Hz spike-waves and polyspike-waves mixed w/classic 3-Hz spike-waves; normal background	Generalized 2- to 3-Hz spike-waves and polyspike-waves; or multifocal spikes; slow background or parietal theta; "Photosensitivity in most cases between 5–15 yrs."
Age at onset	Usually 6 mos; before 1-yr old	4 mos to 3 yrs	1 to 5 yrs	Peaks at 4 years; range 7 mos to 8 yrs.
Sex	M:F 2:1	M:F 2:1	M = F (probands) 1:3 (M:F affected family members)	M:F 2:1
Cognitive development	Normal psychomotor development at onset. Slow development by 2 yrs and behavioral disorders & psychosis.	Normal at onset and course. Rarely, cognitive deficits.	Normal	Variable. From normal to severely impaired.
Family history	Positive in 50%–60%	Positive in 30%	Positive in 60%; More maternal transmission	Positive in 32%, including EEG parietal theta rhythms
Prognosis	Unfavorable course: drug resistance, low IQ, ataxia, tremors, poor coordination, dysarthria. Deaths in 16% mainly from status epilepticus, accidents, infections, and sudden unexplained death due to epilepsy.	Favorable with early treatment. Myoclonic seizures remit. In 18%, tonic-clonic or absences appear during adolescence.	Favorable with early treatment. Persisting up to adulthood.	*Subvariety #1:* Poor outcome with neurologic deficits & developmental delay; frequent status epilepticus of myoclonic, astatic or absence varieties associated cognitive deficits. *Subvariety #2:* Favorable course; Rarely, spontaneous remission.
Diagnosis	Severe myoclonic epilepsy of infancy (SMEI) or Dravet syndrome	Benign myoclonic epilepsy of infancy (BMEI)	Idiopathic early childhood myoclonic astatic epilepsy (IECMAE)	Myoclonic astatic epilepsy (Doose syndrome)

TABLE 1–5. *Myoclonic epilepsies in childhood and adolescence*

	Myoclonic seizures and absences in childhood and adolescence			
Seizure types	Frequent daily long-lasting (10–60 sec) absences with rhythmic symmetric myoclonus of shoulders/arms/legs less in chin/mouth and none in eyelids, elevating and abducting arms, staggering or rarely falling, are the only or preponderant seizures. Variable impairment of consciousness during absences. Tonic-clonic in 1/3 of cases. Rare febrile seizures.	Eyelid myoclonia with jerking/fluttering of eyelids and eye deviation upwards. They appear upon eye closure and may be associated with short-lasting unresponsiveness. Usually evoked by photic stimulation & worse in light. May indulge in self-inducing behavior. In 55%, infrequent myoclonias of the upper limbs, whereas 50% may have generalized tonic-clonic seizures.	Pyknoleptic absences start during childhood; associated with eyelid myoclonia in 30%. 98% have grand mal and 100% with myoclonias during adolescence. Persisting chief complaints during course are absences and tonic-clonic grand mal.	Adolescent onset myoclonic seizures (all) followed by, or simultaneous with, grand mal (95%). Rare absences in 1/3 of patients whereas 5% have myoclonic seizures as the only phenotype.
EEG	Ictal 3-Hz spike-wave, easily triggered by hyperventilation. Normal background; 14% have focal or multifocal abnormalities. Generalized spike-waves of variable duration, sometimes with myoclonias, during sleep stages 1, 2, & 3.	Ictal/interictal: short bursts (0.5–2 secs) of 3–6 Hz spike waves. Rare polyspike-waves	In 78%, 3-Hz single spike-waves. In 54%, 4- to 6-Hz spike & polyspike-waves. In 22%, 15- to 25-Hz diffuse fast rhythms in awake and sleep EEG.	4- to 6-Hz spike- and polyspike-waves in all untreated. Ictal: rapid 16–30-Hz high-amplitude diffuse polyspikes during myoclonus.
Age onset	Mean, 7 yrs Range, 11 months–12 yrs	Mean, 5.8 yrs Range, 2–14 yrs	Mean, 6.9 yrs Range, 1–11 yrs	Mean, 15.1 yrs Range, 7–28 yrs
Sex	M > F 69% : 31%	F > M 80% : 20%	F > M 64% : 36%	F (55%) = M (45%)
Family history	Positive in 20%	Positive in 28%	Positive in 72%. Male and female family members equally affected. More maternal transmission (2:1).	Positive in 49%. 17% of relatives are asymptomatic and have 4–6-Hz polyspike-waves or spike-waves (F > M at 2:1). Maternal equal to paternal transmission
Prognosis	*Pure myoclonic absence (38%):* favorable response to treatment and remission. *Myoclonic absence with tonic-clonic seizures (62%):* variable and may have poor outcome with developmental delay in 50%.	Poor response to antiepileptic drugs (AEDs). Persists into adulthood.	Partial response to sodium valproate (VPA) and other AEDs in 80% with frequent breakthrough convulsions, myoclonias and absence. Only 7% are seizure free on VPA alone. 13% had no response to polytherapy.	59% are seizure free (38% on VPA alone, 16% on polytherapy). Seizures persist in 41%.
Diagnosis	Epilepsy with myoclonic absences	Eyelid myoclonia and absence	Childhood absence persisting with tonic clonic and myoclonic seizures	Classic juvenile myoclonic epilepsy

varies, ranging between normal (asymptomatic) and very severe—namely, pleomorphisms. It is clear that the role played by modifying genes, or by specific clusters or association of genes or even haplotypes, has yet to be elucidated, but the function-modifying and disease-producing effect of *SCN1A, SCN1B,* and *SCN2A* mutations have now been well characterized.

MYOCLONIC EPILEPSIES: THE SCOPE OF THE PROBLEM

The myoclonic nature of seizures often remains unrecognized, and myoclonic epilepsies commonly remain underdiagnosed, especially in infancy and childhood. However, they amount to a significant proportion of all epilepsies seen in clinical practice. Various incidents and prevalence data have been reported for each of the syndromes discussed in this volume, and the reader is referred to the chapters dealing with the myoclonic epilepsies found in infants, children, and adolescents. There are no clear global data based on epidemiological surveys. It is highly probable that numbers would differ according to geographical and ethnic factors; moreover, the "detection rate" for precise epileptic syndromes depends largely on the local level of awareness. The number of cases reported from one area may, indeed, reflect more a specific interest than an actual increased prevalence. It is also true that the prevalence of the rarer syndromes will always be highest in hospital- or tertiary center-based studies than in other, less sophisticated settings, like field studies. Although it had been recognized, under different names, in Europe, for nearly a century, JME did not exist in North America before the first descriptions following Delgado–Escueta and Enrile–Bacsal in 1984 (17): Thus, the prevalence of JME there went from 0 to something by reason of "cultural" factors alone!

Overall, the prevalence of myoclonic epilepsies (including the nonidiopathic forms) has been recently evaluated from a personal, long-standing specialized outpatient clinic at 6.3%, representing 408 out of 6,450 consecutive patients with epilepsy seen in Barcelona, Spain (53). In an epidemiological, population-based study of the prevalence and etiology of epilepsy

in the context of a Latin American tropical country, Honduras, Medina et al. (54) found that myoclonic epilepsies represented only 2.2% of all epilepsies. The discrepancy between these two extremes (2.2% vs. 6.3%) may be explained in the largest part by (a) the selection of cases in an established, urban, Western European epilepsy clinic and (b) the higher prevalence in tropical countries of symptomatic epilepsies (e.g., due to neurocysticercosis in Honduras), which would reduce the proportion of idiopathic myoclonic epilepsies. However, these numbers are actually quite close, because the overall prevalence of epilepsy was high at 23/1,000 in Honduras, which is threefold the prevalence found in industrialized countries. It thus appears that a reasonable estimate of the actual population-based prevalence of myoclonic epilepsies is at least 6% among all epilepsies. These reports on population-based prevalence should be contrasted with hospital- and clinic-based prevalence studies of the more common myoclonic epilepsies. Excluding the very rare syndromes of severe myoclonic epilepsy of infancy, benign myoclonic epilepsy of infancy, myoclonic absence, absence with eyelid myoclonia, photosensitive epilepsies, and familial adult myoclonic epilepsy, the more common syndromes of JME (6.3%), and idiopathic myoclonic-astatic-epilepsy (2.8%) could conservatively account for 9% of all epilepsies (Tables 1–2 and 1–3).

Whatever the true prevalence of myoclonic epilepsies are, they represent a challenge that confronts the clinician–practitioner. For these reasons, the editors have provided two tables (Tables 1–4 and 1–5) differentiating these myoclonic syndromes. As a guide to treatment are algorythms in Chapters 23 and 25.

REFERENCES

1. Friedreich N. Paramyoclonus multiplex. *Virchows Archiv* 1881:86.
2. Unverricht H. *Die myoklonie.* Leipzig, Vienna: Franz Deuticke, 1891.
3. Rabot L. *De la myoclonie épileptique.* [medical thesis]. Paris, 1899.
4. Genton P, Gélisse P. Seminal citations: juvenile myoclonic epilepsy. *Arch Neurol* 2001 Sep;58(9):1487–1490.
5. Janz D, Christian W. Impulsiv Petit-Mal. *Dtsch Z*

Nervenheilk 1957;176:346–386. (English translation by P. Genton. In: Malafosse A, Genton P, Hirsch E, Marescaux C, Broglin D, Bernasconi M, eds. *Idiopathic generalized epilepsies.* London: John Libbey, 1994:229–251).

6. Castells C, Mendilaharsu C. La epilepsia mioclónica bilateral y consciente. *Acta Neurol Latinoamer* 1958;4:23–48.

7. Gastaut H, Rémond H. Etude électroencéphalographique des myoclonies. *Rev Neurol (Paris)* 1952;86:596–609.

8. Gastaut H. "Benign" of "Functionnal" (versus "Organic") epilepsies in different stages of life: an analysis of the corresponding age-related variations in the predisposition to epilepsy. In: Broughton RJ, ed. Henri Gastaut and the Marseilles school's contribution to the neurosciences. *Electroencephal Clin Neurophysiol* 1982[Suppl 35]:17–44.

9. Doose H. Das akinetische Petit Mal. *Arch Psychiatr Nervenk* 1964;205:625–654.

10. Tassinari CA, Lyagoubi S, Santos V, et al. Etude des décharges de pointes ondes chez l'homme. II: Les aspects cliniques et électroencéphalographiques des absences myocloniques. *Rev Neurol* 1969;121:379–383.

11. Tassinari CA, Bureau M. Epilepsy with myoclonic absences. In: Roger J, Dravet C, Bureau M, Dreifuss F, Wolf P, eds. *Epileptic syndromes in infancy, childhood and adolescence.* London: John Libbey, 1985:121–129.

12. Cappovilla G, Rubboli G, Beccaria F, et al. A clinical spectrum of the myoclonic manifestations associated with typical absences in childhood absence epilepsy. A video-polygraphic study. *Epileptic Disord* 2001;3:57–61.

13. Jeavons PM. Nosological problems of myoclonic epilepsies in childhood and adolescence. *Dev Med Child Neurol* 1977;19:3–8.

14. Panayiotopoulos CP, Ferrie CD, Giannakodimos SE, Robinson RO. Perioral myoclonias with absences: a new syndrome. In: Wolf P, ed. *Epileptic seizures and syndromes.* London: John Libbey, 1994:143–155.

15. Chaix Y, Daquin G, Monteiro F, Villeneuve N, Laguitton V, Genton P. Absence epilepsy with onset before age three years: a heterogeneous and often severe condition. *Epilepsia* 2003: Jul;44(7):944–949.

16. Lund M, Reintoft H, Simonsen N. En kontrolleret social og psychologisk undersøgelse af patienten med juvenil myoclon epilepsi. *Ugeskr Laeg* 1975;137:2400–2402.

17. Delgado–Escueta AV, Enrile-Bacsal F. Juvenile myoclonic epilepsy of Janz. *Neurology.* 1984;34:285–294.

18. Lennox WG. The petit mal epilepsies. Their treatment with tridione. *JAMA* 1945;129:1069–1074.

19. Chevrie JJ, Aicardi J. Childhood epileptic encephalopathy with slow spike-wave. A statistical study of 80 cases. *Epilepsia* 1972;13:259–271.

20. Sole Segarra J. Epilepsie myoclonique maligne familiale. *Schweiz Arch Neurol* 1952;79:259.

21. Dravet C. *Encéphalopathie épileptique de l'enfant avec Pointe-Onde lente diffuse ("Petit Mal Varian")* [Thesis]. Marseille, France, 1965.

22. Gastaut H, Roger J, Soulayrol R, et al. Childhood epileptic encephalopathy with diffuse spike-waves (otherwise known as "petit mal variant") or Lennox syndrome. *Epilepsia* 1966;7:139–149.

23. Genton P, Guerrini R, Dravet C. The Lennox–Gastaut syndrome. In: Vinken Pierre J, Bruyn George W, eds.

Handbook of clinical neurology. Amsterdam: Elsevier, 2000;73(23):211–222.

24. Beaumanoir A, Blume WT. The Lennox–Gastaut syndrome. In: Roger J, Bureau M, Dravet C, Genton P, Tassinari CA, Wolf P, eds. *Epileptic syndromes in infancy, childhood and adolescence,* 3rd ed. London: John Libbey, 2002.

25. Dravet C. Les épilepsies graves de l'enfant. *Vie Méd* 1978;8:543–548.

26. Dravet C, Bureau M. L'Epilepsie myoclonique bénigne du nourrisson. *Rev Electroencephalogr Neurophysiol* 1981;11:438–44.

27. Commission on Classification and Terminology of the International League Against Epilepsy. Proposal for revised classification of epilepsies and epileptic syndromes. *Epilepsia* 1989;30:389–399.

28. Engel, J. A Proposed diagnostic scheme for people with epileptic seizures and with epilepsy: Report of the ILAE Task Force on Classification and Terminology. *Epilepsia* 2001;42:796–803.

29. Steinlein OK, Mulley JC, Propping P, et al. A missense mutation in the neuronal nicotinic acetylchoine receptor alpha 4 subunit is associated with autosomal dominant nocturnal frontal lobe epilepsy. *Nat Genet* 1995;11:201–203.

30. Singh NA, Charlier C, Stauffer D, et al. A novel potassium channel gene, KCNQ2, is mutated in an inherited epilepsy of newborns. *Nat Genet* 1998;18:25–29.

31. Charlier C, Singh NA, Ryan SG, et al. A pore mutation in a novel KQT-like potassium channel gene in an idiopathic epilepsy family. *Nat Genet* 1998;18:53–55.

32. Durner M, Zhou G, Fu D, et al. Evidence for linkage of adolescent-onset idiopathic generalized epilepsies to chromosome 8 and genetic heterogeneity. *Am J Hum Genet* 1999;64:1411–1419.

33. Zara F, Labuda M, Garofalo PG, et al. Unusual EEG pattern linked to chromosome 3p in a family with idiopathic generalized epilepsy. *Neurology* 1998;51:493–498.

34. Escayg A, MacDonald BT, Meisler MH, et al. Mutations of SCN1A, encoding a neuronal sodium channel, in two families with GEFS+2. *Nat Genet* 2000;24:343–345.

35. Wallace RH, Wang DW, Singh R, et al. Febrile seizures and generalized epilepsy associated with a mutation in the Na+-channel beta1 subunit gene SCN1B. *Nat Genet* 1998;19:366–370.

36. Sugawara T, Tsurubuchi Y, Agarwala KL, et al. A missense mutation of the Na+ channel alpha II subunit gene Na(v)1.2 in a patient with febrile and afebrile seizures causes channel dysfunction. *Proc Natl Acad Sci USA* 2001;98:6384–6389.

37. Baulac S, Huberfeld G, Gourfinkel-An I, et al. First genetic evidence of GABA(A) receptor dysfunction in epilepsy: a mutation in the gamma2-subunit gene. *Nat Genet* 2001;28:46–48.

38. Wallace RH, Marini C, Petrou S, et al. Mutant GABA(A) receptor gamma2-subunit in childhood absence epilepsy and febrile seizures. *Nat Genet* 2001;28:49–52.

39. Cossette P, Liu L, Brisebois K, et al. Mutation of GABRA1 in an autosomal dominant form of juvenile myoclonic epilepsy. *Nat Genet* 2002;31:184–189.

40. Kalachikov S, Evgrafov O, Ross B, et al. Mutations in LGI1 cause autosomal-dominant partial epilepsy with auditory features. *Nat Genet* 2002;30:335–341.

41. Sato N, Imaizumi K, Manabe T, et al. Increased production of beta-amyloid and vulnerability to endoplasmic

reticulum stress by an aberrant spliced form of presenilin 2. *J Biol Chem* 2001;276:2108.

42. Xu X, Shi YC, Gao W, et al. The novel presenilin-1-associated protein is a proapoptotic mitochondrial protein. *J Biol Chem* 2002;277:48,913–48,922.

43. Burke JR, Roses AD. Genetics of Alzheimer's disease. *Int J Neurol* 1991–1992;25–26:41–51.

44. Fullerton SM, Bartoszewicz A, Ybazeta G, et al. Geographic and haplotype structure of candidate type 2 diabetes susceptibility variants at the calpain-10 locus. *Am J Hum Genet* 2002;70:1096–1106.

45. Bonadona V, Sinilnikova OM, Lenoir GM, Lasset C. Pretest prediction of BRCA1 or BRCA2 mutation by risk counselors and the computer model BRCAPRO. *J Natl Cancer Inst* 2002;94:1582–1583.

46. Claes L, Del–Favero J, Ceulemans B, Lagae L, Van Broeckhoven C, De Jonghe P. De novo mutations in the sodium-channel gene SCN1A cause severe myoclonic epilepsy of infancy. *Am J Hum Genet* 2001;68:1327–1332.

47. Dalla Bernardina D, Zara F. Severe myoclonic epilepsy. Presented at National Congress of the Italian League Against Epilepsy; June 2–5, 2002; Bolgna, Italy.

48. Sugawara T, Mazaki-Miyazaki E, Fukushima K, et al. Frequent mutations of SCN1A in severe myoclonic epilepsy in infancy. *Neurology* 2002;58:1122–1124.

49. Haug K, Warnstedt M, Alekov AK, et al. Mutations in *CLCN2* encoding a voltage-gated chloride channel are associated with idiopathic generalized epilepsies. *Nat Genet* 2003;33:527–532.

50. Heils A, Haug K, Sander T, Cid P, Elger C. Mutations of *CLCN2* encoding a voltage-gated chloride channel causing common forms of epilepsy [Abstract]. *Epilepsia* 2001:42[Suppl 7]:22.

51. Delgado–Escueta AV, Medina MT, Bai DS, et al. Genetics of idiopathic myoclonic epilepsies: an overview. *Adv Neurol* 2002;89:161–184.

52. Scheffer IE, Berkovic SF. Generalised epilepsy with febrile seizures plus. A genetic disorder with heterogeneous clinical phenotypes. *Brain* 1997;120:479–490.

53. Ferrer-Vidal LO. Severity and epidemiology of myoclonic epilepsy. *Rev Neurol* 1999 (Feb 1–15);28(3):269–271.

54. Medina MT, Duron R, Osorio JR, Martinez L. Las epilepsias en Honduras. In: Medina MT, Chaves-Sell F, Chinchilla-Calix N, Gracia F, eds. *Las epilepsias in Centroamerica.* Scancolor: Tegucigalpa, 2002:23–31.

55. Janz D. *Die epilepsien.* Stuttgart, Germany: Georg Thieme Verlag; 1969.

56. Tsuboi T, Christian W. *Epilepsy: A clinical, electroencephalograpic and statistical study of 466 patients.* New York: Springer, 1976.

57. Asconapé J, Penry JK. Some clinical and EEG aspects of benign juvenile myoclonic epilepsy. *Epilepsia* 1984;25:108–114.

58. Gooses, R. *Die Beziehung der Fotosensibilität zu den verschiedenen epileptischen Syndromen.* [Thesis]. West Berlin, 1984.

59. Kramer U, Nevo Y, Neufeld MY, et al. Epidemiology of epilepsy in childhood: a cohort of 440 consecutive patients. *Pediatr Neurol* 1998 Jan;18(1):46–50.

60. Kun LN, Ling LW, Wah YM, Lian TT. Epidemiologic study of epilepsy in young Singaporean men. *Epilepsia* 1999;40:1384–1387.

61. Fong GCY, Mak W, Cheng TS, et al. A prevalence study of epilepsy in Hong Kong. *Hong Kong Med J* 2003;9:252–257.

62. Jain S, Tripathi M, Srivastava AK et al. Phenotypic analysis of juvenile myoclonic epilepsy in Indian families. *Acta Neurol Scand* 2003;107:356–362.

63. Manonmani V. A study of newly diagnosed epilepsy in Malaysia. *Singapore Med J* 1999;40:32–35.

64. Murthy JM, Yangala R, Srinivas M. The syndromic classification of the International League Against Epilepsy: a hospital-based study from South India. *Epilepsia* 1998;39:48–54.

65. Panayiotopoulos CP, Obeid T, Tahan AR. Juvenile myoclonic epilepsy: A 5-year prospective study. *Epilepsia* 1994;35:285–296.

66. Manford M, Hart YM, Sander JW, et al. The National General Practice Study of Epilepsy. The syndromic classification of the International League Against Epilepsy applied to epilepsy in a general population. *Arch Neurol* 1992;49:601–808.

67. Figueredo R, Trevisol-Bittencourt PC, Ferro JB. Clincial-epidemiological study of patients with juvenile myoclonic epilepsy in Santa Catarina State, Brazil. *Arq Neuropsiquiatr* 1999;57:401–404.

68. Reutens DC, Berkovic S. Idiopathic generalized epilepsy of adolescence: Are the syndromes clinically distinct? *Neurology* 1995;45:1469–1476.

69. Jha S, Mathur VN, Mishra VN. Pitfalls in Diagnosis of Epilepsy of Janz and its complications. *Neurol India* 2002;50:467–469.

70. Pazzaglia P, Giovanardi R, Cirignotta F, et al. Nosografia delle epilessie miocloniche. *Rivista Italiana di EEG e Neurofisiología Clinica* 1978;2:245–252.

71. Doose H, Sitepu B. Childhood epilepsy in a German city. *Neuropediatrics* 1983:14:220–224.

72. Oguni H, Tanaka T, Hayashi K, et al. Treatment and long-term prognosis of myoclonic-astatic epilepsy of early childhood. *Neuropediatrics* 2002;122–132.

73. Medina, MT, Durón R, Martínez L, et al. Prevalence, incidence and causes of epilepsy in rural Honduras: the Salamá study. *Epilepsia* (in press, 2004).

2

Ontogeny of the Reticular Formation: Its Possible Relation to the Myoclonic Epilepsies

Harvey B. Sarnat

Alberta Children's Hospital, Pediatrics (Neurology) and Pathology (Neuropathy), Calgary, Alberta, Canada

INTRODUCTION

The reticular formation (RF) is a central core of polysynaptic ascending and descending circuits of interneurons, extending caudally from the thalamus and through the periaqueductal grey matter of the midbrain and the tegmentum of the pons and medulla oblongata to the spinal cord (1,2). The initial connection of the reticular formation with the forebrain is at the marginal zone of the early telencephalon and includes the Cajal–Retzius neurons that form a preplate plexus before the arrival of the first wave of radial migrations of neuroblasts from the subventricular zone. Its influence on spinal cord function is through the reticulospinal pathway and, as with other bulbospinal tracts, axons decussate before or during their longitudinal descent. The fundamental cell of the reticular formation is the interneuron. No primary afferent sensory of efferent motor neurons to or from the reticular formation exit from the central nervous system to project into the periphery.

From an anatomical viewpoint, the RF is unlike any other region of the central nervous system (CNS). It is difficult to visualize in sections of brainstem because it forms discrete anatomic nuclei with histologically defined margins only in some portions. Most of the reticular formation is a diffuse irregular longitudinal column of structures with indistinct boundaries filling the space between more distinctive nuclei of the brainstem. Both magnocellular and parvocellular regions are identified. Many of these regions at different levels of the brainstem have been assigned arbitrary names, based on position and size of the neurons, such as the nucleus paramedianus and the nucleus gigantocellularis dorsalis. In some places, such as the thalamus and midbrain, the bilaterality of the RF is obvious; but even in other regions where it may appear continuous across the midline, it remains a bilateral, symmetrical structure. The descending reticulospinal tracts decussate, as with other bulbospinal axonal projections. Despite its multisynaptic nature, in which neurons have only short axons, the synaptic organization of the RF is not random or unpredictable; rather, it is as precise as in any other part of the brain (3). The number of neuroanatomical and neuroembryological studies on the reticular formation is small, reflecting the difficulty in studying such a heterogeneous and often apparently nebulous anatomic structure. The structures included in the reticular formation vary according to different authors. Many include the locus ceruleus, median raphé nuclei, substantia nigra, and structures adjacent to more defined brainstem nuclei, such as the nucleus and fasciculus solitarius and nucleus ambiguus (3); the latter should be excluded, however, because it contains primary motor neurons. Some authors include portions of the limbic system, including the amygdala and hippocampal formation, as components of the ascending reticular formation. Reciprocal fiber connections with the majority of brainstem structures make it a very complex system and the neurotransmitters synthesized and secreted by reticular formation neurons are multiple and include serotonin, monoamines including dopamine and norepinephrine, γ-aminobutyric acid (GABA), and a variety of neuropeptides. This diversity underscores that the reticular formation is really a heterogeneous group and not a single, unitary entity.

Consistent with the diversity of anatomical structure and neurochemical projections, the functions of the reticular formation are diverse and include coordination of movements of the head and body, alternation of respiration and blood pressure, a gate to block certain sensory inputs such as pain, arousal and attention, sleep states, and influence on emotion in the limbic system (3).

Because of the implication of the RF as a possible site of origin of subcortical epilepsies, and the myoclonic epilepsies of infancy and early childhood, in particular, its ontogenetic, and indeed its phylogenetic, development should be considered in the context of the evolution of subcortical epilepsy, as well as in the context of alterations that the reticular formation may undergo in various cerebral malformations.

WHAT IS AN INTERNEURON?

The essence of the RF is the interneuron, generally one with a long axon and many collateral branches along its length as it descends in the brainstem. An interneuron is a neuron in which afferent and efferent connections remain entirely within the central nervous system and do not project dendrites or axons peripherally. The predominance of interneurons is one of the principal differences distinguishing a ganglion and a brain (Table 2–1) (4). Even the so-called "cephalic ganglion" of very simple invertebrates, such as the flatworm, is a true brain. There is no evidence that, in the embryonic development of humans or any other animals, the initial rostral neural folds of neuroepithelium are ever a cerebral ganglion that later becomes a brain. The interneuron, therefore, is primordial in the development of a CNS in both phylogeny and ontogeny; the reticular formation is one of the fundamental and earliest structures to develop.

The definition of the *interneuron* has itself evolved because of the integration of the neurophysiologic with the initial morphologic criteria. This more modern definition began with the concept that interneurons were inhibitory cells with short axons that regulated excitability in local circuits, by contrast with excitatory principal cells with long axons projecting information to distant regions within the CNS. However, this oversimplification must be further modified, because some reticulospinal axons are long and some nonreticular long pathways within the CNS are mainly inhibitory (e.g., corticospinal tract and corpus callosum) whereas other interneurons with short axons are excitatory (e.g., cholinergic interneurons of the corpus striatum) (5). Most, but not all, interneurons are indeed inhibitory, synthesizing and secreting GABA as their neurotransmitter, but exceptions to this rule also are documented (e.g., the glycenergic inhibitory

TABLE 2–1. *Comparison of brain and ganglion*[a]

Brain	Ganglion
Cephalic site only	Variable sites in body
Serves entire body	Serves limited regions or segments
Bilobar with commissures	Alobar without commissures
Neurons form surface; fibers (axons) form core	Homogeneous mixture of neurons and fibers
Interneurons predominate	Interneurons sparse
Multisynaptic intrinsic circuits	Monosynaptic relays predominate
Specialized local functions	No local specialization of function

[a]Reproduced from Sarnat HB, Netsky MG. When does a ganglion become a brain? Evolutionary origin of the central nervous system. *Sem Pediatr Neurol* 2002; 9:240–253. With permission.

Renshaw cells of the ventral horn of the spinal cord) (6). Nearly all interneurons of the hippocampus and cerebral neocortex release GABA (5–7). These interneurons are electrically coupled with paravalbumen-containing basket cells that are essential for gamma and theta oscillations physiologically, and a highly modifiable syncytium of cholecystokinin-containing interneurons in the neocortex carries impulses from subcortical pathways, related to emotion and motivation; impairment of this inhibitory mechanism may result in disorders of mood, such as anxiety (8). It is evident that there is a much greater diversity in the morphology and connectivity of local circuit interneurons in the mammalian brain than of the primary neurons, including the decussating interneurons with long axons, such as the pyramidal cells of the cerebral cortex, which are more uniform and have much less plasticity (5). Synaptic plasticity, similar to that observed in primary pyramidal neurons, and the presence or absence of long-term potentiation in interneurons are important determinants of their function (7).

The neuroanatomical distribution of the reticular formation is illustrated in Fig. 2–1 (9).

PHYLOGENY OF THE RETICULAR FORMATION

We may infer much from the study of comparative neuroanatomy that is relevant to understanding the relations of different structures of the central nervous system. Those structures that differ substantially in each class and species denote the *evolution* of the nervous system. The forebrain of reptiles and birds, compared with that of mammals, is a good example. Structures identified in all vertebrates and that have changed little except for somewhat more elaborate development in more complex brains tell not about evolution, but rather about the *origin* of the nervous system. The ventricular system is an example, the reticular formation is another good example.

Phylogeny is a perspective of development that compliments and sometimes helps explain ontogeny (10). The reticular formation is present in all vertebrates from the simplest species of jawless fishes and salamanders to humans, with a fundamental similarity in all species. Its connections, with progressively more highly evolved structures, implies that the reticular system itself also evolves. This evolution is reflected in changing functions while retaining some of its basic, universal functions.

The status of the reticular formation in protochordates, such as amphioxus, provides insight into the importance of the interneuron in the development of the brain and in setting a pattern of contralateral ascending and descending projections that becomes almost invariable in all vertebrates and without which the laterality of function cannot be ensured. Amphioxus is a bilaterally symmetrical animal, as with all chordates. It possesses only a few simple reflexes. A stimulus on one side of the body is indiscriminately interpreted as a potential threat, and the animal coils away from it to protect itself. This response is the opposite of the trunk incurvation reflex of Galant in human premature and term neonates, in which the trunk curves toward the side of tactile stimulation, a reflex that is already evident as early as 24 weeks gestation. To develop the "coiling reflex," amphioxus or its ancestor needed a neuron that connected primary sensory neurons on one side of the body with primary motor neurons on the other side, to effect a muscular contraction resulting in coiling away from the threatening stimulus. Unlike the sensory and motor neurons, the interconnecting cell did not require processes that passed outside the CNS, but did require that its axon cross the midline to innervate a motor neuron on the opposite side. This was the first "decussating interneuron" (11–15) and with further cephalization of functions made possible by the development of progressively more rostral nuclei in the brain. All ascending and descending connections had to be decussating interneurons to provide constancy of the lateralizing information and responses (13). Hence, the reticulospinal, vestibulospinal, olivospinal, tectospinal, and corticospinal tracts all evolved as crossed pathways. The cerebellar pathways are an apparent exception, but only because of a double decussation. The decussating interneuron of a primitive chordate or prevertebrate, such as amphioxus, thus provides a phylogenetic basis for explaining the crossing of pathways in the CNS,

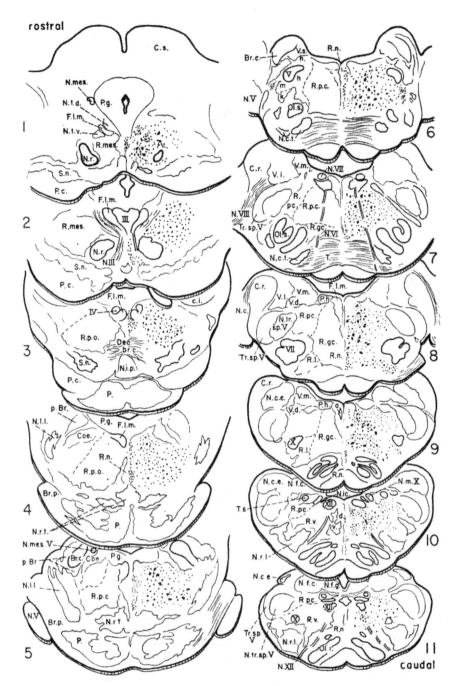

FIG. 2–1. Drawing of the reticular formation in transverse sections of human brain, based on work by Brodal in 1957 and modified by Van der Kooy. (From Van der Kooy D. The reticular core of the brainstem and its descending pathways: Anatomy and function. In: Fromm GH, Faingold CL, Browning RA, Burnham WM, eds. *Epilepsy and the reticular formation: the role of the reticular core in convulsive seizures.* New York: Liss, 1987:9–23(9). With permission.).

an arrangement not found in any other system of the body (13).

Another type of interneuron does not send its axon across the midline. This interneuron developed as motor or sensory neurons with collateral axons that branched to innervate others in the vicinity. With the specialization of function, such neurons with both peripheral and central branches of its axons lost one or the other of these collaterals, and thus became pure motor neurons or, if the peripheral branch of the

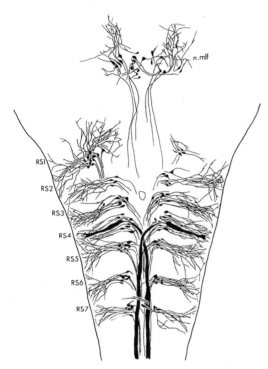

FIG. 2–2. Drawing of reticulospinal tract in a horizontal section of the brainstem of an adult fish. This descending pathway is similar in all vertebrates, including humans. The axons arise at many levels and decussate before descending, reproducing the pattern of the decussating interneuron of protochordates, such as amphioxus, and establishing the crossed pattern for all later longitudinal pathways in the CNS. They also are arranged in a segmental pattern corresponding to the embryonic rhombomeres (RS1–RS7). The most rostral portion (at the top) is the midbrain. [From Lee RKK, Eaton RC, Zottoli SJ. Segmental arrangement of reticulospinal neurons in the goldfish hindbrain. *J Comp Neurol* 1993;329:539–556 (16). With permission.].

axon was lost, became interneurons with short axons for local ipsilateral connections. The proliferation of such interneurons provided for local circuitry and incorporated some decussating interneurons for longer projections to influence more distant parts of the CNS. This proliferation and organization was the earliest reticular formation and a model for the evolutionary development of many other nuclei of the neuraxis.

In comparing the RF of various classes of vertebrates, a fundamental similarity in all vertebrates becomes evident, with elaborations and refinements in more complex species, but the RF is essentially a stable feature of the brain throughout evolution (3). In addition to the decussation made by those interneurons with long ascending or descending axons within the CNS, these decussating interneurons also have a segmental arrangement derived from embryonic rhombomeres (see Fig. 2–2) (16). Local interneurons with short axons do not decussate, by contrast.

ONTOGENY OF THE RETICULAR FORMATION

The interneurons of the brainstem reticular formation exhibit maturation with neuropeptide and neurotransmitter synthesis during the neural tube stage of ontogenesis, at 5 to 6 weeks gestation. This maturation occurs before differentiation of either sensory or motor cranial nerve nuclei is complete and long before the cerebellum is more than an undifferentiated rhombic lip of His. Reticulospinal projections are the earliest bulbospinal axons to descend. Various components of the RF are formed in all eight rhombomeres of the hindbrain, the mesencephalic neuromere, and in at least the diencephalic prosomeres. It is not, therefore, dependent on a gene that is expressed only in a limited number of specific neuromeres and almost certainly has many genes interacting to generate its neurons. The decussating interneurons with long axons that form the reticulospinal part of the bulbospinal tracts exhibit a segmental arrangement in the adult derived from their segmental rhombomeric origin (16).

The early telencephalic plexus may be a rostral extension of the reticular formation because cells of origin of axons forming the initial marginal zone plexus are from deep regions of the mesencephalon (17,18). Indeed, the Cajal–Retzius neurons may be the earliest connection of the forebrain with subcortical reticular structures. These neurons are integral parts of the preplate plexus and present at 5 weeks gestation, before the first wave of radial migration of neuroblasts from the subventricular zone of the telencephalon. They form much earlier than do the first thalamocortical connections at 7 to 8 weeks gestation. The morphology of Cajal–Retzius neurons, with their long axons and a series of ventrally projecting collaterals, bear a striking resemblance to the typical RF neurons in the brainstem and are unlike any other neuron. The origin of the Cajal–Retzius neurons is speculated by some authors to be from the ganglionic eminence because they are GABAergic cells and there is a tangential migratory pathway from that telecephalic structure (19). Another possibility is that they migrate rostrally from the mesencephalic neuromere, with which they are continuous in the embryo (18). Regardless of whichever hypothesis is correct, the Cajal–Retzius neuron and its plexus provides the continuity of the brainstem RF with the telecephalon in the embryo and fetus. It is then replaced as the connection between the cerebral cortex and the brainstem RF by the reciprocal thalamocortical projections in the infant.

RELATION OF THE RETICULAR FORMATION TO MYOCLONIC EPILEPSY

Some epilepsies, particularly the myoclonic epilepsies, are believed to either originate in subcortical structures or at least involve a major participation of subcortical structures. The old term "centrencephalic epilepsy" was formerly used to emphasize this concept in "petit mal lapse (absence) with 3 per second wave and spike rhythm, myoclonic petit mal with multiple spike and wave, sporadic or irregular 1 to 3 per second in bursts, akinetic or atonic 'drop' seizures with irregular spike and wave in short bursts, and petit mal–grand mal with wave and spike or multiple spike and wave" (20). The *centrencephalon*, however, is not really an anatomical structure and

its closest anatomical correlate is the reticular formation. The role of the reticular formation in the pathogenesis of epilepsy, including the modulation of cortical "irritability" or depolarization threshold is still not well understood. The RF is strongly implicated in "brainstem reticular reflex myoclonus," an exaggerated hyperactivity of the nervous system (21).

In the classification of paroxysmal myoclonus, the reticular formation most likely plays an active role in those believed to arise in the cerebral cortex, thalamocortical systems, or brainstem, such as positive or negative cortical myoclonus, reticular reflex myoclonus, startle, palatal, and ocular myoclonus; or in the spinal cord such as segmental, propriospinal, and peripheral myoclonus. Reticular participation in cortical myoclonus is less certain and probably only secondary in its propagation. The basis for the hypothesis that thalamocortical circuits integrate both hemispheres and are responsible for generalized synchronous epileptiform discharges started with the demonstration of recruiting waves during rhythmic, slow electrical stimulation of the intralaminar portion of the thalamus of the cat by Morrison and Dempsey in 1942 (22). These results were confirmed and extended by Jasper and Droogleever–Fortuyn in 1947, who reproduced spike-wave electroencephalographic (EEG) patterns by stimulating the intralaminar thalamus of a somnolent, lightly anesthetized cat at 3 Hz (23). Subsequent 3-Hz midline or intralaminar thalamic stimulation by Hunter and Jasper in 1949 produced an arrest reaction similar to absences in unanesthetized cats and monkeys (24). In 1969, Prince and Farrell discovered that intramuscular doses of penicillin also induced spike-wave paroxysms in cats, together with eye blinking, facial twitching, and myoclonic jerks (25). Later, authors produced evidence diminishing the primary role of the thalamus. However, Gloor (26), Gloor and Testa (27), and Avoli et al. (28) showed that spike-wave discharges evolve from spindles as penicillin-induced depolarizations, and powerful recurrent intracortical inhibitory mechanisms are recruited. They also showed quick recruitment of the thalamus, particularly the midline nucleus centralis medialis and intralaminar nuclei, and proposed that oscillations and reverberations in the thalamocorticothalamic reentrant loop sustain the spike-wave discharges. Coulter, Huguenard, and Prince in 1989 (29) and Huguenard and Prince in 1992 (30) explained self-synchronized thalamic discharges on the basis of phasic T-type calcium-dependent bursts of action potentials in nucleus reticularis thalami. Reciprocal connections between nucleus reticularis thalami and thalamic relay nuclei then provide the anatomic basis for synchronized thalamic discharges. These concepts about the pathogenesis of spike-wave rhythmical discharges await testing in humans with proved channelopathies (31), receptoropathies (32), and nonchannel-mediated mutations (33), whose clinical syndromes include generalized convulsions, myoclonus, and myoclonic epilepsies (34).

There is good reason to suspect that abnormal ontogenesis of the reticular formation plays a role in some of the myoclonic epilepsies, particularly cortical myoclonus, reticular reflex myoclonus, and epileptic syndromes with secondarily generalized epileptic myoclonus, like Dravet syndrome (severe myoclonic epilepsy of infancy) (31). Similarly, abnormal subcortical connections to the cortex that shift from the Cajal–Retzius neurons and preplate plexus to the thalamocortical projections could be a factor in the generation or spread of myoclonic seizures. Little hard evidence is available to support or refute these hypotheses. The reason for the lack of evidence is that there are almost no histopathological studies focused on these issues. The use of special histochemical and immunocytochemical techniques and nonstandard sections of brain (e.g., parasagittal rather than transverse sections of upper brainstem) would be required to demonstrate or negate such evidences. Data derived from clinical and genetic studies, neuroimaging, or electrophysiological examination in the living patient are increasingly available but cannot substitute for direct microscopic tissue examination with special techniques. This article thus ends with an appeal to clinicians to (a) obtain autopsy permission for patients who die with myoclonic epilepsies, despite the best of clinical care; and (b) ensure that the brain is properly examined postmortem by a neuropathologist who is interested in these disorders and experienced with the special techniques required. Ordinary histologic examination is not likely to yield conclusive results. Fixed brain tissue always can be sent to neuropathologists in other instutitions, if the pathologists in a particular hospital do not possess the expertise to study it for this special purpose.

REFERENCES

1. Crosby EC, Humphrey T, Lauer EW. *Correlative anatomy of the nervous system.* New York: MacMillan, 1962:157,212–213,264,273,290,298,498–501.
2. Parent A. *Carpenter's human neuroanatomy.* 9th ed. Baltimore: Williams & Wilkins, 1996:434–436,452–461.
3. Butler AB, Hodos W. *Comparative vertebrate neuroanatomy. evolution and adaptation.* New York: Wiley–Liss, 1996:164–179.
4. Sarnat HB, Netsky MG. When does a ganglion become a brain? Evolutionary origin of the central nervous system. *Sem Pediatr Neurol* 2002;9:240–253.
5. Maccaferri G, Lacaille J-C. Hippocampal interneuron classifications: making things as simple as possible, not simpler. *Trends Neurosci* 2003;26:564–571.
6. Mott DD, Dingledine R. Interneuron research: challenges and strategies. *Trends Neurosci* 2003;26:484–488.
7. McBain CJ, Maccaferri G. Synaptic plasticity in hippocampal interneurons? A commentary. *Can J Physiol Pharmacol* 1997;75:488–494.
8. Freund TF. Rhythm and mood in perisomatic inhibition. *Trends Neurosci* 2003;26:489–495.
9. Van der Kooy D. The reticular core of the brain-stem and its descending pathways: anatomy and function. In: Fromm GH, Faingold CL, Browning RA, Burnham WM, eds. *Epilepsy and the reticular formation: the role of the reticular core in convulsive seizures.* New York: Liss, 1987:9–23.
10. Sarnat HB. *Cerebral dysgenesis: embryology and clinical expression.* New York: Oxford University Press, 1992:66.
11. Bone Q. The central nervous system in amphioxus. *J Comp Neurol* 1960;115:241–270.
12. Guthrie DM. The physiology and structure of the nervous system of amphioxus (the lancelet) Brachiostoma lanceolatum Pallia. *Symp Zool Soc Lond* 1975;36:43–80.
13. Sarnat HB, Netsky MG. *Evolution of the nervous system.* 2nd ed. New York: Oxford University Press, 1981.
14. Fritzsch B. Similarities and differences in lancelet and craniate nervous systems. *Isr J Zool* 1996;42:S147–S160.
15. Holland LZ, Holland ND. Chordate origins of the vertebrate central nervous system. *Curr Opin Neurobiol* 1999;9:596–602.
16. Lee RKK, Eaton RC, Zottoli SJ. Segmental arrangement of reticulospinal neurons in the goldfish hindbrain. *J Comp Neurol* 1993;329:539–556.
17. Marín-Padilla M. Early ontogenesis of the human cerebral cortex. In: Peters A, Jones EG, eds. *Cerebral cortex.* New York: Plenum Publishing, 1988;7:1–34.
18. Sarnat HB, Flores-Sarnat L. Cajal–Retzius and subplate

neurons: their role in cortical development. *Eur J Paediatr Neurol* 2002;6:91–97.

19. Maricich SM, Gilmore EC, Herrup K. The role of tangential migration in the establishment of the mammalian cortex. *Neuron* 2001;31:175–178.

20. Penfield W, Jasper H. *Epilepsy and the functional anatomy of the human brain.* Boston: Little, Brown and Company, 1954:622.

21. Hallett M. Neurophysiology of brainstem myoclonus. *Adv Neurol* 2002;89:99–102.

22. Morrison RS, Dempsey EW. A study of thalamo-cortical relations. *Am J Physiol* 1942;135:281–292.

23. Jasper HH, Droogleever–Fortuyn J. Experimental studies of the functional anatomy of petit mal epilepsy. *Assoc Res Nerve Ment Dis Proc* 1947;26:272–298.

24. Hunter J, Jasper HH. Effects of thalamic stimulation in unanesthetized animals. *Electroencephalogr Clin Neurophysiol* 1949;1:305–324.

25. Prince DA, Farrell D. Centrencephalic spike-wave discharges following parenteral penicillin injections in the cat. *Neurology* 1969;19:309–310.

26. Gloor P. Generalized cortico-reticular epilepsies: some considerations on the pathophysiology of generalized bilaterally synchronous spike and wave discharge. *Epilepsia* 1968;9:249–263.

27. Gloor P, Testa G. Generalized penicillin epilepsy in the cat: effects of intracarotid and intervertebral pentylenetetrazol and amobarbital injections. *Electroencephalogr Clin Neurophysiol* 1974;36:499–515.

28. Avioli M, Gloor P, Kostopoulos G, Gotman J. An analysis of penicillin-induced generalized spike and wave discharges using simultaneous recordings of cortical and thalamic single neurons. *J Neurophysiol* 1983;50:819–837.

29. Huguenard JR, Prince DA. A novel T-type current underlies prolonged Ca^{2+}-dependent burst firing in GABAergic neurons of rat thalamic reticular nucleus. *J Neurosci* 1992;12:3804–3817.

30. Coulter DA, Huguenard JR, Prince DA. Calcium currents in rat thalamocortical relay neurons: Kinetic properties of the transient, low-threshold current. *J Physiol (Lond)* 1989;414:587–604.

31. Claes L, Del Favero J, Cuelemans B, et al. De novo mutations in the sodium-channel gene SCN1A cause severe myoclonic epilepsy of infancy. *Am J Hum Genet* 2001;68:1327–1332.

32. Baulac S, Huberfield G, Gourfinkel-An I, et al. First genetic evidence of GABA(A) receptor dysfunction in epilepsy: A mutation in the gamma 2 subunit gene. *Nat Genet* 2001;28:46–48.

33. Minassian BA, Ianzano L, Delgado–Escueta AV, et al. Identification of new and common mutations in the EPM2A gene in Lafora disease. *Neurology* 2000;55:488–490.

34. Scheffer IE, Berkovic SF. Generalized epilepsy with febrile seizures plus. A genetic disorder with heterogenous clinical phenotypes. *Brain* 1997;120:479–490.

3

Pathophysiology of Myoclonic Epilepsies

Renzo Guerrini,* Paolo Bonanni,* Lucio Parmeggiani,* Mark Hallett,†
and Hirokazu Oguni‡

*Epilepsy, Neurophysiology, Neurogenetics Unit, University of Pisa and Research Institute 'Stella
Maris' Foundation, Pisa, Italy; †Human Motor Control Section, National Institute of Neurological
Disorders and Stroke, National Institutes of Health, Bethesda, Maryland, ‡Department of Pediatrics,
Tokyo Women's Medical University, Tokyo, Japan

INTRODUCTION

Relationship between Myoclonus and Epilepsy

Myoclonus can be defined as an involuntary movement, which is brief and jerky and involves antagonist muscles. It can either originate from abnormal muscle activation in the form of brief electromyographic (EMG) bursts (positive myoclonus) or, more rarely, from brief interruptions of ongoing electromyographic activity (negative myoclonus).

Myoclonus and its association with epilepsy was first described by Dubini (1) in 1846. He described a cohort of patients with possibly different conditions who had as a common feature involuntary jerky movements that he named "electric chorea." The first attempt at classification of myoclonus came much later, when Lundborg (1903) (2) recognized three etiological categories: (a) symptomatic myoclonus, (b) essential myoclonus, and (c) familial myoclonic epilepsy (subdivided into nonprogressive and progressive forms). Later, Muskens (1928) (3) highlighted a close nosologic link between myoclonus and epilepsy and coined the term "fragments of epilepsy" to designate the myoclonic jerks of patients with epilepsy. Since then, many other conditions in which myoclonus is a significant symptom have been reported, allowing the following etiological classification of myoclonus

(4,5): (a) physiologic myoclonus (sleep related, hiccup, and myoclonus induced by anxiety or exercise), (b) essential myoclonus (subjects without other neurologic signs), (c) epileptic myoclonus (conditions in which the predominant element is epilepsy), and (d) symptomatic myoclonus (conditions in which the predominant element is encephalopathy). According to Marsden et al. (4) and Fahn et al. (5), the category of epileptic myoclonus comprises "fragments of epilepsy" and includes forms that originate from an isolated spike discharge in the motor cortex. Concepts on nosology of myoclonic epilepsies have evolved considerably in recent years (6,7), but the use of the term "epileptic myoclonus" is still confusing. Some authors define epileptic myoclonus as that which occurs within the setting of epilepsy and has the epileptic spike as the neurophysiologic hallmark (8). Others define epileptic myoclonus as those forms in which a paroxysmal depolarization shift is thought to be the underlying neurophysiologic substrate, irrespective of which population of neurons (cortical or subcortical) is primarily involved (9) and of the possibility of obtaining a time-locked electroencephalographic (EEG) correlate. Frequently, however, the EEG correlate of myoclonus can only be detected by using jerk-locked [EEG or magneto encephalographic (MEG)] averaging or coherence analysis. Considering the limitations related to these technical difficulties, it has recently been suggested

23

that epileptic myoclonus could be comprehensively defined as an elementary electroclinical manifestation of epilepsy involving descending neurons, whose spatial (spread) or temporal (self-sustained repetition) amplification can trigger overt epileptic activity (9).

EPILEPTIC MYOCLONUS

Epileptic myoclonus includes positive and negative cortical myoclonus, thalamocortical myoclonus, and reticular myoclonus (Fig. 3–1) (10).

Clinically, epileptic myoclonus may be positive or negative. It is focal if it involves a restricted, usually distal, group of muscles; multifocal, when asynchronous focal jerks involve different body areas; or generalized, when jerks involve most body segments in an apparently synchronous manner. Furthermore, it may be spontaneous; or reflex, if induced by movement or by sensory or visual stimuli. Finally, as regards periodicity, epileptic myoclonus may be rhythmic or arrhythmic.

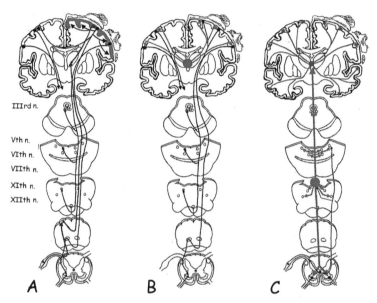

IIIrd n.

Vth n.
VIth n.
VIIth n.
XIth n.
XIIth n.

A   B   C

FIG. 3–1. Schematic drawing showing three main neurophysiological mechanisms of myoclonus. **A:** Cortical myoclonus. Myoclonic-related cortical activity emanates directly or via reflex sensory pathway activation (*upward arrow*), from a hyperexcitable sensorimotor cortex (*gray shading*). A descending volley then activates different muscles through brainstem and spinal motor neurons, according to a rostrocaudal pattern. Myoclonic-related cortical activity can intracortically spread within the same hemisphere or to the contralateral hemisphere through the corpus callosum (*black arrows*). **B:** Idiopathic (primary) generalized epileptic myoclonus. Myoclonic-related cortical activity originates subsequent to afferent volleys from subcortical structures (*gray shading*) that act synchronously on a diffusely hyperexcitable cortex. As a consequence, muscles from both sides are activated synchronously and muscles innervated by the cranial nerves are involved through a rostrocaudal pattern of activation, as in cortical myoclonus. This suggests that a descending volley passes through the brainstem. However, it is also possible for the descending volley to pass through a polysynaptic, thalamo-reticular pathway (see text, Thalamo-Cortical myoclonus—Neurophysiologic Findings). **C:** Reticular reflex myoclonus. Myoclonic-related activity originates from the reticular formation in the medulla (*gray dot and upward gray arrows*). Surface EMG recordings show an initial activation of the trapezius muscle (XIth cranial nerve), followed by the sternocleidomastoid (XIth cranial nerve), then the orbicularis oris (VIIth cranial nerve), and finally the masseter (Vth cranial nerve). EEG recordings show diffuse abnormalities, widely projected over both hemispheres, which are not time locked to the myoclonic EMG burst and often follow muscle activation. This supports the fact that they are not related to myoclonus generation.

The neurophysiological characteristics of epileptic myoclonus (8–10) are (a) duration of the myoclonic electromyography (EMG) burst ranging between 10 and 100 msec; duration of the EMG silent period of negative myoclonus, ranging from 50 to 400 msec; (b) synchronous EMG bursts or silent periods on antagonist muscles; (c) presence of an EEG correlate detectable by routine surface EEG or burst-locked EEG averaging. The EEG correlate is time locked in cortical reflex myoclonus and in primary generalized epileptic myoclonus. Secondarily generalized epileptic myoclonus, as defined in this chapter, has a time-locked EEG correlate, but the temporal relationships between EEG and EMG event may vary according to the pattern of muscle spread. Reticular reflex myoclonus may have an EEG correlate, which, however, is not time locked.

CORTICAL MYOCLONUS

Clinical Findings

Cortical myoclonus can be positive or negative; focal, multifocal, or generalized; spontaneous or reflex; and rhythmic or arrhythmic.

Neurophysiologic Findings

Origin

Cortical myoclonus originates from abnormal neuronal discharges in the sensorimotor cortex. Abnormally firing motoneurons may be primarily hyperexcitable or may be driven by abnormal inputs originating from hyperexcitable parietal (11) or occipital (12) neurons. Each jerk represents the discharge from a small group of cortical motoneurons somatotopically connected to a group of contiguous muscles. A cortical potential that is temporally and consistently correlated with the myoclonic potential, and localized on the contralateral sensorimotor region, can be demonstrated by EEG, MEG, or jerk-locked averaging (JLA) (13–16). In some patients with focal myoclonus, epilepsia partialis continua, and focal motor seizures, excision of a small cortical region, identified by electrophysiological recordings as the area of origin of

the myoclonic discharges, leads to remission of symptoms (17–19). However, in epilepsia partialis continua, the cortical site of origin of the myoclonic discharges and the site of origin of the associated focal seizures do not necessarily coincide (7).

In patients with progressive myoclonus and epilepsy (PMEs), the polarity of the premyoclonic potential as detected by JLA is positive (14,15,20–26). In contrast, in patients with Alzheimer's disease, Down syndrome, and in some patients with Lennox–Gastaut syndrome LGS, there is a negative sharp wave associated with myoclonus (27–29). Mima and coworkers (16) used MEG and EEG to study patients with cortical myoclonus caused by PMEs, familial cortical myoclonic tremor (see specific section, "Rhythmic or Arrhythmic Recurrence" of cortical myoclonus), corticobasal degeneration, Alzheimer's disease, and LGS. In all patients, jerk-locked MEG averaging revealed cortical activities associated with myoclonic jerks. The estimated generator of the earliest peak of the premyoclonus cortical activity was localized at the contralateral precentral gyrus. As judged from the direction of the electric current, surface-positive activity was detected in PMEs, familial cortical myoclonic tremor, and corticobasal degeneration; and negative activity, in Alzheimer's disease and LGS. According to Mima and colleagues (16), the negative premyoclonic potential may be generated by a hyperexcitable motor cortex, through a mechanism of epileptogenesis [i.e., in the motor cortex, the paroxysmal depolarization shift (PDS) is widely distributed]. The positive polarity potential is thought instead to be generated by a PDS restricted to the deep layers (probably in lamina V) of the motor cortex (16,22). However, there is good evidence from other authors (18,19) that cortical hyperexcitability may reside in sensory or parietal regions rather than in the motor cortex. If this were the case, then it is conceivable that premyoclonic potentials of opposite polarity could occur simply because of the reversal in anatomic orientation of pyramidal cells in motor and sensory parts of the central sulcus. Jerk-locked MEG is more sensitive than jerk-locked EEG averaging, at least in some patients, in detecting cortical activity associated with myoclonus (22), possibly because the magnetic fields are not attenuated by the skull.

Induction Mechanisms

In patients with cortical reflex myoclonus, appropriate stimuli administered to a resting somatic segment produce a reflex muscle response (jerk), which, in normal subjects, can only be detected during voluntary contraction. The normal reflex pattern from mixed nerve stimulation consists of an H response after ~28 msec and a long latency reflex (LLR II) at ~50 msec. An earlier reflex component at ~42 msec (LLR I) is present in 30% of normal subjects, and at ~70 msec an additional LLR III may occur (30). The reflex jerk was originally called a C- (cortical) reflex, as it was presumed to be cortically mediated (31). Electric or mechanic stimulation of a relevant nerve produces a reflex response that has a latency of 30 to 50 msec for the upper limb and 60 to 70 msec for the lower limb. If the afferent [N20 of somatosensory evoked potentials (SEPs)] and efferent motor-evoked potentials (MEPs) from transcranial magnetic stimulation (TMS) conduction times are subtracted from these latencies, the cortical relay time (CRT) is obtained, corresponding to the intracortical transmission time of myoclonic activity. SEPs of giant amplitude are often observed in patients with cortical reflex myoclonus (CRM) (Fig. 3–2). The giant components are most often P25/P30 (P1) and N35 (N2) (32), and their generators are localized close to the central sulcus (26,33). Because the subcortical components and the first cortical component (N20) have normal amplitude, an abnormality of intracortical inhibition following arrival of the first volley of thalamocortical activity could be the cause both of the abnormal enlargement of the giant SEP components and of activation of descending motor outputs leading to the C-reflex (32). The striking resemblance in latency and morphology of the giant SEPs to the myoclonus-related cortical spike suggests that both originate from common cortical mechanisms (15).

In the typical forms of CRM, the reflex jerk in the hand has a latency of ~50 msec and the CRT has a mean duration of 7 msec (34). Typical CRM can be observed in patients with focal cortical lesions (31), spinocerebellar degeneration

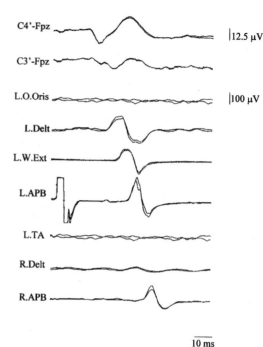

FIG. 3–2. Patient with autosomal dominant cortical myoclonus and epilepsy. Cortical SEP after electrical stimulation of the left median nerve at wrist. An enlarged N20–P30–N35 complex is followed by C-reflex in the left deltoid, wrist extensors, and abductor pollicis brevis. The ipsilateral muscular response precedes a contralateral response by ~8 msec. This delay is consistent with interhemispheric transcallosal spread. *L.*, left; *O. Oris*, orbicularis oris; *Delt*, deltoid; *W. Ext*, wrist extensors; *APB*, abductor pollicis brevis; *TA*, tibialis anterior; *R*, right.

(14,22,35), multiple system atrophy (22,36,37), cerebral anoxia (14,38), childhood metabolic degenerations, such as neuronal ceroid lipofuscinosis and sialidosis (30,33), Alzheimer's disease, Down syndrome (27,28), and mitochondrial disorders (39–41).

If the latency of the reflex myoclonus is reduced to ~40 msec, that is to say ~10 msec shorter than usual and ~2 msec longer than the sum of the afferent and efferent times to and from the cortex, CRM is defined as atypical. Atypical forms have been observed in patients with epilepsia partialis continua (21,42), postanoxic myoclonus (35), PMEs (30,33), neuronal ceroid lipofuscinosis (32), Huntington disease (42), and corticobasal degeneration (33).

It has been hypothesized that the different patterns of abnormality in CRM might be explained by differences in the processing and relay of sensory information in thalamocortical pathways (30,34). In the typical forms, CRM may involve abnormal relays through the sensory cortex to the motor cortex, either directly or via cerebellar–thalamocortical projections (32,34). In the atypical forms, myoclonus may represent enhancement of a direct sensory input to the motor cortex (34).

A form of CRM characterized by more prolonged C-reflex latency has been described in Rett syndrome (44). Clinically, myoclonus is multifocal, predominating distally, and arrhythmic. A positive potential, localized on the contralateral centroparietal area, precedes myoclonus with a latency of 34 ± 7 msec for the forearm muscle. This is compatible with corticomotoneuronal conduction. The N20–P30 and P30–N35 components of the SEPs have significantly increased amplitude. In addition, the latency of the N20 component is delayed and the N20–P30–N35 interval is significantly increased and has expanded morphology. The latency between electric stimulation (median nerve) and onset of reflex myoclonus is 65 ± 5 msec when the recording is made from the abductor pollicis brevis (APB) muscle. Topographic mapping of the SEP voltage shows, for the P30 component, a field distribution very similar to that of the premyoclonic potential. The CRT has a duration of 28 ± 4 msec—a value that is three- to four-fold higher than that observed in PMEs (34). It is, therefore, probable that in Rett syndrome the following sequence of events occurs: slight delay in central conduction of the impulse afferent to the sensorimotor cortex (N20), slowing of the processing of the afferent impulse (interval N20–P30; mean = 11 msec), delay in corticocortical transmission to the precentral neurons subserving movement of the stimulated body segment (latency increase P30-C-reflex; mean = 32 msec), and rapid descending volley to the spinal motoneurons. Thus, the premyoclonic EEG and the corresponding P30 wave would represent a discharge arising from the postcentral neurons, subsequently slowly activating the motor efferences through connections with the precentral neurons (45). Intracortical conduction time could

be particularly prolonged due to the synaptic abnormalities present in the brain of Rett patients with mutation in *MECP2* gene (46).

One particular form of CRM may be induced by photic stimuli, in idiopathic generalized epilepsies (benign myoclonic epilepsy, juvenile myoclonic epilepsy), in idiopathic generalized photosensitive epilepsies, or in some forms of cryptogenic epilepsies (myoclonic-astatic epilepsy and severe myoclonic epilepsy). The most active frequency of stimulation is between 10 and 20 Hz. The ratio between stimulus (flash) and reflex response (jerk) is not constant and is only partly time locked. Responses are usually symmetric and predominate in the upper limbs. In most cases, they are mild, only producing head-nodding and slight arm abduction. More generalized jerks, involving the face, trunk, and legs, may occasionally cause the patient to fall. Isolated myoclonic jerks occur without loss of consciousness. However, generalized jerks may be repeated, especially if the stimulus is protracted. In this situation consciousness may be impaired and a generalized tonic–clonic seizure may follow. The relationship of myoclonic jerks to the stimulus is complex. Sometimes there is no definite time relationship. On other occasions, the jerks may be repeated rhythmically with the same frequency as the stimulus or at one of its subharmonics (47). If the triggering stimulus is prolonged, the clinical response may translate into a generalized convulsion (48).

In patients with diffuse degenerative brain damage (49,50) or with occipital lesions (11), when intermittent photic stimulation (IPS) is performed at low frequencies (0.5–3 Hz), each flash may provoke a frontal giant potential, which is time locked to the stimulus and precedes by ~15-msec myoclonic jerk localized in the face or spreading from the face in a rostrocaudal pattern. Further repetition of the stimulus may induce a generalized tonic–clonic seizure (50). The potential evoked on the occipital cortex may be normal or giant. Because the occipital response precedes the giant frontocentral response by ~4 msec, which may correspond to the time required for the impulse to pass from the occipital to the frontal cortex, long pathways of occipitofrontal intracortical transfer have been hypothesized (51). Study of the recovery cycles of the

EEG components in response to a pair of flash stimuli has shown that components on the central regions recover more rapidly than those on the occipital regions. Brain-mapping analysis indicates that the frontal activity correlated with the myoclonus originates in the premotor and motor cortices. Therefore, hyperexcitability of the visual cortex was not considered an essential prerequisite in this type of myoclonus by some authors (49,50).

The orbitofrontal photomyoclonic response, which is widely described in the EEG literature, in adults undergoing IPS (synonyms: frontopolar response, recruiting response, photooculoclonic response), is probably a form of photic CRM which may also be observed in normal individuals. The frequency of flashes that is effective in triggering this response is usually between 8 and 20 Hz. Patients present with rapid myoclonic jerking of the periorbital muscles producing fluttering of the eyelids and blinking, which is synchronous with the flashes. There may be vertical oscillations of the eyeballs. Amplitude of the response increases progressively during the first flashes, reaching a maximum within a few seconds. The maximal amount of muscle activity is initially observed in the inferior orbicularis oculi muscles with subsequent irradiation to other facial muscles, the frontal and occipital areas, and the neck (52). Further spread may be seen if IPS stimulation is protracted. The response is blocked by opening of the eyes or cessation of IPS. Although the pathophysiology and significance of the orbitofrontal photomyoclonic response have long been disputed, our current understanding indicates it to be an expression of cortical origin (53) within the spectrum of photic CRM (50).

Photic CRM provides a clear example of how a single jerk (fragment of epilepsy) can gradually translate into overt seizure activity, through a temporal summation effect of the triggering stimuli.

Rhythmic or Arrhythmic Recurrence

A focal spike generated in the sensorimotor cortex can produce a focal myoclonic jerk. Rhythmic or arrhythmic jerk recurrence may lead to epilepsia partialis continua (4). The cortical origin of myoclonus in epilepsia partialis continua has been widely demonstrated (18,19,22,54–56). However, a subcortical origin has also been proposed, at least in some patients showing basal ganglia or cerebellar lesions and no jerk-locked EEG activity (56–60).

Bilateral, rhythmic, virtually continuous myoclonus at 11 to 18 Hz is typically observed in Angelman syndrome (61). The jerks are spontaneous at rest and, if particularly intense, may produce dystonic posturing of the upper limbs or the feet. A cortical transient in the contralateral sensorimotor cortex precedes each EMG burst by an interval consistent with rapid corticomotoneuronal conduction (20–30 msec). Clinical and neurophysiological characteristics suggest a high propensity for intrahemispheric and interhemispheric cortical spread of myoclonic activity that can be manifested as apparently generalized myoclonic jerks (Fig. 3–3). There is no giant SEP and lack of C-reflex hyperexcitability correlates with the absence of reflex jerks. The post-MEP silent period has short duration and testifies to a deficit of inhibitory cortical mechanisms (62). The pattern of myoclonus observed in Angelman syndrome suggests that small areas within the motor cortex are able to independently produce hypersynchronous, rhythmic neuronal discharges recruiting muscle activity similar to tremor. Distal myoclonic jerks can convert into overt generalized myoclonic status (61). As this pattern of myoclonus is observed in all patients with Angelman syndrome, irrespective of their genetic class, mutations in the *UB3A* gene must play a direct role in its genesis. Transition to overt seizure activity in Angelman syndrome may in turn be facilitated by reduced representation of GABAA subunit receptors, as demonstrated by the much more frequent and severe epilepsy observed in patients bearing a chromosome 15q11-13 deletion, leading to reduction of gene product.

A rhythmic pattern of cortical myoclonus, bearing some similarities to that seen in Angelman syndrome, may be observed in association with different clinical conditions. Schulze–Bonhage and Ferbert (63) described a patient who developed cortical action tremor and focal motor seizures of the left hand, following a right

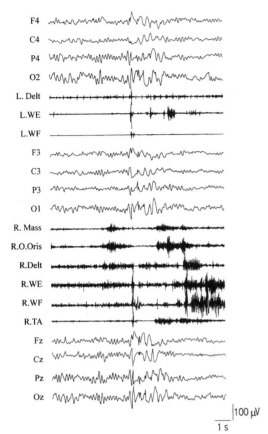

FIG. 3–3. Patient with Angelman syndrome (age; 1 year). Myoclonic seizure. Note that a generalized polyphasic EMG potential of ~80-msec duration is followed by a transient suppression of normal tonic activity, lasting ~200 msec. On EEG tracings, a myoclonic jerk is associated with a generalized burst of irregular spike-waves. *Delt*, deltoid; *L.*, left; *Mass.*, masseter; *O. Oris*, orbicularis oris; *R.*, right; *TA*, tibialis anterior; *WE*, wrist extensors; *WF*, wrist flexors.

parietal infarction. Wang and co-workers (64) reported cortical tremor appearing after surgical removal of a frontal lobe meningioma.

A similar rhythmic pattern was produced as a reflex response to tapping on the forehead or by sudden acoustic stimuli in some patients with Down syndrome (65) and tuberous sclerosis (9). Cortical tremor, in the form of postural or action tremor, and showing the neurophysiological characteristics of reflex cortical myoclonus, can also be observed in patients with PMEs

(24, 25) or with familial adult myoclonic epilepsy (FAME) (66–68) and autosomal dominant cortical reflex myoclonus and epilepsy (ADCME) (see Chapter 21).

In rhythmic cortical myoclonus, EEG–EMG frequency analysis (69,70) proved superior to jerk-locked backaveraging in detecting cortical correlates of rhythmic myoclonic jerks. Repetitive myoclonic jerks can produce a sort of rhythmic, almost synousoidal EEG correlate on backaveraged data, with the maximum amplitude coincident to the applied trigger point (Fig. 3–4). In this situation, the definition of the proper EEG peak from which latency to EMG bursts can be measured becomes arbitrary. Therefore, application of frequency analysis by means of discrete Fourier transform to both EEG and EMG signals appears appropriate to overcome the methodological limitation of backaveraging. The linear association of different rhythmic signals can then be estimated using coherence analysis. Coherence measures the linear association between two signals and can take values from 0 to 1, where 0 indicates no linear association and 1 indicates a perfect linear association. Coherence between scalp EEG and surface EMG activity has been used to detect functional coupling between oscillatory activity in the motor cortex and that in muscle in physiologic and pathologic conditions (71,72). Grosse and co-workers (70) applied EEG–EMG and EMG–EMG coherence analysis to the study of rhythmic cortical myoclonus (ADCME, Angelman syndrome, LGS, and celiac disease) and compared results with those generated by traditional backaveraging. Coherence analysis proved more sensitive than traditional backaveraging and showed an exaggerated coherence between EEG and contralateral EMG and between pairs of ipsilateral, distal EMG signals in the band that corresponded to the more represented frequencies on EMG channels. These findings support a cortical driving for rhythmic EMG activity (70).

In conclusion, different clinical conditions can be associated with rhythmic cortical myoclonus. Their etiologies range from genetic disorders such as Angelman syndrome to cases with acquired lesions. Rhythmic cortical generators are observed within layers IV and V of the

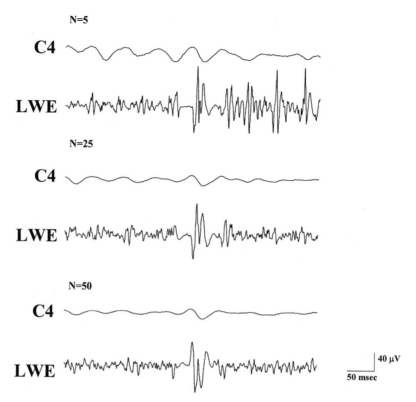

FIG. 3–4. EEG activity is backaveraged using the onset of myoclonic jerks in left wrist extensor (*LWE*) muscle as a trigger in a patient with Angelman syndrome. Letter *N* indicates the number of replications. A positive–negative–positive transient gradually emerges from background noise after increasing the number of averaged EEG epochs. However, other EEG transients are observed and appear time locked to other EMG bursts. This is due to the repetitive, rhythmical appearance of cortical myoclonus in Angelman syndrome. A different approach is needed to better assess the correlation between EEG and EMG activity.

normal motor cortex (73). Therefore, the translation of this physiological activity into rhythmic myoclonus can be unveiled by various mechanisms that produce hyperexcitability, such as lack of γ-aminobutyric acid-GABAergic inhibition in Angelman syndrome or deafferentation in cases with gross lesions.

Mechanisms of Spread

Facilitation of inter- and intrahemispheric spread of cortical myoclonic activity through transcallosal or intrahemispheric corticocortical pathways seems to play a major role in producing generalized or bilateral myoclonus (74). Spread

of cortical myoclonic activity can also underlie the transition from a "fragment of epilepsy" to epilepsy. In patients with cortical myoclonus, bilateral jerks are not synchronous. EMG activity in ipsilateral muscles under stimulation or during movement precedes that in the contralateral muscles by a delay ($\sim$10 msec) that is appropriate for transcallosal transfer of the excitation (Fig. 3–2) (20,28). The latencies pertaining to EMG activity of the muscles on a given side are consistent not only with the length of the descending motor pathway, but also with an extra delay due to spread within the motor cortex itself (74). Intrahemispheric spread follows a somatotopic pattern and could be attributed to corticocortical connections (74). Interhemispheric spread of myoclonic activity is also observed in Angelman syndrome, in which the myoclonic jerks usually start in one hand and spread to the contralateral hand (61) with a stable interside latency.

In some patients with cortical reflex myoclonus with various etiologies, myoclonic activity remains localized in the segment stimulated (74). Lack of any spread is particularly evident in Rett syndrome (44) and might be evidence of severely reduced horizontal corticocortical connectivity.

Rothwell and Brown (75) and Brown and colleagues (76) demonstrated impairment of ipsilateral and transcallosal inhibition, which could facilitate the spread of myoclonic activity. Patients with multifocal myoclonus were defined as "nonspreaders," and patients with generalized myoclonus, as "spreaders." Motor thresholds to single transcranial magnetic shocks were higher in "nonspreaders" than in "spreaders" or controls. This increase in the motor threshold was attributed to an increase in corticocortical inhibitory mechanisms. In addition, paired transcranial magnetic stimuli showed that "spreaders" had less ipsilateral inhibition at interstimulus intervals of 1–6 msec and less transcallosal inhibition across inhibitory timings (10–14 msec) compared with "nonspreaders." Although abnormalities in corticocortical and transcallosal inhibition may facilitate spreading of myoclonic activity, they do not appear to play a role in the production of generalized seizures, which were present to the same extent in both groups. There was no difference in inhibitory mechanisms between patients with and those without epilepsy (76).

It is likely that myoclonic activity descends from the sensorimotor cortex through the rapid conduction pyramidal pathways (9). This hypothesis is supported by the fact that (a) the time interval separating activation of two muscles involved in the spontaneous or reflex myoclonic jerk is similar to the time interval measurable between the same muscles by TMS; (b) the latency separating the premyoclonic EEG potential and the P30 component of the onset of the myoclonic jerks is similar to the latency of the MEP for that muscle obtained by TMS (77).

EPILEPTIC NEGATIVE MYOCLONUS

Brief (50–200 msec) and irregular muscle inhibitions during maintenance of a posture, visible as EMG silent periods, give rise to asterixis (78), a phenomenon observed in patients with metabolic encephalopathies or with focal lesions of the sensorimotor cortex (78,79). Asterixis is one of the expressions of negative myoclonus (4). Asterixis is usually multifocal in distribution but may affect a single somatic segment. In some patients with asterixis, jerk-locked EEG averaging shows a contralateral cortical transient time locked with the EMG silent period (80,81). Shibasaki and colleagues (82) have described cortical reflex negative myoclonus limited to muscles of one limb in patients with PMEs.

A similar clinical phenomenon is epileptic negative myoclonus, in which 50 to 400-msec periods of muscle inhibition with focal, multifocal, or bilateral distribution are time locked to sharp waves or spike-wave discharges on the contralateral central areas [(83,84; reviewed in Guerrini et al. (85)]. Clinically, it may be difficult to differentiate positive and negative epileptic myoclonus, as silent periods of sufficient duration may cause sudden lapses in posture, followed by brisk jerky movements that represent attempts to resume the original posture. Epileptic negative myoclonus is etiologically heterogeneous and may be observed in idiopathic epilepsy, in association with cortical dysplasia, or may be precipitated by adverse reaction to antiepileptic drugs (83,86,87). Shewmon and Erwin (88) studied a visual-related task in patients with occipital spike-and-wave discharges as a model aimed at demonstrating that each "interictal" paroxysmal EEG discharge may disrupt a specific cortical function for a length of time corresponding to its duration. According to this model, epileptic negative myoclonus is the clinical counterpart of spike-and-wave discharges involving neurons in the sensorimotor cortex. When the paroxysmal abnormalities are very frequent, anatomic-specific dysfunction of the higher cortical functions may also appear (89).

EMG silence, in selected muscles, with a duration of 50 to 300 msec, may be triggered either by stereotaxic stimulation of the boundary region between the thalamus and the capsula interna (90) or by transcutaneous electric or transcranial magnetic stimulation of the motor cortex (91). Rubboli et al. (1995), from the result of a computer based EEG analysis, concluded that a central epileptic focus secondarily involving the frontal area is responsible for ENM. In particular, they suggested an involvement of the supplementary motor area where a localized inhibitory area had been identified by cortical stimulation (Luders et al., 1995). Baumgartner et al. (1996) confirmed that the premotor cortex is responsible for ENM by combined ictal EEG-ictal single-photon emission computer tomography study in a 17 year-old patient with epilepsy and ENM refractory to various anticonvulsant drugs. In contrast a recent study suggested that the contralateral parietal or post-central cortex is important to produce ENM as demonstrated by subdurally implanted electrodes in patients with paracentral cerebral dysgenesis and ENM (Ikeda et al., 2000), Most recently, Matsunaga et al. (2000) studied ENM in a patient with Creutzfeldt-Jakob disease and suggested that inhibition in the motor cortex is enhanced. Shibasaki (2002), reviewing several papers on ENM and adding personal data, showed that the inhibitory activity of the primary motor cortex is enhanced in patients with ENM. He postulated that an excessive input arising from pre-motor or post-central regions to the primary motor cortex results in increasing inhibition of the motor system, leading to ENM. Therefore, interpretation of such inhibitory motor phenomenona does not necessarily require disinhibitory (98) ictal activation of "negative" motor areas (99). It is sufficient to assume hypersynchronous ictal inhibition in "primary" motor cortex neurons. The myoclonic jerks produced by the postural lapses and subsequent postural recovery, typical of epileptic negative myoclonus, seems to be different from postmyoclonic atonic phenomena, which are usually generalized (100). Gastaut and Regis (101) showed that "inhibition of muscle tonus can immediately follow the my-oclonias of Petit Mal and may be so pronounced as to cause a fall" and that "myoclonia always corresponds to the polyspikes, whereas the tonic inhibition corresponds to the slow waves which follow them." We now know that several epileptic syndromes featuring violent myoclonic jerks, followed by a transient (100–400 msec) inhibition, are characterized by myoclonoatonic falls (e.g., myoclonoastatic epilepsy).

THALAMOCORTICAL MYOCLONUS/ IDIOPATHIC (PRIMARY) GENERALIZED EPILEPTIC MYOCLONUS

Clinical Findings

This type of myoclonus is common to various epileptic syndromes, in which it may be observed either as the sole manifestation or in association with other seizure types. Clinically, myoclonus presents as generalized, spontaneous, predominantly arrhythmic jerks, with inconstant axial predominance. Depending on severity, patients may present with simple head nodding or raised shoulders, or may stagger or fall.

Neurophysiologic Findings

The generalized jerks appear to originate from afferent volleys from subcortical structures that act synchronously on a hyperexcitable cortex (8,102). As a consequence, muscles from both sides are activated synchronously, as in reticular myoclonus, and muscles innervated by the cranial nerves are involved through a rostrocaudal pattern of activation, as in cortical myoclonus. This suggests that the impulse generating the myoclonus descends through the brainstem. The EEG correlate is a generalized spike-wave, in which the negative peak of the spike precedes the generalized jerks by 20 to 75 msec (7). Duration of the EEG transient is 30 to 100 msec and that of the myoclonic potential is less than 100 msec. Okino et al. (1997), studying patients with both idiopathic and symptomatic myoclonic seizures, found latencies between the spike of the spike-and-wave complex and the myoclonic potential ranging from 21 to 80 ms (mean = 38 ms). They argued that these latencies are longer than the time required for passing through the piramidal tract and proposed a polysynaptic, thalamo-reticular, descending pathway.

However, reported neurophysiological data do not provide conclusive evidences in favour of either pathophysiological hypotheses. EEG-EMG and EMG-EMG coherence analysis (see Cortical Myoclonus—Rhythmic or Arrhythmic Recurrence section) could eventually prove a cortical or thalamo-reticular origin for the descending pathway.

RETICULAR REFLEX MYOCLONUS

Reticular myoclonus presents most of the clinical and neurophysiological characteristics of epileptic myoclonus, although it lacks a time-locked EEG correlate (9).

Clinical Findings

Clinically, myoclonic jerks are generalized, with greater involvement of proximal and flexor muscles, spontaneous, or induced by somatosensory, auditory and visual stimuli, or by movement (9,104).

Neurophysiologic Findings

Reticular myoclonus is believed to originate from the brainstem reticular formation. This hypothesis is supported by the finding that when there is involvement of muscles innervated by the cranial nerves, the surface EMG shows activation, initially, of the trapezius muscle (XIth cranial nerve), followed by the sternocleidomastoid (XIth cranial nerve), the orbicularis oris (VIIth cranial nerve), and, finally, the masseter (Vth cranial nerve). The initial activation of the trapezius muscle suggests that the impulse generating the myoclonus originates from the medulla (104). In addition, EEG or JLA allows demonstration of an EEG potential with wide distribution over the hemispheres and greater amplitude at the vertex, which is not time locked with the myoclonic potential, but often follows muscle activation. These observations suggest that the spike is projected and is not directly responsible for the myoclonus (9).

The SEPs do not have increased amplitude. When the myoclonus is of the reflex type, it is possible to estimate the speed of conduction of the efferent bulbospinal motor pattern. The difference in latency between the different muscles activated may be similar to that between the same muscles when activation is obtained through TMS of the motor cortex (105) when rapidly conducting bulbospinal motor pathways mediate the reflex jerks. However, slower conduction has also been observed, suggesting that there could be various subtypes of reticular reflex myoclonus, given that there are several descending reticular spinal systems with different conduction velocities (32). Patients have been described with postanoxic encephalopathy, and with a combination of cortical myoclonus and brainstem reticular reflex myoclonus (14,35,105). Clinically, there are both multifocal and generalized jerks.

Cantello and co-workers (106) found that in a series of patients with myoclonic epilepsy with ragged-red fiber disease (MERRF) and Unverricht–Lundborg disease, the sum of afferent and efferent times to and from the cortex was longer than the latency of the reflex or spontaneous myoclonus. These authors hypothesized that the short-latency myoclonic discharge originated subcortically, at a site with sufficient somatotopic organization, to spread upward to produce a cortical potential, and downward to the spinal cord to produce the jerk. Such a subcortical mechanism would be additional and not alternative to cortical reflex myoclonus. Although no hypothesis was formulated about the specific subcortical site of origin of myoclonus, a reticular origin was considered unlikely because of its focal nature. The patients studied had multifocal spontaneous, action and reflex jerks, but none presented with generalized jerks, which is a frequent expression of action myoclonus. However, in a subsequent study the same pattern of myoclonus was also observed in patients showing reflex generalized jerks consistent with reticular reflex myoclonus, in response to somatosensory stimulation (R. Cantello, *personal communication*, 2000). One wonders whether a predominantly multifocal or generalized expression of reticular myoclonus is possible according to the underlying pathologic substrate.

Neurophysiologic study of reticular reflex myoclonus is difficult, especially because of the coexistence of cortical myoclonus. Only a few patients have been reported. As a consequence, its neurophysiologic correlates and relationships with epilepsy are not fully understood. The presence of seizures in most reported patients indicates a close clinical association with epilepsy. Although an EEG spike is often associated with the myoclonic jerks, EEG and EMG events are not time locked, suggesting that the spike is projected, does not originate primarily in the cortex, and is not directly responsible for the myoclonus (9).

Myoclonus produced in the cat after urea infusion (107) has been proposed as an animal model for reticular reflex myoclonus. Electrophysiologic recording demonstrated this to be generated by neuronal activity resembling paroxysmal depolarization shifts in the nucleus reticularis gigantocellularis. Cobalt injection at this level also causes myoclonus (108). According to such a model, in humans paroxysmal depolarization shifts in the caudal brainstem reticular formation would generate a volley-producing muscle recruitment down the spinal cord and up the brainstem, as well as a projected EEG discharge.

Reticular reflex myoclonus must be distinguished from hyperekplexia, in which the reflex jerks represent an exaggerated normal startle reflex. Neurophysiologic investigation has shown that the origin of startle response is in the caudal brainstem, but, unlike reticular reflex myoclonus, utilizes slowly conducting bulbospinal motor pathways (32).

CLASSIFICATION OF MYOCLONIC EPILEPSIES ACCORDING TO THE PATHOPHYSIOLOGY OF EPILEPTIC MYOCLONUS

The Nosologic Problem of the Myoclonic Epilepsies

The term *myoclonic epilepsies* has been often used to collectively designate a large group of epilepsies characterized by repeated, brief seizures often responsible for multiple falls, by a severe course that frequently is resistant to antiepileptic drugs, and by their usual association with mental retardation (109,110). As a result, confusion has arisen as this wide group clearly includes several different syndromes with different seizure types only superficially similar.

Part of the difficulty arises from the fact that there exist several types of brief seizures manifested by sudden, brief jerks. Although these seizures are superficially similar and, as a consequence, are often loosely termed myoclonic, they correspond to different neurophysiologic mechanisms. Precise analysis of the ictal manifestations by combined clinical, EEG, EMG, and videomonitoring permits distinction of different types of seizures: (a) "true" myoclonic seizures, (b) atonic seizures, (c) tonic seizures or spasms (Fig. 3–5). "True" myoclonic seizures are manifested as biphasic or polyphasic EMG potentials of 20- to 150-msec duration that may be followed by a tonic contraction of affected muscles or by a transient suppression of normal tonic activity, lasting up to 400 msec and may, therefore, be termed myoatonic seizures (111,112). On EEG tracings, myoclonic seizures are associated with generalized bursts of polyspike-and-waves or spike-waves. During atonic seizures, the patient may fall to the ground suddenly or slump in a rhythmic, step-by-step fashion (113), or may have only a brief nodding of the head or a sagging of the body. Atonic seizures are accompanied on EEG recordings by slow spike-waves (114,115), 3-Hz spike–waves (116), polyspike-waves (117, 118), or fast recruiting rhythms (117,119). The EMG shows suppression of normal tonic activity in the involved muscles (101,118). Tonic seizures involve the tonic contraction of certain muscle groups without progression to a clonic phase (113,120). They also can cause the patient to fall to the ground when the lower limbs are forcibly flexed or the patient is thrown off balance, especially when the tonic contraction is asymmetrical. The EMG, during a tonic seizure, shows an interferential muscle discharge similar to that in voluntary contraction. The EEG may show simple flattening of all activity throughout the attack, a very fast activity ($\sim$20 Hz) of increasing amplitude, or a discharge of 10-Hz rhythm with a high amplitude from onset but otherwise similar to the

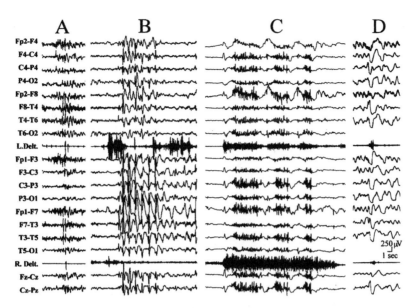

FIG. 3–5. Polygraphic characterization of different brief seizures, clinically manifested as jerks. **A:** Myoclonic seizure. Note that the EMG burst is very brief (<100 msec) and it is time locked to a polyspike-and-wave discharge. **B:** Atonic seizure. The spike-and-wave discharge is accompanied by an EMG silent period, lasting as long as the discharge on left deltoid. Note that the onset of the silent period is progressive. **C:** Tonic seizure. A polyspike discharge is associated to a tonic contraction that has a crescendo pattern at onset but remains sustained subsequently. **D:** Epileptic spasm. A brief, diamond shaped EMG burst, lasting around 500 msec, is correlated to a high-amplitude, diffuse polyphasic slow transient on EEG channels.

"epileptic recruiting rhythm" (118,119,121,122). Spasms that are, in fact, very similar to brief tonic seizures can also occur and are an important cause of sudden falls (123).

In conclusion, "true" myoclonic seizures are characteristic of myoclonic epilepsy. They can rarely represent the only seizure type as in benign myoclonic epilepsy of infancy, but they are usually associated to other seizure types, namely, absence seizures and generalized tonic-clonic seizures in most of the other myoclonic epilepsies.

EPILEPTIC SYNDROMES AND NEUROLOGIC DISORDERS WITH CORTICAL MYOCLONUS

Cortical Action/Reflex Myoclonus

Progressive Myoclonus Epilepsies

This group of diseases is characterized by progressive myoclonus, generalized, tonic-clonic seizures, and neurologic deterioration (5). Onset is most frequent in late childhood or adolescence (124). Different forms are known, such as Unverricht–Lundborg disease, Lafora disease, neuronal ceroid–lipofuscinosis, type III Gaucher disease, infantile and juvenile GM2-gangliosidosis, some mitochondrial encephalopathies, sialidosis, and dentatorubropallidoluysian atrophy (124). Specific mutations have been defined in some (125). Onset features comprise myoclonus and rare generalized tonic-clonic seizures, as in idiopathic myoclonic epilepsies (86,124). Tonic-clonic seizures can occur without any warning or after a long build-up of myoclonus. The EEG shows generalized polyspike and spike-and-wave discharges frequently precipitated by photic stimulation. Background EEG activity becomes progressively slower (124). CRM is common to all PME syndromes, in which it is manifested with the classic combination of action myoclonus, spontaneous jerks, giant SEPs, C-reflex at rest, and the premyoclonus spike. Initially mild, myoclonus becomes increasingly disabling during its course.

Rhythmic Fast-Bursting Cortical Myoclonus

Angelman Syndrome

Angelman syndrome is a neurogenetic disorder caused by a defect in maternal chromosome 15q11-q13. A molecular deletion including three genes coding for the $\alpha 5$, $\beta 3$ and $\gamma 3$ subunits of the GABAA (*GABRB3, GABRA5,* and *GABRG3*) and for the *UBE3A* gene is present in 70% of patients (126). Less frequently, Angelman syndrome is caused by uniparental paternal disomy (UPD), or mutations in the imprinting center or in the *UBE3A* gene. Patients present with severe mental retardation, absence of language, microbrachicephaly, inappropriate paroxysmal laughter, epilepsy, EEG abnormalities, ataxic gait, tremor, and jerky movements. Neurophysiologic and polygraphic investigations reveal a spectrum of myoclonic manifestations (61). All patients present with rapid distal jerking of fluctuating amplitude, which causes a sort of coarse distal tremor combined with dystonic limb posturing. Jerks occur at rest in prolonged runs. In addition, the majority of patients have myoclonic and absence seizures, as well as episodes of myoclonic status. Bilateral jerks of myoclonic absences show rhythmic repetition at ~2.5 Hz and are time locked with a cortical spike. Interside latency of both spikes and jerks is consistent with transcallosal spread, and spike-to-jerk latency indicates propagation through rapid conduction corticospinal pathway. Epilepsy is much more severe in patients with a deletion than in those without. It is therefore likely that in addition to *UBE3A*, other genes in 15q11-13 (especially *GABRB3*) could play a major role in epileptogenesis (127).

Familial Autosomal Dominant Myoclonus and Autosomal Dominant Cortical Reflex Myoclonus and Epilepsy

Familial autosomal dominant myoclonus has been described in several families of mostly Japanese origin (66,67,128–130). Affected patients present very homogeneous characteristics: (a) autosomal dominant inheritance; (b) adult onset (mean age 38 years, range: 19–73); (c) nonprogressive course; (d) distal, rhythmic myoclonus, enhanced during posture maintenance; (e) rare, apparently generalized seizures often preceded by worsening of myoclonus; (f) absence of other neurologic signs; (g) generalized interictal spike-and-wave discharges; (h) photoparoxysmal response; (i) giant SEPs; (j) hyperexcitability of the C-reflex; and (k) cortical EEG potential time locked to the jerks. Linkage analysis in the original Japanese families indicated that the disease was linked to chromosome 8q23.3-q24 locus (131,132). However, the European families with a similar phenotype did not link to the same locus (130,133).

Autosomal dominant cortical reflex myoclonus and epilepsy (134) (see also Chapter 21) patients present with a homogeneous syndromic core including an association of nonprogressive cortical reflex myoclonus, expressed with semicontinuous rhythmic distal jerking (cortical tremor), generalized tonic-clonic seizures (GTCSs) preceded in some patients by generalized myoclonic jerks, and generalized EEG abnormalities. Age at onset of cortical tremor and of GTCSs overlap in a given individual, but vary among individuals, ranging from 12 to 50 years. This clinical picture shares some features with FAME (131,132), however, all ADCME patients have in addition focal frontotemporal EEG abnormalities and some individuals also have focal seizures. They start at around the same age as the other manifestations and are either intractable or, alternatively, go into remission after several years.

The pattern of inheritance is autosomal dominant with high penetrance and linkage analysis identified a critical region on chromosome 2p11.1-q12.2. The exclusion of the locus for FAME on chromosome 8q23.3-q24 from linkage to ADCME family and the new localization of the responsible gene to chromosome 2, together with the different phenotype, defines a new epilepsy syndrome (134). Interestingly, the two Italian families with FAME, described earlier by De Falco and colleagues (133) show linkage to chromosome 2p11.1-q12.2 and suggest a possible allelism with ADCME.

Epileptic Syndromes With Secondarily Generalized Epileptic Myoclonus

Severe Myoclonic Epilepsy

Severe myoclonic epilepsy (SME) is observed in 6% to 7% of children with seizure onset in the first 3 years of life (135). Genetic factors play an important role in SME. Claes et al. (136) described *de novo* truncating mutations of the *SCN1A* gene in seven consecutive children with SME. However, frequency and types of *SCN1A* mutations are variable. Some groups found a mutation rate of 77% to 82%, with truncating mutations being the most frequent (137–139). Other authors indicate that *SCN1A* mutations, including missense mutations, which do not result in severe loss of the protein product, are observed in only about 35% of patients with SME. In about 10% of cases they are inherited from parents who are either asymptomatic or suffer from a mild form of epilepsy (140). These observations suggest genetic heterogeneity and imply the possibility that involvement of a second gene is required for the syndrome to manifest.

Onset of epilepsy occurs during the first year of life with prolonged seizures (generalized or unilateral, clonic or tonic-clonic, often evolving to status) during fever. They rapidly become associated with similar nonfebrile attacks. By the fourth year of life, resistant myoclonic, focal seizures, and atypical absences also appear. EEG, normal at the beginning, subsequently shows multifocal and generalized abnormalities. Early photosensitivity is seen in some children. Neurologic development appears delayed from the second year of life onward. Two main types of myoclonus are observed. Almost all children show arrhythmic, distal jerks, manifested as twitching of fingers, whereas some also have generalized jerks preceded by clear-cut spike-and-wave discharges (Fig. 3–6). Although distal jerks are not accompanied by a premyoclonic potential on JLA, generalized jerks appear to originate from spread of CM activity (86). SME is an epileptic encephalopathy whose evolution is constantly severe. Both different seizure types and the characteristic of generalized myoclonus, shifting generator from one hemisphere to the other in sequential discharges, support a diffuse hyperexcitability of the brain and can explain why this syndrome is so difficult to treat.

Lennox–Gastaut Syndrome

LGS has a prevalence of 2% to 3% in children with epilepsy and is usually observed in children with diffuse brain damage (141). Typical seizures start at 3 to 5 years of age as tonic, atonic, or atypical absences (141), but a previous form of epilepsy, especially West syndrome, is frequently observed. Other associated seizure types are myoclonic, generalized tonic-clonic, and focal. Epilepsy is drug resistant and episodes of status are frequent. Interictal EEG shows abnormal background activity, slow (1.5–2.5 Hz) generalized spike-waves, and, often, multifocal abnormalities. During sleep, all patients show typical rhythmic discharges at around 10 Hz, accompanying tonic seizures or without apparent clinical correlate. Myoclonus is not a prominent feature of LGS (142), but some patients exhibit generalized myoclonic jerks. They seem to be produced by a secondary generalization of focal CM (86,143). Minipolymyoclonus, presenting with distal, small focal jerks, frequently leading to individual tiny finger movements, is observed in different symptomatic conditions, including LGS (28). Backaveraged EEG shows, in some patients, a bifrontal negative slow wave, with a 20- to 500-msec latency from myoclonus onset, whereas in other patients a sharper bifrontal negativity leading the jerks by 40 to 70 msec (29). Minipolymyoclonus is strongly similar to the pattern of distal myoclonus observed in patients with SME, LGS, or Angelman syndrome (61).

EPILEPTIC SYNDROMES AND NEUROLOGIC DISORDERS WITH THALAMOCORTICAL MYOCLONUS
Idiopathic Generalized Epilepsies

Benign Myoclonic Epilepsy of Infancy

Benign myoclonic epilepsy of infancy (BMEI) affects 0.4% to 2% of all children with seizure

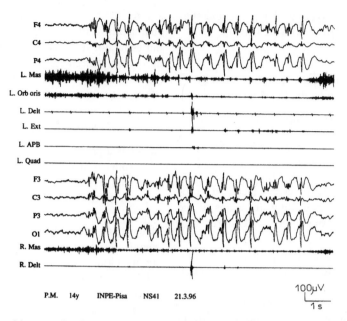

FIG. 3–6. Polygraphic recording in a 14-year-old boy affected by SME (or Dravet syndrome), showing a generalized, 2.5 to 3-Hz polyspike-and-wave discharge, lasting around 6–7 sec. A single, whole body jerk, time locked to a polyspike-and-wave complex is recorded on EMG channels. Note the presence of repetitive, almost rhythmic myoclonic jerks on left masseter. Each potential is time locked to a polyspike-and-wave discharge and is followed by a postmyoclonic silent period. *APB*, abductor pollicis brevis; *Delt*, deltoid; *Ext*, wrist extensor; *L.*, left; *Mass*, masseter; *Orb oris*, orbicularis oris; *Quad*, quadriceps; *R.*, right.

onset by age 3 years (144–146). Age at onset ranges between 4 months and 3 years in children with normal development. Some patients, however, can have mild mental retardation (145,147,148). Seizures consist of generalized myoclonic jerks, brief, isolated or repeated in series of two or three. If the child is standing or sitting, the jerks often cause nodding with upward gaze deviation and eyelid myoclonus, accompanied by slight arm abduction or elbow bending. Staggering may occur, especially up to the second year of life, when walking is still unstable. If falls occur, the child collapses on his or her buttocks and then gets up immediately. In most cases, the jerks occur many times per day. A few patients may have generalized tonic-clonic seizures in adolescence after therapy withdrawal (145). About 10% of children with BME have photic-induced jerks (145,146). Some have both spontaneous and reflex myoclonus, the latter triggered by tactile or sudden acoustic stimuli (149–151). Neurophysiol-

ogy of myoclonus reveals symmetric, rostrocaudal muscle activation and a premyoclonus negative spike preceding jerks by 30 ± 2 msec (9). Duration of the myoclonic jerk is roughly 100 msec.

In general, BMEI is a benign syndrome, in which myoclonic seizures represent the only seizure type. Its evolution, in particular for patients presenting with stimulus-triggered seizures, is age dependent with remission within a few years from onset. However, the definition of BMEI was based on retrospective selection of patients who presented a good outcome. Following children with myoclonic seizures as the main or only seizure type, there are patients who present with a less favorable evolution either in terms of seizure control or in terms of cognitive outcome. These patients share features of both BMEI and myoclonic-astatic epilepsy (MAE). In a review of 103 cases reported under the heading of BMEI, Dravet et al. (152) slightly modified the initial concepts. They acknowledged that age at onset may be as late as 5 years (146), that the term "benign" is questionable according to the most recent ILAE definitions (153), and that the differentiation of BMEI from the milder cases of MAE, may not be entirely clear. It seems likely that epilepsies with prominent myoclonic activity, including BMEI, MAE, and other unclassifiable cases (but excluding SME and LGS that clearly belong to separate categories) are part of a continuum in which, despite different degrees of severity and a different outcome, the clinical presentation and etiological factors (e.g., genetics) may be closely related.

Juvenile Myoclonic Epilepsy (JME)

JME has a prevalence of between 3.4% and 11.9% (154) and represents 23.3% of all idiopathic generalized epilepsies (154). Although a gene involved has been linked to chromosome 6p, JME is genetically heterogeneous (155). Onset occurs at around age 14, with generalized myoclonus and generalized tonic-clonic seizures. Myoclonic jerks constitute the initial symptom in 54% of patients and are bilateral, single, repetitive (37 vs. 63%, Oguni et al., 1994), or arrhythmic, and more pronounced in the upper limbs. Video analysis showed that either distal or proximal muscle involvement of upper limbs predominate. In the former, there is mild bilateral flexion and external rotation of the forearms; in the latter, flexion of both arms at the elbow, flexion and abduction of the thighs and extension of the back (Oguni et al., 1994). When the patient keeps both arms outstretched, the arms drop out and, on polygraphy, this clinical event is correlated to a sudden interruption of ongoing EMG activity. If intense, this may result in falls but do not seem to be accompanied by loss of consciousness. They are characteristically concentrated in the minutes following awakening. In 5% of patients, generalized jerks are also triggered by intermittent photic stimulation. In 7% of patients, there may be episodes of myoclonic status (156), at times precipitated by inappropriate drug use, especially carbamazepine. Generalized tonic-clonic seizures are present in 84% of patients and represent the initial symptom in 35% of cases. They are often preceded by generalized myoclonic jerks. In 27% of patients, absences are also present, occurring infrequently (less than several times per week). Treatment with valproic acid in monotherapy or in association with clonazepam leads to total control of seizures in 80% of patients (154). Discontinuation of drug therapy is followed by a high rate of relapse (90%) (154).

Neurophysiologic analysis of myoclonus indicates that muscles from both sides are activated synchronously and muscles innervated by the cranial nerves are involved through a rostrocaudal pattern of activation. The EEG correlate is a generalized spike- or polyspikes-wave at 3–5 Hz, in which the negative peak of the spike precedes the generalized jerks by 30 msec (8). Duration of the EEG transient is ~100 msec and that of the myoclonic potential is less than 100 msec.

Myoclonic-Astatic Epilepsy (MAE)

Epilepsy with myoclonic-astatic seizures is a generalized cryptogenic or symptomatic form with onset between 7 months and 6 years. Children with MAE have several types of seizures, including atypical absences, generalized clonic or tonic-clonic seizures, massive myoclonus, and episodes of status epilepticus with erratic myoclonus, and clouding of consciousness. Since the classification was published (6), there has been growing evidence that among children with MAE, there is a large subgroup with idiopathic epilepsy or "primarily generalized seizures" (157). Although the distinction between MAE and LGS is now accepted (141,158), among patients previously included under the heading of MAE there still appears to be an overlap with other syndromes that feature myoclonus.

In children whose only clinical feature is severe myoclonus and whose prognosis is favorable, the likely diagnosis is BMEI. Children who have frequent and prolonged unilateral alternating febrile and afebrile clonic seizures from the first year of life and myoclonic attacks after some years probably have severe myoclonic epilepsy in infancy (135). However, there continues to be a rather large subgroup of patients with "true myoclonic-astatic epilepsy" (7,159) who share some distinct electroclinical features but may have a variable outcome.

The neurophysiology of myoclonus in MAE confirms this nosologic interpretation (9,143). Thus, myoclonus may manifest in the form of bilateral synchronous single whole body jerks. As with myoclonus in BMEI and JME, this is consistent with the hypothesis of a thalamocortical volley. The jerks, which have a duration of ~100 msec, are preceded by a negative EEG potential of ~30 msec. These children also show a peculiar form of myoclonic status, with the neurophysiologic characters of erratic cortical myoclonus with multifocal jerking, increase in basic muscle tone, and clouding of consciousness. Status may occur spontaneously or be precipitated by carbamazepine (9).

EPILEPTIC SYNDROMES WITH MYOCLONUS OF UNCLEAR NEUROPHYSIOLOGIC CHARACTERIZATION

Early Myoclonic Encephalopathy

Early myoclonic encephalopathy is a rare syndrome classified among the generalized symptomatic epilepsies with nonspecific etiology (6). Some inborn errors of metabolism can provoke early myoclonic encephalopathy, such as methylmalonic acidemia and nonketotic hyperglycinemia. Onset is neonatal or during the first month of life with severe myoclonus, followed by focal seizures and tonic spasms. Myoclonus involves the muscles of the face and the extremities, with a multifocal distribution, leading to the description of "erratic." Neurologic development is severely delayed, with marked hypotonia, impaired alertness, and, often, vegetative state (160). The EEG is characterized by suppression bursts: Bursts of spikes, sharp waves and slow waves, are irregularly separated by periods of electric silence. Erratic myoclonus generally does not have an ictal EEG correlate (160).

Myoclonic Status in Fixed Encephalopathies

This condition is seen exclusively in severe encephalopathies with profound cognitive deficit and hypotonia and is characterized by recurrent, prolonged, and drug-resistant episodes of myoclonic status (161). About half the cases, reported by Dalla Bernardina et al. (161) turned out to have Angelman syndrome. Associated seizure types include partial motor, myoclonic absences, generalized myoclonias, and, rarely, unilateral or generalized clonic seizures.

Myoclonic status is characterized by almost continuous absences accompanied by erratic, distal, multifocal, frequent myoclonias, which sometimes become more rhythmic and diffuse. This condition may be insidious, because reduced awareness may be diffcult to recognize in severely mentally retarded children and associated jerks may be very mild, and become clearly detectable only during polygraphic EEG/EMG recordings.

When the myoclonic jerks are rhythmic and bilateral, in bursts or continuous, they are closely related to 1.5-to 2.5-Hz spike-and-wave discharges (61). Sometimes, myoclonias are continuous, but asynchronous, in the different muscles involved. In this case, the relationship between myoclonic jerks and paroxysmal EEG discharges is more difficult to appreciate on surface EEG (161). It is extremely important to recognize this condition, which can mimic a progressive encephalopathy.

Epilepsy with Myoclonic Absences

Epilepsy with myoclonic absences is currently classified among cryptogenic or symptomatic generalized epilepsies (6). Onset is at about age 7 years with absences recurring many times a day, accompanied by bilateral rhythmic jerks, involving the shoulders, arms or legs. There may be concomitant mild axial tonic contraction. Consciousness is cloudy (162) but not completely interrupted. Bilateral, synchronous, and symmetric spike-wave discharges at 3 Hz accompany the absences. Myoclonic jerks have the same frequency as the EEG discharges. Absences are often resistant to treatment. Other types of seizures are observed only rarely. Evolution is variable: cognitive deterioration, evolution toward a different type of epilepsy, at times full recovery without sequelae.

The physiology of myoclonus in epilepsy with myoclonic absences is difficult to study, as this condition is rare, and in the majority of patients the jerks appear against a background of increased muscle tone (9). Tassinari and co-workers (163) found a close and constant relationship between the spike-and-wave complex and the jerk, in that the positive spike of the spike-and-wave complex is followed by a myoclonic jerk with a latency of 15 to 40 msec (proximal muscles).

CONCLUSIONS

Epileptic myoclonus can be divided on a neurophysiologic basis into cortical, positive and negative, thalamocortical, and reticular. Cortical epileptic myoclonus constitutes a fragment of partial or symptomatic generalized epilepsy; thalamocortical epileptic myoclonus is a fragment of idiopathic generalized epilepsy (91). Reflex reticular myoclonus, which does not have a time-locked EEG correlate, represents the clinical counterpart of fragments of hypersynchronous epileptic activity of neurons in the brain stem reticular formation.

Attempts have been made to elaborate a specific classification of childhood epilepsies in which myoclonus constitutes the clinically most relevant element (6,7,164). However, considerable confusion still persists in clinical practice, as many cases prove difficult to classify.

Available data on epileptic syndromes with prominent myoclonic seizures indicate that three main subgroups can be identified on the basis of the neurophysiologic characteristics of epileptic myoclonus (Table 1): (a) syndromes with prominent cortical epileptic myoclonus; (b) syndromes with thalamocortical epileptic myoclonus; (c) syndromes in which myoclonus is neurophysiologically difficult to classify.

Using neurophysiologic criteria, in addition to classical clinical and EEG observations, may certainly help determine diagnosis and treatment in uncertain cases. Specific epileptic syndromes, such as SME, LGS and MAE, which have in the past been lumped together and confused with one another under the definition of myoclonic epilepsies, show different neurophysiologic patterns of myoclonus, in addition to specific clinical features, and different responses to treatment.

TABLE 3–1. *Classification of myoclonic epilepsies according to the pathophysiology of epileptic myoclonus*

A) EPILEPTIC SYNDROMES AND NEUROLOGICAL DISORDERS WITH CORTICAL MYOCLONUS

Cortical reflex myoclonus

Progressive myoclonus epilepsies
Photic induced eyelid myoclonia

Rhythmic fast bursting cortical myoclonus

Angelman syndrome
FAME
ADCME
Fixed encephalopathies of various etiology
(tuberous sclerosis, Down syndrome, post traumatic)
Progressive myoclonus epilepsies

Secondarily generalized epileptic myoclonus

Severe myoclonic epilepsy
Lennox-Gastaut syndrome
Progressive myoclonus epilepsies

B) EPILEPTIC SYNDROMES OR DISORDERS WITH PRIMARY GENERALIZED EPILEPTIC (THALAMO-CORTICAL) MYOCLONUS

Benign myoclonic epilepsy of infancy
Myoclonic-astatic epilepsy
Juvenile myoclonic epilepsy
Other unclassified "myoclonic" epilepsies

C) EPILEPTIC SEIZURES/SYNDROMES WITH MYOCLONUS OF UNCLEAR NEUROPHYSIOLOGIC CHARACTERIZATION

Early Myoclonic Encephalopathy
Myoclonic Status in Fixed Encephalopathies
Myoclonic absences
Photic-induced generalised myoclonus

REFERENCES

1. Dubini A. Primi cenni sulla corea electrica. *Annali Universali di Medicina (Milano)* 1846;117:5–50.
2. Lundborg H. *Die progressive mioklonus-epilepsie.* Upsalla: Almquist and Wiksell, 1903.
3. Muskens LJJ. *Epilepsy: comparative pathogenesis, symptoms, treatment.* New York: William Wood.
4. Marsden CD, Hallett M, Fahn S. The nosology and pathophysiology of myoclonus. In: Marsden CD, Fahn S, eds. *Movement disorders,* London: Butterworths Scientific, 1982: 196–249.
5. Fahn S, Marsden CD, Van Woert MH. Definition and classification of myoclonus. *Adv Neurol* 1986; 43:1–5.
6. Commission on classification and terminology of the international league against epilepsy. Proposal for revised classification of epilepsies and epileptic syndromes. *Epilepsia* 1989;30:389–399.
7. Commission on pediatric epilepsy of the international league against epilepsy. Myoclonus and epilepsy in childhood. *Epilepsia* 1997;38:1251–1254.

8. Patel VM, Jankovic J. *Myoclonus. Curr Neurol* 1988; 8:109–156.

9. Hallett M. Myoclonus: relation to epilepsy. *Epilepsia* 1985;26[suppl. 1]:67–77.

10. Guerrini R, Bonanni P, Rothwell J, et al. Myoclonus and epilepsy. In: Guerrini R, Aicardi J, Andermann F, Hallett M, eds. *Epilepsy and movement disorder.* Cambridge: Cambridge University Press, 2002:165–210.

11. Deuschl G, Ebner A, Hammers R, et al. Differences of cortical activation in spontaneous and reflex myoclonias. *Electroencephalogr Clin Neurophysiol* 1991;80:326–328.

12. Kanouchi T, Yakota T, Kamata T, Ishii K, Senda M. Central pathway of photic reflex myoclonus. *J Neurol Neurosurg Psychiatry* 1997;62:414–417.

13. Shibasaki H, Kuroiwa Y. Electroencephalographic correlates of myoclonus. *Electroencephalogr Clin Neurophysiol* 1975;39:455–463.

14. Hallett M, Chadwick D, Marsden CD. Cortical reflex myoclonus. *Neurology* 1979;29:1107–1125.

15. Shibasaki H, Kakigi R, Ikeda A. Scalp topography of giant SEP and pre-myoclonus spike in cortical reflex myoclonus. *Electroencephalogr Clin Neurophysiol* 1991;81:31–37.

16. Mima T, Nagamine T, Ikeda A, Yazawa S, Kimura J, and Shibasaki, H. Pathogenesis of cortical myoclonus studied by magnetoencephalography. *Ann Neurol* 1998;43:598–607.

17. Kugelberg E, Widén L. Epilepsia partialis continua. *Electroencephalogr Clin Neurophysiol* 1954;6:503–506.

18. Cowan JMA, Rothwell JC, Wise RJS, et al. Electrophysiologic and positron emission studies in a patient with cortical myoclonus, epilepsia partialis continua and motor epilepsy. *J Neurol Neurosurg Psychiatry* 1986;49:796–807.

19. Legatt AD, LaSala PA, Mitnick R, et al. Electrophysiologic studies and intraoperative localization in a child with epilepsia partialis continua. *J Epilepsy* 1996;9:192–197.

20. Shibasaki H, Yamashita Y, Kuroiwa Y. Electroencephalographic studies of myoclonus. Myoclonus-related cortical spikes and high amplitude somatosensory evoked potentials. *Brain* 1978;101:447–460.

21. Kelly JJ, Shorbrough FW, Daube JR. A clinical and electrophysiologic evaluation of myoclonus. *Neurology* 1981;31:581–589.

22. Obeso J, Rothwell JC, Marsden CD. The spectrum of cortical myoclonus: from focal reflex jerks to spontaneous motor epilepsy. *Brain* 1985;108:193–224.

23. Kakigi R, Shibasaki H. Generator mechanisms of giant somatosensory evoked potentials in cortical reflex myoclonus. *Brain* 1887;110:1359–1373.

24. Ikeda A, Kakigi R, Funai N, et al. Cortical tremor: a variant of cortical reflex myoclonus. *Neurology* 1990;40:1561–1565.

25. Toro C, Pascual-Leone A, Deuschl G. Cortical tremor: a common manifestation of cortical myoclonus. *Neurology* 1993;43:2346–2353.

26. Ikeda A, Shibasaki H, Nagamine T, et al. Peri-rolandic and fronto-parietal components of scalp-recorded giant SEPs in cortical myoclonus. *Electroencephalogr Clin Neurophysiol* 1995;96:300–309.

27. Ugawa Y, Kkohara N, Hirasawa H, et al. Myoclonus in Alzheimer disease. *J Neurol* 1987;235:90–94.

28. Wilkins DE, Hallett M, Berardelli A, et al. Physiologic analysis of the myoclonus of Alzheimer disease. *Neurology* 1984;34:898–903.

29. Wilkins DE, Hallett M, Erba G. Primary generalized epileptic myoclonus: a frequent manifestation of minipolymyoclonus of central origin. *J Neurol Neurosurg Psychiatry* 1985;48:506–516.

30. Deuschl G, Schenck E, Lücking CH, et al. Cortical reflex myoclonus and its relation to normal long-latency reflexes. In: Benecke R, Conrad B, Marsden CD, eds. *Motor disturbances,* London: Academic Press, 1987:305–319.

31. Sutton GG, Mayer RF. Focal reflex myoclonus. *J Neurol Neurosurg Psychiatry* 1974;7:207–217.

32. Rothwell JC, Obeso JA, Marsden CD. Electrophysiology of somatosensory reflex myoclonus. *Adv Neurol* 1986;43:385–398.

33. Shibasaki H, Yamashita Y, Neshige R, Tobimatsu S, Fukui R. Pathogenesis of giant somatosensory evoked potentials in progressive myoclonic epilepsy. *Brain* 1985;108:225–240.

34. Thompson PD, Day BL, Rothwell JC, et al. The myoclonus in corticobasal degeneration. Evidence for two forms of cortical reflex myoclonus. *Brain* 1994;117:1197–1207.

35. Chadwick D, Hallett M, Harris R, Jenner P, Reynolds EH, Marsden CD. Clinical, biochemical, and physiologic features distinguishing myoclonus responsive to 5-hydroxy-tryptophan, tryptophan with a monoamine oxidase inhibitor, and clonazepam. *Brain* 1977;100:455–487.

36. Chen R, Ashby P, Lang AE. Stimulus-sensitive myoclonus in akinetic-rigid syndromes. *Brain* 1992;115:1875–1888.

37. Rodriguez ME, Artieda AJ, Zubieta JL, Obeso JA. Reflex myoclonus in olivopontocerebellar atrophy. *J Neurol Neurosurg Psychiatry* 1994;57:316–319.

38. Rosing HS, Hopkins LC, Wallace DC, et al. Maternally inherited mitochondrial myopathy and myoclonic epilepsy. *Ann Neurol* 1985;17:228–237.

39. Young RR, Shahani BT. Clinical neurophysiological aspects of post-hypoxic intention myoclonus. *Adv Neurol* 1979;26:85–105.

40. So N, Berkovic S, Andermann F, et al. Myoclonus epilepsy and ragged-red fibres (MERFF). Electrophysiologic studies and comparison with other progressive myoclonus epilepsies. *Brain* 1989;112:1261–1276.

41. Thompson PD, Hammans SR, Harding AE. Cortical reflex myoclonus in patients with the mitochondrial DNA transfer RNALys(8344) (MERRF) mutation. *J Neurol* 1994;241:335–340.

42. Chauvel P, Louvel J, Lamarche M. Transcortical reflexes and focal motor epilepsy. *Electroencephalogr Clin Neurophysiol* 1978;45:309–318.

43. Carella F, Scaioli V, Ciano C, Binelli S, Oliva D, Girotti F. Adult onset myoclonic Huntington's disease. *Mov Disord* 1993;8:210–215.

44. Guerrini R, Bonanni P, Parmeggiani L, et al. Cortical reflex myoclonus in Rett syndrome. *Ann Neurol* 1998;43:472–479.

45. Uesaka Y, Terao Y, Ugawa Y, et al. Magnetoencephalographic analysis of cortical myoclonic jerks. *Electroencephalogr Clin Neurophysiol* 1996;9:141–148.
46. Armstrong DD. Neuropathology of Rett syndrome. *Ment Retard Develop Disabil Res Rev* 2002;8:72–76. Review.
47. Walter WG. The central effects of rhythmic sensory stimulation. *Electroencephalogr Clin Neurophysiol* 1949;1:57–86.
48. Gastaut H, Tassinari CA. Triggering mechanisms in epilepsy. The electroclinical point of view: *Epilepsia* 1966;7:85–138.
49. Shibasaki H, Neshige R. Photic cortical reflex myoclonus. *Ann Neurol* 1987;22:252–257.
50. Artieda J, Obeso JA. The pathophysiology and pharmacology of photic cortical reflex myoclonus. *Ann Neurol* 1993;34:175–184.
51. Pandya DN, Kuypers HGJM. Cortico-cortical connections in the rhesus monkey. *Brain Res* 1969;13:13–36.
52. Bickford RG, Sem-Jacobsen CV, White PT, Daly D. Some observations on the mechanism of photic and photo-Metrazol activation. *EEG Clin Neurophysiol* 1952;4:275–282.
53. Chatrian GE, Perez–Borja C. Depth electrographic observations in two cases of photo-oculoclonic response. *Electroencephalog Clin Neurophysiol* 1964;17:71–75.
54. Thomas IE, Raegan TJ, Klass DW. Epilepsia partialis continua. A review of 32 cases. *Arch Neurol* 1977;34:266–275.
55. Chauvel P, Trottier S, Vignal JP, et al. Somatomotor seizures of frontal origin. (Review) *Adv Neurol* 1992; 57:182–232.
56. Cockerell OC, Rothwell J, Thompson PD, et al. Clinical and physiologic features of epilepsia partialis continua. Cases ascertained in the UK. *Brain* 1996;119:393–407.
57. Juul-Jensen P, Denny-Brown D. Epilepsia partialis continua. *Arch Neurol* 1966;15:563–578.
58. Kristinasen K, Henriksen GF. Epilepsia partialis continua. *Epilepsia* 1971;12:263–267.
59. Botez MI, Brossard L. Epilepsia partialis continua with well-delimited subcortical frontal tumor. *Epilepsia* 1974;15:39–43.
60. Colamaria V, Plouin P, Dulac O, et al. Kojewnikow's epilepssia partialis continua: two cases associated with striatal necrosis. *Neurophysiologie Clinique (Paris)* 1988;18:525–530.
61. Guerrini R, DeLorey T, Bonanni P, et al. Cortical myoclonus in Angelman syndrome. *Ann Neurol* 1996;40:39–48.
62. Inghilleri M, Mattia D, Berardelli A, Manfredi M. Asymmetry of cortical excitability revealed by transcranial stimulation in a patient with focal motor epilepsy and cortical myoclonus. *Electroencephalogr Clin Neurophysiol* 1998;109:70–72.
63. Schulze–Bonhage A, Ferbert A. Cortical action tremor and focal motor seizures after parietal infarction. *Mov Disord* 1998;13:356–358.
64. Wang HC, Hsu WC, Brown P. Cortical tremor secondary to a frontal cortical lesion. *Mov Disord* 1999;14:370–374.
65. Guerrini R, Genton P, Bureau M, et al. Reflex seizures are frequent in patients with Down syndrome and epilepsy. *Epilepsia* 1990;31:406–417.
66. Terada K, Ikeda A, Mima T, et al. Familial cortical tremor as a unique form of cortical reflex myoclonus. *Mov Disord* 1997;12:370–377.
67. Okuma Y, Shimo Y, Shimura H, Hatori K, Hattori T, Tanaka S, Kondo T, Mizuno Y. Familial cortical tremor with epilepsy: an under-recognized familial tremor. *Clin Neurol Neurosurg* 1998;100:75–78.
68. Elia M, Musumeci S, Ferri R, et al. Familial cortical tremor, epilepsy, and mental retardation. *Arch Neurol* 1998;55:1569–1573.
69. Brown P, Marsden CD. Rhythmic cortical and muscle discharge in cortical myoclonus. *Brain* 1996;119:1307–1316.
70. Grosse P, Guerrini R, Parmeggiani L, et al. Abnormal corticomuscular and intermuscular coupling in high-frequency rhythmic myoclonus. *Brain* 2003;126[Pt 2]: 326–342.
71. Mima T, Hallett M. Corticomuscular coherence: a review. *J Clin Neurophysiol* [Review] 1999;16(6):501–511.
72. Leocani L, Comi G. EEG coherence in pathological conditions. *J Clin Neurophysiol* [Review] 1999;16(6): 548–555.
73. Connors BW, Amitai Y. Making waves in the neocortex. *Neuron* 1997;18:347–349.
74. Brown P, Day BL, Rothwell JC, et al. Intrahemispheric and interhemispheric spread of cerebral cortical myoclonic activity and its relevance to epilepsy. *Brain* 1991;114:2333–2355.
75. Rothwell JC, Brown P. The spread of myoclonic activity through sensorimotor cortex in cortical reflex myoclonus. *Adv Neurol* 1995;67:143–155.
76. Brown P, Ridding MC, Werhahn KJ, Rothwell JC, Marsden CD. Abnormalities of the balance between inhibition and excitation in the motor cortex of patients with cortical myoclonus. *Brain* 1996;119:309–317.
77. Toro C, Hallett M. Pathophysiology of myoclonic disorders. In: Watts RL, Koller WC, eds. *Movement disorders. Neurologic principles and practice.* New York: McGraw-Hill, 1997:551–560.
78. Young RR, Shahani BT. Asterixis: one type of negative myoclonus. *Adv Neurol* 1986;43:137–156.
79. Degos JD, Verroust J, Bouchareine A, et al. Asterixis in focal brain lesions. *Arch Neurol* 1979;36:705–707.
80. Ugawa Y, Shimpo T, Mannen T. Physiologic analysis of asterixis: silent period locked averaging. *J Neurol Neurosurg Psychiatry* 1989;52:89–93.
81. Artieda J, Muruzabal J, Larumbe R, Garcia de Casasola C, Obeso JA. Cortical mechanisms mediating asterixis. *Mov Disord* 1992;7:209–216.
82. Shibasaki H, Ikeda A, Nagamine T, et al. Cortical reflex negative myoclonus. *Brain* 1994;117:477–486.
83. Guerrini R, Dravet C, Genton P, et al. Epileptic negative myoclonus. *Neurology* 1993;43:1078–1083.
84. Shibasaki H. Pathophysiology of negative myoclonus and asterixis. *Adv Neurol* 1995;67:199–210.
85. Guerrini R, Parmeggiani L, Shewmon A, et al. Motor dysfunction resulting from epileptic activity involving the sensori-motor cortex. In: Guerrini R, Aicardi J, Andermann F, Hallett M, eds. *Epilepsy and movement disorder.* Cambridge: Cambridge University Press, 2002;77–96.
86. Guerrini R, Belmonte A, Genton P. Antiepileptic

drug-induced worsening of seizures in children. *Epilepsia* 1998;39[Suppl. 3]:2–10.

87. Parmeggiani L, Seri S, Bonanni P, et al. Electrophysiological characterization of spontaneous and carbamazepine-induced epileptic negative myoclonus in benign childhood epilepsy with centro temporal spikes. *Clin Neurophysiol* 2004, 115:50–8.

88. Shewmon DA, Erwin RJ. Focal spike-induced cerebral dysfunction is related to the after-coming slow wave. *Ann Neurol* 1988;23:131–137.

89. Seri S, Cerquiglini A, Pisani F. Spike-induced interference in auditory sensory processing in Landau-Kleffner syndrome. *Electroencephalogr Clin Neurophysiol* 1998;108:506–510.

90. Pagni CA, Ettorre G, Infuso L, Marossero F. EMG responses to capsular stimulation in the human. *Experientia* 1964;20:691–692.

91. Marsden CD, Merton PA, Morton HB. Is the human stretch reflex cortical rather than spinal? *Lancet* 1973;1:759–761.

92. Rubboli G, Parmeggiani L and Tassinari CA (1995). Frontal inhibitory spike component associated with epileptic negative myoclonus. *Electroenceph Clin Neurophysiol* 95,201–205.

93. Lüders HO, Dinner DS, Morris HH, Wyllie E and Comair YG (1995). Cortical electrical stimulation in humans. The negative motor areas. *Adv Neurol* 67, 115–129.

94. Baumgartner C, Podreka I, Olbrich A, Novak K, Serles W, Aull S, Almer G, Lurger S, Pietrzyk U, Prayer D and Lindinger G (1996). Epileptic negative myoclonus: an EEG-single-proton emission CT study indicating involvement of premotor cortex. *Neurology* 46, 753–758.

95. Ikeda A, Ohara S, Matsumoto R, Kunieda T, Nagamine T, Miyamoto S, Kohara N, Taki W, Hashimoto N and Shibasaki H (2000). Role of primary sensorimotor corticies in generating inhibitory motor response in human. *Brain* 123, 1710–1721.

96. Matsunaga K, Uozumi T, Akamatsu N, Nagashio Y, Qingrui L, Hashimoto T, Tsuji S (2000). Negative myoclonus in Creutzfeldt-Jakob disease. *Clin Neurophysiol* 111, 471–476.

97. Shibasaki H (2002). Physiology of Negative Myoclonus. *Adv Neurol* 89, 103–113.

98. Engel J, Jr. Inhibitory mechanisms of epileptic seizure generation. *Adv Neurol* 1995;67:157–171.

99. Hallett M. Transcranial magnetic stimulation. Negative effects [Review]. *Adv Neurol* 1995;67:107–113.

100. Guerrini R, Dravet C, Genton P, et al. Epileptic negative myoclonus. [Replay from the Authors], [letter] *Neurology* 1994;44:989–990.

101. Gastaut H, Regis H. On the subject of Lennox's "akinetic" petit mal. *Epilepsia* 1961;2:298–305.

102. Gloor P. Generalized epilepsy with spike-and-wave discharge: a reinterpretation of its electrographic and clinical manifestations. *Epilepsia* 1979;20:571–588.

103. Okino S (1997). Familial benign myoclonus epilepsy of adult onset; a previously unrecognized myoclonic disorder. *J Neurol Sci,* 145, 113-8,

104. Hallett M, Chadwick D, Adam J, et al. Reticular reflex myoclonus: a physiologic type of human posthypoxic myoclonus. *J Neurol Neurosurg Psychiatry* 1977;40:253–264.

105. Brown P, Thompson PD, Rothwell JC, et al. A case of postanoxic encephalopathy with cortical action and brainstem reticular reflex myoclonus. *Mov Disord* 1991b;6:139–144.

106. Cantello R, Gianelli M, Civardi C, Mutani R. Focal subcortical reflex myoclonus. A clinical and neurophysiological study. *Arch Neurol* 1997;54:187–196.

107. Zuckermann EG, Glaser GH. Urea induced myoclonic seizures. *Arch Neurol* 1972;27:14–28.

108. Cesa-Bianchi M, Mancia M, Mutani R. Experimental epilepsy induced by cobalt powder in lower brain-stem and thalamic structures. *Electroencephalog Clin Neurophysiol* 1967;22:525–536.

109. Aicardi, J. Childhood epilepsies with brief myoclonic, atonic or tonic seizures. In: Laidlaw J, Richens A, eds. *A textbook of epilepsy.* Edinburgh: Churchill Livingstone, 1982:88–96.

110. Aicardi J. Myoclonic epilepsies in childhood. *Int Pediatr* 1991;6:195–200.

111. Gastaut H, Tassinari CA. Ictal discharges in different types of seizures. In: Remond A, ed. *Epilepsies: handbook of electroencephalography and clinical neurophysiology,* Vol. 13, Part A. Amsterdam: Elsevier 1975;13–45.

112. Niedermeyer E, Fineyre F, Riley T, Bird B. Myoclonus and the electroencephalogram: A review. *Clin Electroenceph* 1979;10:75–96.

113. Erba G, Browne TR. Atypical absence, myoclonic, atonic, and tonic seizures, and the "Lennox–Gastaut syndrome." In: Browne TR, Feldman RG, eds. *Epilepsy: diagnosis and management.* Little Brown, Boston: 1983;75–94.

114. Gastaut H, Roger J, Soulayrol R, et al. Childhood epileptic encephalopathy with diffuse spike-waves (otherwise known as "petit mal variant") or Lennox syndrome. *Epilepsia* 1966;7:139–179.

115. Lombroso CT, Erba G. Myoclonic seizures: Considerations in toxonomy. In: Akimoto H, Kazamatsuri H, Seino M, Ward A, eds. *Advances in epileptology: XIIIth epilepsy international symposium.* New York: Raven Press, 1982:129–134.

116. Aicardi J, Chevrie JJ. Myoclonic epilepsies of childhood. *Neuropediatrie* 1971;3:177–190.

117. Chayasirisobhon S, Rodin EA. Atonic-akinetic seizures. *Electroencephalogr Clin Neurophysiol* 1981; 50:225.

118. Gastaut H, Broughton R, Roger J, et al. Generalized convulsive seizures without local onset. In: Vinken PJ, Bruyn GW, eds. *Handbook of clinical neurology,* Vol. 15: *the epilepsies,* Amsterdam: Elsevier, 1974: 107–129.

119. Fariello RG, Doro JM, Forster FM. Generalized cortical electrodecremental event: clinical and neurophysiological observations in patients with dystonic seizures. *Arch Neurol* 1974:285–291.

120. Gastaut H, Broughton R. *Epileptic seizures.* Springfield, IL: Charles C Thomas, 1972.

121. Brenner RP, Atkinson R. Generalized paroxysmal fast activity: Electroencephalographic and clinical features. *Ann Neurol* 1982;11:386–390.

122. Gastaut H, Roger J, Ouachi S, et al. An electro—clinical study of generalized epileptic seizures of tonic expression. *Epilepsia* 1963;4:15–44.

123. Egli M, Mothersill I, O'Kane M, O'Kane F. The axial spasm—the predominant type of drop seizure in

patients with secondary generalized epilepsy. *Epilepsia* 1985;26:401–415.

124. Roger J, Genton P, Bureau M, et al. In: Roger J, Bureau M, Dravet C, Dreifuss FE, Perret A, Wolf P, eds. *Epileptic syndromes in infancy, childhood and adolescence,* 2nd ed. London and Paris: John Libbey, 1992:381–400.

125. Delgado-Escueta AV, Ganesh S, Yamakawa K. Advances in the genetics of progressive myoclonus epilepsy. *Am J Med Genet* 2001;106:129–138.

126. Guerrini R, Carrozzo R, Rinaldi R, et al. Angelman syndrome: etiology, clinical features, diagnosis, and management of symptoms. *Paediatr Drugs* 2003;5:647–661.

127. Minassian BA, DeLorey TM, Olsen RW, et al. Angelman syndrome: correlations between epilepsy phenotypes and genotypes. *Ann Neurol* 1998;43:485–493.

128. Kuwano A, Takakubo F, Morimoto Y, Uyama E, Uchino M, Ando M, Yasuda T, Terao A, Hayama T, Kobayashi R, Kondo I. Benign adult familial myoclonus epilepsy (BAFME): an autosomal dominat form not linked to the dentatorubral pallidoluysian atrophy (DRPLA) gene. *J Med Genet,* 1996;33:80–81.

129. Okino S. Familial benign myoclonus epilepsy of adult onset: a previously unrecognized myoclonic disorder. *J Neurol Sci* 1997;145:113–118.

130. Labauge P, Amer LO, Simonetta-Moreau M. et al. Absence of linkage to 8q24 in a European family with familial adult myoclonic epilepsy (FAME). *Neurology* 2002;58:941–944.

131. Mikami M, Yasuda T, Terao A, et al. Localization of a gene for benign adult familial myoclonic epilepsy to chromosome 8q23. 3-q24.1. *Am J Hum Genet,* 1999; 65:745–751.

132. Plaster NM, Uyama E, Uchino M, et al. Genetic localization of the familial adult myoclonic epilepsy (FAME) gene to chromosome 8q24. *Neurology* 1999;53:1180–1183.

133. De Falco FA, Striano P, De Falco A, et al. Benign adult familial myoclonic epilepsy: Genetic heterogeneity and allelism with ADCME. *Neurology* 2003;60:1381–1385.

134. Guerrini R, Bonanni P, Patrignani A, et al. Autosomal dominant cortical myoclonus and epilepsy (ADCME) with complex partial and generalized seizures: A newly recognized epilepsy syndrome with linkage to chromosome 2p11. 1-q12.2. *Brain* 2001;124:2459–2475.

135. Dravet C, Bureau M, Guerrini R, et al. Severe myoclonic epilepsy in infants. In: Roger J, Bureau M, Dravet C, Dreifuss FE, Perret A, Wolf P, eds. *Epileptic syndromes in infancy, childhood and adolescence,* 2nd ed. London and Paris: John Libbey, 1992:75–88.

136. Claes L, Del-Favero J, Ceulemans B, et al. De novo mutations in the sodium-channel gene SCN1A cause severe myoclonic epilepsy of infancy. *Am J Hum Genet* 2001;68:1327–1332.

137. Sugarawa T, Mazaki-Miyazaki E, Fukushima K, et al. Frequent mutation of SCN1A in severe myoclonic epilepsy in infancy. *Neurology* 2002;58:1122–1124.

138. Ohmori I, Ouchida M, Ohtsuka Y, Oka E, Shimizu K. Significant correlation of the SCN1A mutations and severe myoclonic epilepsy in infancy. *Biochem Biophys Res Commun* 2002;295:17–23.

139. Fujiwara T, Sugarawa T, Mazaki-Miyazaki E, et al. Mutations of sodium channel a subunit type 1 (SCN1A) in intractable childhood epilepsies with frequent generalized tonic-clonic seizures. *Brain* 2003;126:531–546.

140. Nabbout R, Gennaro E, Dalla Bernardina B, et al. Spectrum of SCN1A mutations in severe myoclonic epilepsy of infancy. *Neurology* 2003;60:1961–1967.

141. Beaumanoir A, Dravet C. The Lennox-Gastaut syndrome. In: Roger J, Bureau M, Dravet C, Dreifuss FE, Perret A, Wolf P, eds. *Epileptic syndromes in infancy, childhood and adolescence.* 2nd ed. London and Paris: John Libbey, 1992:115–132.

142. Gastaut H. The Lennox–Gastaut syndrome: comments on the syndrome's terminology and nosological position amongst the secondary generalized epilepsies of childhood. *Electroencephalogr Clin Neurophysiol* 1982;35[Suppl.]:71–84.

143. Bonanni P, Parmeggiani L, Guerrini R. Different neurophysiologic patterns of myoclonus characterize Lennox–Gastaut syndrome and myoclonic astatic epilepsy. *Epilepsia* 2002;43:609–615.

144. Dalla Bernardina B, Colamaria V, Capovilla G, et al. Nosological classification of epilepsies in the first three years of life. In: Nisticò G, Di Perri R, Meinardi H, *Iepsy an update on research and therapy.* New York: Liss, 1983:165–183.

145. Dravet C, Bureau M, Roger J. Benign myoclonic epilepsy in infants. In: Roger J, Bureau M, Dravet C, Dreifuss FE, Perret A, Wolf P, eds. *Epileptic syndromes in infancy, childhood and adolescence,* 2nd ed. London: John Libbey, 1992:67–74.

146. Guerrini R, Dravet C, Gobbi G, et al. Idiopathic generalized epilepsies with myoclonus in infancy and childhood. In: Malafosse A, Genton P, Hirsch E, Marescaux C, Broglin D, Bernasconi R, eds. *Idiopathic generalized epilepsies: clinical, experimental and genetics aspects.* London: John Libbey, 1994:267–280.

147. Dravet C. Les épilepsies myocloniques bénignes du nourrisson. *Epilepsies* 1990;2:95–101.

148. Dravet C, Bureau M, Genton P. Benign myoclonic epilepsy of infancy: electroclinical symptomatology and differential diagnosis from the other types of generalized epilepsy in infancy. In: Degen R, Dreifuss F, eds. *The benign localized epilepsies in early childhood,* (Epilepsy Research). Amsterdam: Elsevier, 1992 [Suppl 6]:131–135.

149. Revol M, Isnard H, Beaumanoir A, et al. Touch evoked myoclonic seizures in infancy. In: Beaumanoir A, Naquet R, Gastaut H, eds. *Reflex seizures and reflex epilepsies.* Genève: Médecine et Hygiène, 1989:103–105.

150. Deonna T, Despland PA. Sensory-evoked (touch) idiopathic myoclonic epilepsy of infancy. In: Beaumanoir A, Naquet R, Gastaut H, eds. *Reflex seizures and reflex epilepsies,* Genève: Médecine et Hygiène, 1989:99–102.

151. Ricci S, Cusmai R, Fusco L, et al. Reflex myoclonic epilepsy in infancy: a new age-dependent idiopathic epileptic syndrome related to startle reaction. *Epilepsia* 1995;36:342–348.

152. Dravet C, Bureau M. Benign myoclonic epilepsy in infancy. In: Roger J, Bureau M, Dravet C, Genton P,

Tassinari CA, Wolf P, eds. *Epileptic syndromes in infancy childhood and adolescence,* 3rd ed. London, Paris: John Libbey, 2002:69–79.

153. Engel J, Jr. A proposed diagnostic scheme for people with epileptic seizures and with epilepsy: report of the ILAE Task Force on Classification and Terminology. *Epilepsia* 2001;42:1–8.

154. Genton P, Salas-Puig X, Tunon A, et al. Juvenile myoclonic epilepsy and related syndromes: clinical and neurophysiological aspects. In: Malafosse A, Genton P, Hirsch E, Marescaux C, Broglin D, Bernasconi R. *Idiopathic generalized epilepsies: clinical, experimental and genetics aspects.* London: John Libbey, 1994;253–266.

155. Delgado-Escueta AV, Liu A, Serratosa J, et al. Juvenile myoclonic epilepsy: is there heterogeneity? In: Malafosse A, Genton P, Hirsch E, Marescaux C, Broglin D, Bernasconi R, eds. *Idiopathic generalized epilepsies: clinical, experimental and genetics aspects,* London: John Libbey Eurotext Ltd, 1994:281–286.

155a. Oguni H, Mukahira K, Oguni M, et al. A video-EEG analysis of myoclonic seizures in juvenile myoclonic epilepsy. *Epilepsia* 1994;35:307–316.

156. Salas-Puig X, Camara da Silva AM, Dravet C. et al. L'épilepsie myoclonique juveénile dans la population du Centre Saint Paul. *Epilepsies* 1990;2:108–113.

157. Doose H. Myoclonic astatic epilepsy of early childhood. In: Roger J, Bureau M, Dravet C, Dreifuss FE, Perret A, Wolf P, eds. *Epileptic syndromes in infancy,* *childhood and adolescence,* 2nd ed. London and Paris: John Libbey Eurotext Ltd, 1992:103–114.

158. Dulac O, N' Guyen T. The Lennox-Gastaut syndrome. *Epilepsia* 1993;34[Suppl 7]:S7–S17.

159. Dulac O, Plouin P, Chiron C. Forme "bénigne" d' épilepsie myoclonique chez l'enfant. *Neurophysiol Clin (Paris)* 1990;20:115–129.

160. Aicardi J. Early myoclonic encephalopathy (neonatal myoclonic encephalopathy) In: Roger J, Bureau M, Dravet C, Dreifuss FE, Perret A, Wolf P, eds. *Epileptic syndromes in infancy, childhood and adolescence.* 2nd ed. London and Paris: John Libbey, 1992:13–23.

161. Dalla Bernardina B, Fontana E, Sgro' V, et al. Myoclonic epilepsy ('myoclonic status') in nonprogressive encephalopathies. In: Roger J, Bureau M, Dravet C, Dreifuss FE, Perret A, Wolf P. eds. *Epileptic syndromes in infancy, childhood and adolescence,* 2nd ed. London: John Libbey, 1992:89–96.

162. Tassinari CA, Bureau M, Thomas P. Epilepsy with myoclonic absences. In: Roger J, Bureau M, Dravet C, Dreifuss FE, Perret A, Wolf P, eds. *Epileptic syndromes in infancy, childhood and adolescence,* 2nd ed. London: John Libbey, 1992:151–160.

163. Tassinari CA, Michelucci R, Rubboli G, et al. Myoclonic absence epilepsy. In: Duncan JS, Panayiotopoulos CP, eds. *Typical absences and related epileptic syndromes,* London: Churchill Communications Europe, 1995;187–195.

164. Aicardi J. Myoclonic epilepsies. *Res Clini Forums* 1980;2:47–55.

4

Progressive Myoclonus Epilepsies: *EPM1, EPM2A, EPM2B*

Elayne M. Chan,* Danielle M. Andrade,* Silvana Franceschetti,[†]
and Berge Minassian[‡]

*Program in Genetics and Genomic Biology, The Hospital for Sick Children, Toronto, Canada;
[†]Department of Clinical Neurophysiology, Instituto Nazionale Neurologico Carlo Besta, Milan, Italy;
[‡]Division of Neurology, The Hospital for Sick Children, Toronto, Canada

INTRODUCTION

The differential diagnosis of progressive my-oclonus epilepsy (PME) with onset between late childhood and late adolescence includes neu-ronal ceroid lipofuscinosis, type I sialidosis, and myoclonic epilepsy with ragged red fibers. How-ever, the two most common forms of PME in this age group are Lafora disease and Unverricht–Lundborg disease (ULD). This chapter reviews the clinical and pathologic features, molecular genetics, and animal models of these two disor-ders. As will be seen, in both, the promise of great insights following disease gene discovery has in-deed materialized, but with it has also the realiza-tion that much work lays ahead. It is hoped that a clear understanding of pathophysiology will uncover therapeutic entry points to allow better treatments, or cures, for these disorders.

UNVERRICHT–LUNDBORG DISEASE

Clinical Characteristics and Neurophysiology

Unverricht–Lundborg disease (ULD) is an auto-somal recessive PME. Onset is between ages 6 and 15 years, after a period of apparent normal development. The disease is principally charac-terized by stimulus-sensitive myoclonus (1–4).

These are sudden, brief, shocklike muscle con-tractions that become generalized and interfere with routine activities such as writing, swallow-ing, speaking, and walking. They can be precip-itated by the simple intention to move. Tonic-clonic and myoclonic seizures also appear early in the clinical picture, but other types of seizures may present later. The disease progresses slowly, with ataxia, action tremor, and emotional labil-ity, and patients demonstrate a slow decline in intelligence.

In recent years, it has become evident that the clinical course is greatly influenced by antiepileptic medications. Phenytoin is exqui-sitely neurotoxic to these patients and appears to have been a major contributor to the severe pro-gressive myoclonus and cerebellar ataxia docu-mented in previous years. In correctly managed patients, dementia can be averted, myoclonus and seizures can be minimized, and life span can be normal (5). Valproic acid, zonisamide, and levetiracetam are preferred anticonvulsants, and piracetam is helpful against the myoclonus. *N*-Acetylcysteine (NAC) improves tremor, gait, and myoclonus in some patients (6). Its mechanism of action is poorly understood and has been related to protection against oxidative stress. However, NAC is also antiapoptotic in cultured neurons deprived of nerve growth factor (7) and may be protective against the apoptotis recently shown to characterize ULD neurodegeneration (see the following section).

Electroencephalographic (EEG) recordings are abnormal in ULD, even before symptom onset (4). Background activity is disorganized and slow, EEG paroxysms of fast spike-waves or polyspike-waves with larger amplitudes in central regions are present, and photosensitivity is prominent. The frequency of EEG paroxysms diminishes with rational antiepileptic treatment (8). The stimulus sensitive myoclonus lacks a visible EEG correlate, but backaveraging analysis demonstrates time-locked cortical spikes preceding the myoclonic jerks (9). Giant somatosensory evoked potentials (SEPs) and enhanced long-loop (cortical) reflex (LLR) (9) further implicate cortical hyperexcitability in the myoclonus of ULD. Additional observations derived from comparisons with the neurophysiology of Lafora disease are discussed next.

EPM1, the ULD Gene

The gene responsible for ULD was identified using a positional cloning approach. A genome-wide search for linkage was undertaken in 12 families localizing the gene to 21q22.3 (10). Linkage disequilibrium analysis followed by a systematic search for genes resulted in the identification of the gene for a previously known but unmapped cysteine protease inhibitor called cystatin B (CSTB). Ultimately, the identification of two point mutations in this gene proved it to be responsible for ULD (11). EPM1, the CSTB gene, is composed of three exons and is 674bp in length. To date, a total of six different mutations have been identified in the coding region of EPM1. Three mutations, 1926-1G→C, 2027G→A, and 2355-2A→G affect conserved splice-site sequences and predict severe splicing defects. Two other mutations in exon 3, consisting of a nonsense codon (R68X) or a frameshift (2400delTC), predict a truncated protein. The sixth mutation is a transversion in exon 1 that results in the substitution of a highly conserved glycine by an arginine at amino acid position 4 (G4R)(11–13).

Interestingly, only 10% of EPM1 alleles contain mutations within the transcriptional unit. Southern blot analysis of Pst I-digested ge-nomic DNA revealed the presence of abnormally large EPM1-containing fragments in ULD patients. PCR amplification and sequence analysis demonstrated the expansion to be composed of a CCCCGCCCCGCG dodecamer repeat 175bp upstream from the translation initiation codon of EPM1. Normal alleles contain two to three tandem copies of this dodecamer (although rare normal alleles containing 12–17 repeats have also been reported). ULD patients have 30 to 150 copies, resulting in dramatically reduced, although not completely absent, expression of EPM1 mRNA (13–17).

Preliminary analysis revealed no correlation between the number of repeats and clinical severity of the disease or age of onset (13–17). It is suggested that once the dodecamer repeat expands beyond a critical threshold, EPM1 gene expression is reduced in certain cells with pathological consequences. In vitro studies have demonstrated that altered spacing of transcription factor-binding sites upstream of the dodecamer repeat contribute to the reduction in downstream gene expression (18). However, the two- to fourfold reduction in transcriptional activity observed in this study was not as dramatic as that observed in ULD patients. Further studies are required to determine additional causes for the low expression of EPM1 associated with the dodecamer expansion.

Cystatin B and the Cystatin B-Deficient Mouse

The cystatin superfamily encompasses proteins that contain multiple cystatin-like sequences. Some of the members are active cysteine protease inhibitors, whereas others do not have this inhibitory activity. There are three inhibitory families in the superfamily, including the type 1 cystatins (stefins), type 2 cystatins, and kininogens. CSTB is a stefin that functions as an intracellular protease inhibitor. CSTB is able to inhibit papain and cathepsins B, H, L, and S in vitro (19). This protein is thought to play a role in protecting cellular structures against lysosomal proteases in vivo.

Previous histopathological studies of patients with ULD demonstrated cerebellar granular and Purkinje cell loss, gliosis, and neuronal degeneration of the medial and reticular nuclei of the thalamus. Such studies also reported degenerative changes in the cortex, striatum, mammillary bodies, anterior and lateral thalamic nuclei, multiple brain stem nuclei, and ventral gray matter of the spinal cord (3,20,21). However, until recently it was not clear if these pathological findings were the consequence of a genetic mutation, leading to reduced levels of CSTB, or the result of neurotoxicity from phenytoin, the antiepileptic drug used for many years to treat ULD. This issue was resolved in 1998, when Pennacchio and colleagues reported histopathological findings in *EPM1* knockout mice that did not receive phenytoin treatment (22). Targeted disruption of *EPM1* caused these animals to develop a phenotype that resembles ULD, including myoclonic seizures and ataxia. Histopathological analysis revealed apoptosis of cerebellar granular and Purkinje cells. A more detailed study with nontreated *EPM1* knockout mice demonstrated not only apoptosis of cells in the cerebellum, but also cortical and striatal gliosis and atrophy of cortical neurons (23).

A recent study analyzed transcript levels of brain-expressed genes in CSTB-deficient mice by using modified differential display oligonucleotide microarray hybridization and quantitative reverse transcriptase polymerase chain reaction. Interestingly, levels of the protease cathepsin S were consistently elevated *in vivo*, whereas alterations in the levels of cathepsins B, H, and L were inconsistent (24). Protease activity could be entirely regulated at the level of uninhibited protein availability, but another possibility is that there are feedback loops that alter the levels of protease transcripts in response to the lack of the protease inhibitor CSTB. In this case, the finding of consistently elevated levels of cathepsin S suggests that proteolysis by this protein may be a key trigger event in the initiation of apoptosis in ULD.

Another interesting finding in the study of Lieuallen and colleagues is the elevated mRNA levels of five other genes in the brain of *EPM1*-deficient mice when compared to controls. These genes, encoding for β2-microglobulin, apolipoprotein D, fibronectin 1, Gfap, and C1qB, may have transcript levels elevated as a result of glial activation (24). These gene products have been reported to be increased in reactive astrocytes (β2-microglobulin and apolipoprotein D), secreted by glial cells and involved in astroglial proliferation (fibronectin 1), and expressed in microglia (C1qB and Gfap). Reactive fibrillary astrocytes, capable of producing microglial scars (gliosis) create a physical barrier between damaged and healthy neurons, possibly as a form of adaptation to protect the remaining healthy cells. Glial activation has also been reported in other neurodegenerative diseases including Alzheimer's disease and Creuzfeldt–Jakob's disease (25,26), where it is also thought to be a biological response to neuronal damage.

One more indication that CSTB has a neuroprotective role comes from the study of D'Amato and colleagues (27), who demonstrate that a series of focal and generalized seizures induced by kindling brain stimulation in wild-type mice lead to a transient elevation of *EPM1* mRNA accompanied by transient elevation of CSTB levels in some areas of the brain. It is believed that this is an endogenous neuroprotective mechanism that acts to limit neuronal apoptosis caused by the electric insult.

Currently the greatest challenge in ULD research is the question of whether the known CSTB effect on cathepsins is the pathophysiologically relevant function, or whether alternate CSTB functions exist, yet to be revealed. Paradoxically, in contrast to Lafora disease (LD), discussed next, the absence of genetic heterogeneity in ULD does not allow the genetic unraveling of a second pathway, whose intersection with the CSTB pathway(s) would help establish the biological underpinnings of the disease.

LAFORA DISEASE

Clinical Characteristics

LD is an autosomal recessive PME. Onset is between ages 9 and 18 years, after a period of apparent normal development (28). In retrospect, however, many families describe a certain "slowness" in childhood years compared to their unaffected children. In fact, a subphenotype with learning disabilities in childhood associated with particular mutations has been delineated (29). In addition, febrile and rare afebrile seizures in childhood are more common in LD than in the general population (28).

The LD patient is brought to clinical attention following the appearance of one of five symptoms: myoclonic jerks, a generalized seizure, a decline in school performance, behavioral changes including depression, apathy, disinhibition or delusions, or visual (occipital ictal) hallucinations. At this point, EEG shows slowing of the background with irregular spike-wave discharges, raising the specter of a progressive disease. The disease then accelerates, with worsening of all the above manifestations and additional seizure types. Proper antiepileptic medications have a major effect against generalized convulsions, sometimes resulting in freedom from seizure for many months at a time. In fact, generalized convulsions are rare in treated patients even years after disease onset. Myoclonus also diminishes initially with treatment, but this response is not maintained.

The clinical picture within 2 years of diagnosis is as follows. Myoclonus is frequent during wakeful hours, especially in the early morning, and ceases with sleep. It affects walking, and with cerebellar ataxia and drop attacks, and soon results in wheelchair dependence. It is stimulus sensitive, provoked by movement, intention, light changes, and is exacerbated by emotion. Myoclonus, ataxia, and dysarthria combine with cognitive decline, emotional lability, visual hallucinations, delusions, and disinhibited behavior (with pursuant social rejection) to devastate the young person. Within 5 to 10 years, the patient is bed bound, usually tube fed, and in almost constant myoclonus and ictal confusion. Through the long years in this state, periods of semilucidity and responsiveness to family are maintained, which renders letting go extremely difficult for some parents. Death usually results from status epilepticus and aspiration pneumonia.

The traditional antiepileptic treatment for LD is valproic acid. In recent years, zonisamide has been shown to have a significant effect on seizures and myoclonus (30,31), and is presently the authors' first-line choice. Piracetam and levetiracetam (32) are temporarily helpful against the myoclonus. The ketogenic diet is an important therapeutic modality. The Lafora bodies, which occupy vast numbers of dendrites in LD brain, are carbohydrate accumulations and might diminish in the absence of carbohydrate intake. We have been placing our newly diagnosed cases on the diet. Our observations so far suggest an important slowing of disease progression. Controlled experiments of the diet in animal models are being initiated.

Neurophysiology

The EEG background activity in LD is slow, showing dominant theta-delta components interrupted by recurrent posterior or diffuse multiple spikes discharges (33). Generalized or segmental spontaneous myoclonus, associated with clear EEG paroxysms, is a prominent feature, and the presence of negative myoclonus, associated with polyspike-wave discharges, is common and characteristic (34).

The large amplitude of cortical SEPs components found in LD (and ULD) indicates that in both disorders an aberrant integration of somatosensory stimuli occurs and can subsequently involve motor cortex. In agreement, protocols investigating motor-evoked potentials demonstrated that somatosensory afferent stimuli delivered prior to transcranial magnetic stimulation are capable of abnormally facilitating motor cortex excitability in PME case series (35,36). However, SEPs can be normal in some patients (35,37), or "normalized" by antiepileptic treatment, but action myoclonus usually persists, suggesting that motor cortex "per se" is primarily hyperexcitable. In agreement, enhanced LLR, and central spikes time locked with action myoclonus may occur also in patients with "normal" SEPs.

To better investigate the hyperexcitability of motor cortex, spectral analyses have been applied as a method for detecting the relationship between rhythmic or quasirhythmic myoclonic events and EEG (or magneto-EEG) activity (37,38). The data indicate that highly coherent beta–gamma oscillations occur between motor cortex and muscle during movement-activated myoclonic discharges, and that pathologically exaggerated fast rhythms probably drive the generation of cortical myoclonus. In a recent study (39), performed by applying autoregressive models to the analysis of short EEG–electromyogram (EMG) epochs, a coherent beta activity coupling motor neocortex and contralateral muscles involved in action myoclonus was found in both LD and ULD. However, the coherence profile was more heterogeneous in LD patients, including multiple coherence peaks in subjects with more severe disease progression. This could suggest that a complex distortion of corticosubcortical or corticocortical interaction occurs in LD, probably accounting for the greater heterogeneity of the myoclonus, including spontaneous generalized and focal (positive or negative) negative myoclonus.

Pathology

Lafora bodies (LB) are the prominent finding in LD pathology. They are present in the brain and in almost every other organ including skin. Outside the brain they are most prominent in liver and muscle. In brain, LB are largely found in neurons where they localize in the perikaryal region and in largest amounts in dendrites, but not in axons (40). In the brain [and in liver (41,42)], LB are not usually membrane bound (43–49), unlike in muscle where many are enclosed in a membrane (47). LB stain strongly with periodic acid–Schiff. They are accumulations of a glucose polysaccharide termed polyglucosan (50). Unlike glycogen, polyglucosans lack a regular branching pattern and, as such, more closely resemble starch than glycogen. Newly forming polyglucosan fibrils appear to be in physical association with the endoplasmic reticulum (ER) (51) or ribosomes (52).

Genetics of Lafora Disease

EPM2A, the First LD Gene, and Laforin, Its Encoded Protein

In 1998, mutations in the *EPM2A* gene on chromosome 6q24 were identified using a positional cloning approach (53). The human *EPM2A* gene consists of four exons spanning 130 kb, encoding a 331-amino acid protein, laforin. *EPM2A* encodes two protein isoforms (A and B) that differ in the lengths of their carboxy termini. Isoform A with the longer C-terminus, localizes to the

rough ER and isoform B to the nucleus (54). The presence of a mutation in an LD family that is C-terminus specific to isoform A provided the first evidence that this isoform is the disease-relevant molecule (54a). To date, a total of 36 or more mutations have been found to be responsible for ~48% of LD cases in our study population. Identified sequence changes include homozygous missense, nonsense, frameshift, and deletions, all located within the coding region of the gene (53,55). *EPM2A* homologs are restricted to higher vertebrates. The mouse (56), rat, and dog homologs share greater than 90% sequence identity with the human gene at the amino acid level.

Bioinformatic analysis of the *EPM2A* gene-encoded product laforin revealed the presence of the consensus sequence for the active site of protein tyrosine phosphatases (PTPs), HCXXGXXRS/T (53). *In vitro* assays using generic substrates found laforin to have dual-specificity protein tyrosine phosphatase (DSP) activity (57,58); however, despite efforts by many groups, its *bona fide* phosphoprotein substrate is yet to be identified. DSPs utilize the same catalytic site as PTPs, but are also capable of dephosphorylating phosphoserine/threonine residues, in addition to phosphotyrosine-containing substrates. Sequence analysis of laforin also revealed the presence of a carbohydrate-binding domain of type 4 (CBD-4) at the N-terminus (55). This domain is characteristic of a number of bacterial and lower eukaryotic amylases. *In vivo* and *in vitro* assays have shown that the CBD-4 domain has the ability to target laforin to glycogen particles (59). Subcellular localization studies using a tagged fusion of the laforin protein showed it to be associated with the ER and plasma membrane (57). Studies by Ganesh et al. (58) found laforin to be associated with polyribosomes at the ER through protein–protein interactions.

EPM2B, the Second LD Gene, and Malin, Its Encoded Protein

Following identification of the *EPM2A* gene, genetic locus heterogeneity was demonstrated in LD (60). *EPM2A* mutations were not identified and linkage did not exist at markers in the

6q24 region in a number of families. Among this group was a French-Canadian (F-C) cluster of families, all originating from the same region of eastern Quebec (lower Saint Lawrence, southern shore). A genome-wide linkage scan was performed on this F-C isolate in search for the second LD gene (61). Linkage analysis identified a locus on 6p22.3 that produced a maximum multipoint lod score of 5.37 using markers across the region. Haplotype analysis and homozygosity mapping in the F-C families, in addition to another LD family that did not have mutations in the *EPM2A* gene, resulted in a final critical interval of 0.84 Mb. Genes in the region were sequenced in affected individuals and a previously uncharacterized 1188bp single-exon gene was identified (*EPM2B*, also known as *NHLRC1*) (62). Seventeen mutations were identified in this gene in 26 different LD families and included an insertion, missense and nonsense changes, frameshifts, and deletions in both compound heterozygous and homozygous states. Approximately 40% of our study population have mutations in *EPM2B*. Similar to *EPM2A*, *EPM2B* homologs are also limited to higher vertebrates, and the mouse, rat, and dog homologs share over 75% identity with the human gene. No genotype–phenotype differences are present between patients carrying mutations in the *EPM2B* gene versus patients with *EPM2A* mutations.

The *EPM2B* gene product encodes a 395 amino acid protein named malin containing a zinc finger of the RING type at the N-terminus and six NHL-repeat motifs at the C-terminus (62). The RING-finger motif ($C-X_2-C-X_{16}-C-X_1-H-X_2-C-X_2-C-X_{14}-C-X_2-C$) is characteristic of E3 ubiquitin ligases. The six NHL domains were predicted on the basis of the presence of an approximately 44-residue motif rich in glycine and hydrophobic amino acids seeded with a cluster of charged residues. NHL-repeat motifs are thought to be involved in protein–protein interactions. The subcellular location of *myc*-tagged malin was examined and found to be in the cytoplasm at the ER and within the nucleus. These results were similar to the cellular localization observed for the two alternative transcripts (A and B) of *EPM2A*, which encode isoforms of laforin found in the cytoplasm at the ER and in the nucleus, respectively (54–57).

Further Genetic Heterogeneity

In total, 88% of our LD families can now be accounted for by mutations in *EPM2A* (48%) and *EPM2B* (40%) (62). The presence of further genetic heterogeneity in LD has been established based on linkage analysis and mutation screening of the remaining 12% of families. Results revealed the absence of linkage to microsatellite markers at chromosomes 6q24 and 6p22 in several families with no *EPM2A* or *EPM2B* mutations. Although the number of loci-containing genes that cause LD is not known, a third genome-wide linkage scan is being performed to search for the third gene.

Laforin Protein–Protein Interactors

Following identification of the *EPM2A* gene, three independent yeast two-hybrid experiments investigating putative protein partners of laforin were performed. These results identified three candidate protein partners: EPM2AIP1 (63), HIRIP5 (64), and R5 (65).

EPM2AIP1

The first yeast two-hybrid experiment was performed using a human brain cDNA library (63). Full-length laforin was used as bait and identified a previously uncharacterized protein that was later named *EPM2AIP1*. *In vivo* coimmunoprecipitation binding assays using transfected full-length proteins in Cos-7 cells were able to confirm the interaction. Further analysis using the yeast two-hybrid system was able to show that absence of either the CBD or PTP motifs of laforin abolished interaction with *EPM2AIP1* and, therefore, intact laforin is required for interaction. The protein is encoded by a single exon gene, *EPM2AIP1*, that localizes to chromosome 3p22.1. *In silico* analysis of the 607 amino acid protein sequence revealed no functional domains other than the presence of two coiled-coil domains. Subcellular localization studies of *EPM2AIP1* resulted in a reticular pattern around the nucleus (i.e., ER), similar to that of laforin.

HIRIP5

The second yeast two-hybrid screen using a human fetal brain cDNA library identified the laforin interactor named *HIRIP5* that was also confirmed by *in vivo* interaction experiments (64). The protein contains a NifU-like domain, the only conserved region among nitrogen-fixing proteins, and a putative MurD ligase domain. The mouse and human *HIRIP5* transcripts both appear to be ubiquitously expressed in all subregions of the brain tested, as well as during embryonic development. Analysis of *HIRIP5* expression in the mouse brain using *in situ* hybridization revealed predominant expression in cerebellum and hippocampus, a pattern similar to that of the *Epm2a* gene. Localization experiments to determine the subcellular distribution of *HIRIP5* found an almost complete colocalization with laforin. *In vitro* phosphorylation studies found that laforin was able to dephosphorylate *HIRIP5* on both tyrosine and serine/threonine residues, suggesting that *HIRIP5* may be a potential substrate for laforin. The role that *HIRIP5* plays in the biological mechanism of LD is not clear as is the significance of the NifU and MurD ligase domains to the actual function of *HIRIP5*. When *HIRIP5* was tested *in vitro* for any MurD ligase activity, none was detected. NifU-containing genes appear to have roles in cofactor biosynthesis, amino acid interconversion, and regulation of ammonia storage. However, there are still roles for NifU-containing proteins that have not yet been identified and, as a result, the function of the NifU domain in determining *HIRIP5* function is currently being investigated. Interestingly, a *HIRIP5* ortholog exists in yeast and encodes for a mitochondrial matrix protein that is involved in iron metabolism. The relationship between *HIRIP5* and laforin, and how iron homeostasis may play a role in LD, awaits further exploration in the *Epm2a* knockout mouse, where neurodegenerative changes included mitochondrial abnormalities are observed.

R5, the Glycogen-Targeting Protein

A third very recent study in the search for additional laforin interactors using the yeast two-hybrid approach identified a protein, R5, which has a well-studied role in the known pathways of glycogen metabolism. In these experiments, brain and muscle cDNA libraries were used (65). The interaction between laforin and R5 was confirmed by *in vitro* pull-down and colocalization experiments. An additional interacting protein identified in this study was laforin itself, which was found to self-bind using the C-terminal region of the protein (65).

R5 was first discovered as the protein that permits targeting of protein phosphatase (PP1) to glycogen to induce further glycogen synthesis (66–68). It was since shown to also be involved in transporting other glycogen-metabolizing enzymes to the glycogen particle, including glycogen synthase, glycogen phosphorylase, and glycogen phosphorylase kinase, using an attachment domain for these proteins different from the one used to bind PP1. R5, therefore, likely serves as a scaffold to approximate PP1 with any one of these enzymes at the glycogen particle to allow its regulation by PP1. Laforin binds R5 in the same region as the three enzymes regulated by PP1 mentioned earlier. Whether PP1 regulates laforin, as it does the other proteins, is not known.

To summarize laforin's known relationships with glycogen: laforin binds glycogen (59), and it is targeted to glycogen in the same way as are enzymes of glycogen metabolism (65). What role it plays at the glycogen particle that, when disturbed, results in polyglucosan remains unknown and is the subject of further intense study toward understanding the pathogenesis of LB.

The *Epm2a* Knockout Mouse Model of Lafora Disease

To study the biological mechanism underlying LD and to further understand the associated pathogenesis, a mouse model using the knockout approach was generated (69). The exon containing the PTP domain was deleted. Homozygous null mutants were viable and, starting from as early as 2 months of age, prominent periodic acid–Schiff (PAS)-positive inclusions appeared in neurons throughout the brain. By 4 months, regions of the brain including hippocampus, cerebellum, cerebral cortex, thalamus, and brainstem were saturated with LB. The presence of LB appeared in the brain before any other nonneuronal tissues, including muscle and liver. At the ultrastructural level, LB in the null mice were very similar to those present in humans and were composed of a fibrillar material surrounded by fine punctiform particles. In general, the observed LB were found to increase in size with age.

Ultrastructural analysis in knockout mice brains as early as 2 months of age revealed neuronal cell death in cerebellar Purkinje cells, hippocampal pyramidal and granular cells, and cerebral cortical pyramidal cells. Features of somatic degeneration were observed in the form of dark mitochondria, dilated cisterni of endoplasmic reticulum, and distorted and shrunken cytoplasm. Interestingly, LB were absent in many of the neurons displaying degenerative features.

Phenotypic, including behavioral, analysis revealed that the presence of LB and neurodegeneration at 2 months of age was not accompanied with observable abnormalities. Only at 4 months of age did null mice begin to display an impaired behavioral response. It was at the later age of 9 months when null mice began to exhibit myoclonic seizures, ataxia, and EEG epileptiform activity. These results indicate that the presence of LB accumulations and neurogeneration predates the onset of any phenotypical anomalies in these mice. Many of the LD phenotypic characteristics present in humans were observed in the *Epm2a* null mutant mice. Grand mal tonic-clonic seizures were not observed.

The generation of *Epm2a* knockout mice resulted in a model that mimicked many of the clinical features of LD. Two novel findings resulted from this study that will prove to be invaluable to the understanding of the cellular pathways involved in LD onset. First was the peculiar degeneration of neurons that also did not result in the development of LB. The second interesting finding was that the neurodegeneration and onset of LB inclusions predated any behavioral abnor-

malities. This mouse model will not only allow for further investigation addressing each of these novel findings but also prove invaluable to the design of therapeutic treatments of LD.

Pathogenesis of Lafora Disease

The pathognomonic LB associated with LD are composed of polyglucosans, a glucose polymer with irregular branching. This abnormal branching pattern, unlike glycogen, results in their insolubility and resistance to digestion. The formation of polyglucosans is likely due to defects in one or more enzymes of glycogen metabolism, because this is the only mechanism that exists in animal tissues for the production of glucose polymers.

Formation of polyglucosans occurs in a small number of other conditions. These include Andersen disease (glycogen storage disease type IV), which is caused by loss of function mutations in the gene coding for the glycogen-branching enzyme (BE) (70). In this disease, polyglucosans are present in all tissues, including the brain; however, the disease is usually fatal in early childhood from liver cirrhosis (71). BE is crucial to the regular branching pattern of glycogen. Without this enzyme, glycogen synthase would continue lengthening the chain of glucose polymers without branch formations resulting in polyglucosans (72,73). Milder mutations in the gene encoding BE are the cause of adult polyglucosan body disease (APBD), a neurological disorder where patients develop polyglucosan bodies in the axons or axon hillocks of neurons, but never in the soma or dendrites (74,75). Interestingly, patients with APBD display upper and lower motor neuron signs, as well as dementia, but no seizures or myoclonus.

In the normal process of aging, small numbers of polyglucosans form in tissues including neurons and glia (40). These inclusions, named corpora amylacea (CA), increase in both size and number with advanced aging. Similar to the inclusions seen in APBD, corpora amylacea are also present in axons, but never in soma or dendrites. It is believed that in both cases they are produced in the neuronal somas and then are disposed of via axoplasmic flow to the axons (40).

In contrast, polyglucosans of LD are in the perikaryal region and dendrites, but not in axons (28). LD and APBD are both neurologic disorders and the composition of polyglucosans in both cases is similar. As a result, the differences in clinical presentation are likely due to the distinct intracellular compartment in which the polyglucosan bodies reside. The dendritic accumulations of polyglucosans in LD may affect neuronal signaling resulting in hyperexcitability causing seizures and myoclonus. In the case of APBD, the presence of polyglucosans in the axons specifically may be the cause of the motor defects and neurologic deterioration associated with the disease (75).

Electron microscopic examination of polyglucosans of newly forming LB in LD has found them to be associated with the ER and ribosomes (48,51,52). Interestingly, rough ER is exclusively compartmentalized to the dendrites and perikaryal regions of the neuron. This may be one reason for the localization of LD polyglucosans to these two cellular compartments. Alternatively, one of the pathways defective in LD may be one that is involved in the clearing or disposing of polyglucosans toward axons from where they could be eliminated by axoglial transfer, as appears to occur with CA (40).

The *EPM2B*-encoded product, malin, contains a RING finger domain and, therefore, likely plays the role of an E3 ubiquitin ligase. E3 ligases are required as part of the ubiquitination pathway to target specific substrates for degradation by the 26 S proteosome (76). This process has proved to be important for the regulation of many enzymes. Recently, increasing evidence has shown that ubiquitin can act as a nonproteolytic signal, depending on the type of ubiquitin chain (77,78). Proteins destined for degradation by the 26 S proteosome are usually tagged with a polyubiquitin chain, whereas those proteins with monoubiquitin tags are commonly participants of a signaling or regulatory mechanism similar to that of phosphorylation. How malin plays a role in the LD pathway is still unclear. Laforin and malin interact (2004). It is possbile that laforin regulates malin through phosphorylation or vice versa through ubiquitination. Alternatively, malin may play the more traditional E3 ligase role and target its physiologic substrate for degradation. This substrate may be glycogen synthase or another protein whose overfunction results in polyglucosan formation.

Clearly much remains to be learned before a complete understanding of the pathogenesis of LD is achieved. As has been seen, however, many pieces of the puzzle have been identified. These will lead to further pieces to be revealed and fitted one with the other. Key research goals at this time include identification of the third or more LD genes, understanding the polyglucosan biochemical pathway, exploring the dendritic compartmentalization of LB, examining whether the neurodegeneration is independent of LB accumulation, and determining the role of each of the latter two in the epilepsy of LD.

REFERENCES

1. Harenko A, Toiv Akka EI. Myoclonus epilepsy (Univerricht–Lundborg) in Finland. *Acta Neurol Scand* 1961;37:282–296.
2. Koskiniemi M. Psychological findings in progressive myoclonus epilepsy without Lafora bodies. *Epilepsia* 1974;15:537–545.
3. Koskiniemi M, Donner M, Majuri H, et al. Progressive myoclonus epilepsy. A clinical and histopathological study. *Acta Neurol Scand* 1974;50:307–332.
4. Koskiniemi M, Toivakka E, Donner M. Progressive myoclonus epilepsy. Electroencephalographical findings. *Acta Neurol Scand* 1974;50:333–359.
5. Lehesjoki AE. Clinical features and genetics of Unverricht-Lundborg disease. *Adv Neurol* 2002;89: 193–197.
6. Hurd RW, Wilder BJ, Helveston WR, et al. Treatment of four siblings with progressive myoclonus epilepsy of the Unverricht–Lundborg type with *N*-Acetylcysteine. *Neurology* 1996;47:1264–1268.
7. Ferrari G, Yan, CY, Greene LA. *N*-Acetylcysteine (D- and L-stereoisomers) prevents apoptotic death of neuronal cells. *J Neurosci* 1995;15:2857–2866.
8. Lehesjoki AE, Koskiniemi M. Progressive myoclonus epilepsy of Unverricht-Lundborg type. *Epilepsia* 1999; 40[Suppl 3]:23–28.
9. Shibasaki H. Electrophysiological studies of myoclonus. *Muscle Nerve* 2000;23:321–335.
10. Lehesjoki AE, Koskiniemi M, Norio R, et al. Localization of the EPM1 gene for progressive myoclonus epilepsy on chromosome 21: linkage disequilibrium allows high resolution mapping. *Hum Mol Genet* 1993;2:1229–1234.
11. Pennacchio LA, Lehesjoki AE, Stone NE, et al. Mutations in the gene encoding cystatin B in progressive myoclonus epilepsy (EPM1). *Science* 1996;271:1731–1734.
12. Lalioti MD, Mirotsou M, Buresi C, et al. Identification of mutations in cystatin B, the gene responsible

for the Unverricht–Lundborg type of progressive myoclonus epilepsy (EPM1). *Am J Hum Genet* 1997;60:342–351.

13. Virtaneva K, D'Amato E, Miao J, et al. Unstable minisatellite expansion causing recessively inherited myoclonus epilepsy, EPM1. *Nat Genet* 1997;15:393–396.

14. Lafreniere RG, Rochefort DL, Chretien N, et al. Unstable insertion in the 5′ flanking region of the cystatin B gene is the most common mutation in progressive myoclonus epilepsy type 1, EPM1. *Nat Genet* 1997;15:298–302.

15. Lalioti MD, Scott HS, Antonarakis SE. What is expanded in progressive myoclonus epilepsy? *Nat Genet* 1997;17:17.

16. Lalioti MD, Scott HS, Buresi C, et al. Dodecamer repeat expansion in cystatin B gene in progressive myoclonus epilepsy. *Nature* 1997;386:847–851.

17. Virtaneva K, Paulin L, Krahe R, et al. The minisatellite expansion mutation in EPM1: resolution of an initial discrepancy. Mutatations in brief no. 186. Online. *Hum Mutat* 1998;12:218.

18. Lalioti MD, Scott HS, Antonarakis SE. Altered spacing of promoter elements due to the dodecamer repeat expansion contributes to reduced expression of the cystatin B gene in EPM1. *Hum Mol Genet* 1999;8:1791–1798.

19. Ritonja A, Popovic T, Turk V, et al. Amino acid sequence of human liver cathepsin B. *FEBS Lett* 1985;181:169–172.

20. Haltia M, Kristensson K, Sourander P. Neuropathological studies in three Scandinavian cases of progressive myoclonus epilepsy. *Acta Neurol Scand* 1969;45:63–77.

21. Eldridge R, Iivanainen M, Stern R, et al. "Baltic" myoclonus epilepsy: hereditary disorder of childhood made worse by phenytoin. *Lancet* 1983;2:838–842.

22. Pennacchio LA, Bouley DM, Higgins KM, et al. Progressive ataxia, myoclonic epilepsy and cerebellar apoptosis in cystatin B-deficient mice. *Nat Genet* 1998;20:251–258.

23. Shannon P, Pennacchio LA, Houseweart MK, et al. Neuropathological changes in a mouse model of progressive myoclonus epilepsy: cystatin B deficiency and Unverricht–Lundborg disease. *J Neuropathol Exp Neurol* 2002;61:1085–1091.

24. Lieuallen K, Pennacchio LA, Park M, et al. Cystatin B-deficient mice have increased expression of apoptosis and glial activation genes. *Hum Mol Genet* 2001;10:1867–1871.

25. Cotter RL, Burke WJ, Thomas VS, et al. Insights into the neurodegenerative process of Alzheimer's disease: a role for mononuclear phagocyte-associated inflammation and neurotoxicity. *J Leukoc Biol* 1999;65:416–427.

26. Liberski PP, Brown P, Cervenakova L, et al. Interactions between astrocytes and oligodendroglia in human and experimental Creutzfeldt–Jakob disease and scrapie. *Exp Neurol* 1977;144:227–234.

27. D'Amato E, Kokaia Z, Nanobashvili A, et al. Seizures induce widespread upregulation of cystatin B, the gene mutated in progressive myoclonus epilepsy, in rat forebrain neurons. *Eur J Neurosci* 2000;12:1687–1695.

28. Minassian BA. Progressive myoclonus epilepsy with polyglucosan bodies: Lafora disease. *Adv Neurol* 2002;89:199–210.

29. Ganesh S, Delgado-Escueta AV, Suzuki T, et al. Genotype-phenotype correlations for EPM2A mutations in Lafora's progressive myoclonus epilepsy: Exon 1 mutations associate with an early-onset cognitive deficit subphenotype. *Hum Mol Genet* 2002;11:1263–1271.

30. Yoshimura I, Kaneko S, Yoshimura N, et al. Long-term observations of two siblings with Lafora disease treated with zonisamide. *Epilepsy Res* 2001;46:283–287.

31. Kyllerman M, Ben-Menachem E. Zonisamide for progressive myoclonus epilepsy: long-term observations in seven patients. *Epilepsy Res* 1998;29:109–114.

32. Boccella P, Striano P, Zara F, et al. Bioptically demonstrated Lafora disease without EPM2A mutation: A clinical and neurophysiological study of two sisters. *Clin Neurol Neurosurg* 2003;106:56–60.

33. Tassinari CA, Bureau-Paillas M, Dalla Bernardina B, et al. [Lafora disease (author's transl)]. *Rev Electroencephalogr Neurophysiol Clin* 1978;8:107–122.

34. Shibasaki H. Physiology of negative myoclonus. *Adv Neurol* 2002;89:103–113.

35. Reutens DC, Puce A, Berkovic SF. Cortical hyperexcitability in progressive myoclonus epilepsy: a study with transcranial magnetic stimulation. *Neurology* 1993;43:186–192.

36. Manganotti P, Tamburin S, Zanette G, et al. Hyperexcitable cortical responses in progressive myoclonic epilepsy: a TMS study. *Neurology* 2001;57:1793–1799.

37. Silen T, Forss N, Salenius S, et al. Oscillatory cortical drive to isometrically contracting muscle in Unverricht–Lundborg type progressive myoclonus epilepsy (ULD). *Clin Neurophysiol* 2002;113:1973–1979.

38. Brown P, Farmer SF, Halliday DM, et al. Coherent cortical and muscle discharge in cortical myoclonus. *Brain* 1999;122[Pt 3]:461–472.

39. Panzica F, Canafoglia L, Franceschetti S, et al. Movement-activated myoclonus in genetically defined progressive myoclonic epilepsies: EEG-EMG relationship estimated using autoregressive models. *Clin Neurophysiology* 2003;114:1041–1052.

40. Cavanagh JB, Corpora-amylacea and the family of polyglucosan diseases. *Brain Res Rev* 1999;29:265–295.

41. Nishimura RN, Ishak KG, Reddick R, et al. Lafora disease: Diagnosis by liver biopsy. *Ann Neurol* 1980;8:409–415.

42. Carpenter S, Karpati G. Ultrastructural findings in Lafora disease. *Ann Neurol* 1981;10:63–64.

43. Schwarz GA, Yanoff M. Lafora disease, distinct clinicopathological form of Unverricht's syndrome. *Arch Neurol* 1965;12:172–188.

44. Janeway R, Ravens JR, Pearce LA, et al. Progressive myoclonus epilepsy with Lafora inclusion bodies. I. Clinical, genetic, histopathologic, and biochemical aspects. *Arch Neurol* 1967;16:565–582.

45. Gambetti P, Di Mauro S, Hirt L, et al. Myoclonic epilepsy with lafora bodies. Some ultrastructural, histochemical, and biochemical aspects. *Arch Neurol* 1971;25:483–493.

46. Neville HE, Brooke MH, Austin JH. Studies in myoclonus epilepsy. (Lafora body form). IV. Skeletal muscle abnormalities. *Arch Neurol* 1974;30:466–474.

47. Carpenter S, Karpati G, Andermann F, et al. Lafora's disease: Peroxisomal storage in skeletal muscle. *Neurology* 1974;24:531–538.
48. Van Heycop ten Ham M. Lafora disease, a form of progressive myoclonus epilepsy. *Handb Clin Neurol* 1974;15:382–422.
49. Busard HL, Renier WO, Gabreels FJ, et al. Lafora disease: a quantitative morphological and biochemical study of the cerebral cortex. *Clin Neuropathol* 1987;6:1–6.
50. Sakai M, Austin J, Witmer F, et al. Studies in myoclonus epilepsy (Lafora body form). II. Polyglucosans in the systemic deposits of myoclonus epilepsy and in corpora amylacea. *Neurology* 1970;20:160–176.
51. Collins GH, Cowden RR, Nevis AH. Myoclonus epilepsy with Lafora bodies. An ultrastructural and cytochemical study. *Arch Pathol* 1968;86:239–254.
52. Toga M, Dubois D, Hassoun J. [Ultrastructure of Lafora bodies]. *Acta Neuropathol (Berlin)* 1968;10:132–142.
53. Minassian BA, Lee JR, Herbrick JA, et al. Mutations in a gene encoding a novel protein tyrosine phosphatase cause progressive myoclonus epilepsy. *Nat Genet* 1998;20:171–174.
54. Ganesh S, Suzuki T, Yamakawa K. Alternative splicing modulates subcellular localization of laforin. *Biochem Biophys Res Commun* 2002;291:1134–1147.
54a. Ianzano L, Young EJ, Zhao XC, et al. (2004) Loss of function of the cytoplasmic isoform of the protein laforin (EPM2A) causes Lafora progressive myoclonus epilepsy. *Hum Mutat* 23:170–176.
55. Minassian BA, Ianzano L, Meloche M, et al. Mutation spectrum and predicted function of laforin in Lafora's progressive myoclonus epilepsy. *Neurology* 2000;55:341–346.
56. Ganesh S, Agarwala KL, Amano K, et al. Regional and developmental expression of Epm2a gene and its evolutionary conservation. *Biochem Biophys Res Commun* 2001;283:1046–1053.
57. Minassian BA, Andrade DM, Ianzano L, et al. Laforin is a cell membrane and endoplasmic reticulum-associated protein tyrosine phosphatase. *Ann Neurol* 2001;49:271–275.
58. Ganesh S, Agarwala KL, Ueda K, et al. Laforin, defective in the progressive myoclonus epilepsy of Lafora type, is a dual-specificity phosphatase associated with polyribosomes. *Hum Mol Genet* 2000;9:2251–2261.
59. Wang J, Stuckey JA, Wishart MJ, et al. A unique carbohydrate binding domain targets the lafora disease phosphatase to glycogen. *J Biol Chem* 2002;277:2377–2380.
60. Minassian BA, Sainz J, Serratosa JM, et al. Genetic locus heterogeneity in Lafora's progressive myoclonus epilepsy. *Ann Neurol* 1999;45:262–265.
61. Chan EM, Bulman DE, Paterson AD, et al. Genetic mapping of a new Lafora progressive myoclonus epilepsy locus (EPM2B) on 6p22. *J Med Genet* 2003;40:671–675.
62. Chan EM, Young EJ, Ianzano L, et al. Mutations in NHLRC1 cause progressive myoclonus epilepsy. *Nat Genet* 2003;35:125–127.
63. Ianzano L, Zhao XC, Minassian BA, et al. Identification of a novel protein interacting with laforin, the EPM2A Progressive Myoclonus Epilepsy gene product. *Genomics* 2003;81:579–587.
64. Ganesh S, Tsurutani N, Suzuki T, et al. The Lafora disease gene product laforin interacts with HIRIP5, a phylogenetically conserved protein containing a NifU-like domain. *Hum Mol Genet (advanced access publication)* 2003:10.1093/hmg/ddg253.
65. Fernandez-Sanchez ME, Criado-Garcia O, Heath KE, et al. Laforin, the dual-phosphatase responsible for Lafora disease, interacts with R5 (PTG), a regulatory subunit of protein phosphatase-1 that enhances glycogen accumulation. *Hum Mol Genet* 2003;12:3161–3171.
66. Doherty MJ, Young PR, Cohen PT. Amino acid sequence of a novel protein phosphatase 1 binding protein (R5) which is related to the liver- and muscle-specific glycogen binding subunits of protein phosphatase 1. *FEBS Lett* 1996;399:339–343.
67. Printen JA, Brady MJ, Saltiel AR. PTG, a protein phosphatase 1-binding protein with a role in glycogen metabolism. *Science* 1997;275:1475–1478.
68. Fong NM, Jensen TC, Shah AS, et al. Identification of binding sites on protein targeting to glycogen for enzymes of glycogen metabolism. *J Biol Chem* 2000;275:35,034–35,039.
69. Ganesh S, Delgado-Escueta AV, Sakamoto T, et al. Targeted disruption of the Epm2a gene causes formation of Lafora inclusion bodies, neurodegeneration, ataxia, myoclonus epilepsy and impaired behavioral response in mice. *Hum Mol Genet* 2002;11:1251–1262.
70. Moses SW, Parvari R. The variable presentations of glycogen storage disease type IV: A review of clinical, enzymatic and molecular studies. *Curr Mol Med* 2002;2:177–188.
71. Schochet SS, Jr, McCormick WF, Zellweger H. Type IV glycogenosis (amylopectinosis). Light and electron microscopic observations. *Arch Pathol* 1970;90:354–363.
72. Raben N, Danon M, Lu N, et al. Surprises of genetic engineering: a possible model of polyglucosan body disease. *Neurology* 2001;56:1739–1745.
73. Pederson BA, Csitkovits AG, Simon R, et al. Overexpression of glycogen synthase in mouse muscle results in less branched glycogen. *Biochem Biophys Res Commun* 2003;305:826–830.
74. Ziemssen F, Sindern E, Schroder JM, et al. Novel missense mutations in the glycogen-branching enzyme gene in adult polyglucosan body disease. *Ann Neurol* 2000;47:536–540.
75. Robitaille Y, Carpenter S, Karpati G, et al. A distinct form of adult polyglucosan body disease with massive involvement of central and peripheral neuronal processes and astrocytes: a report of four cases and a review of the occurrence of polyglucosan bodies in other conditions such as Lafora's disease and normal aging. *Brain* 1980;103:315–336.
76. Hatakeyama S, Nakayama KI. U-box proteins as a new family of ubiquitin ligases. *Biochem Biophys Res Commun* 2003;302:635–645.
77. Conaway RC, Brower CS, Conaway JW. Emerging roles of ubiquitin in transcription regulation. *Science* 2002;296:1254–1258.
78. Pickart CM. Ubiquitin enters the new millennium. *Mol Cell* 2001;8:499–504.

5

Myoclonic Status in Nonprogressive Encephalopathies

Bernardo Dalla Bernardina,* Elena Fontana,* and Francesca Darra*

*Servizio Neuropsichiatria Infantile, Policlinico G.B. Rossi, Studi di Verona, Verona, Italy;

INTRODUCTION

The existence in infants and young children, with a nonprogressive encephalopathy, of epilepsies characterized predominantly by myoclonic manifestations and having, in their natural history, a significant risk to develop more or less frequently a myoclonic status is well documented in the literature (1–10).

Nevertheless, the reports outlining the existence of an epileptic syndrome essentially characterized by the recurrence of long-lasting or subcontinuous myoclonic status in children with a nonprogressive encephalopathy are rare (11–18).

Several authors (17–26) describe a quite similar electroclinical picture in children with Angelman syndrome and in some children with 4p-syndrome (27), but few authors have stressed how, in some of these cases, the electroclinical picture was typically that of a "myoclonic status in nonprogressive encephalopathy" (12–15, 27–29).

Following the results of our electroclinical longitudinal study of 51 cases, we describe this peculiar form of epileptic encephalopathy, recently proposed also in the scheme of the ILAE Task Force on Classification and Terminology (30) under the heading "Syndromes in development." This form of epilepsy is characterized by recurrence of long-lasting myoclonic status appearing in infants and young children with a nonprogressive encephalopathy and having a variable poor prognosis.

CLINICAL AND ELECTROENCEPHALOGRAPHIC–POLYGRAPHIC FEATURES

The 51 children studied include 34 females and 17 males with a sex ratio male:female of 1:2; their actual age is between 3 and 19 years (mean age 6 years). Five children (3 females and 2 males) died at the ages of 18, 24, and 30 months, and at 6 and 10 years, respectively. Familial antecedents of epilepsy were reported in 9 cases (17.6%).

The population can be divided into three etiological groups:

1. Genetic: Twenty-four subjects (47%; 17 females and 7 males). In 19 (37%), there was a deficit in chromosome 15q 11-q13, which is testimony to Angelman syndrome (13 females and 6 males). Two females presented a deletion of the short arm of chromosome 4 and the typical phenotype of the Wolf–Hirschhorn syndrome (currently known as 4p- syndrome). Two girls were affected by Rett syndrome and a Prader–Willi syndrome was diagnosed in one boy. No neuroradiologic abnormalities were present.

2. Fetal/neonatal anoxic injury: Eight subjects (15.6%; 2 females and 6 males). On neuroradiologic investigation, significant atrophic abnormalities were recognizable only in 3 subjects.

3. Unknown: Nineteen subjects (37%; 15 females and 4 males) were affected by a

assessed symptomatic nonprogressive encephalopathy of which we were unable to define the etiology. The neuroradiologic picture [magnetic resonance imaging (MRI)] revealed a focal unilateral or bilateral micropolygyria in five subjects, a complete callosum agenesia with microcephalia in one subject, a slight colpocephaly with vermis hypoplasia and microcephalia in two sisters, and a partial callosum agenesia with bilateral hippocampal dysgenesis and vermis hypoplasia in another two sisters from another family. In 10 of 19 cases, therefore, the pathology appears to be constituted by a cortical dysplasia, in most cases, probably genetically determined.

The most constant clinical aspect at onset (38 patients, 75%) was that of an axial hypotonia of variable degree causing, in 23 cases (45%), a simple retardation in postural acquisitions; in 19 (37%), aposturality was associated with polymorphous abnormal movements presenting a picture of hypotonic "ataxic" cerebral palsy with a dystonic–dyskinetic syndrome and severe mental retardation.

Dysmorphisms evoking a probable genetic and/or malformative etiology were present at onset in 13 subjects (25%); slight microcephaly, reported at birth in 3, were present in 11 subjects (22%).

The average age of seizure onset was 10 months (range: 1 day–5 years). In 22 cases, the epilepsy onset was constituted by a myoclonic status characterized by very frequent during the day or subcontinuous "absences," accompanied by periorbital and perioral myoclonias and rhythmic and arrhythmic jerks of distal muscles.

In the others, the initial seizures were mostly partial motor seizures, more or less typical brief myoclonic absences, massive myoclonias, and, more rarely, generalized or unilateral clonic seizures recurring in some patients only during cases of a febrile illness. Furthermore, the recurrence of brief massive startles was frequently reported at rest and during drowsiness.

The average age when myoclonic status was recognized was 14 months (range: 3 months–5 years). Because of severe mental retardation and continuous abnormal movements, both the paroxysmal attention disturbances ("absences") and the myoclonias could remain hidden for several months in many cases. Considering the insidious appearance and probably the age at onset of myoclonias, the status, in many cases, may be unrecognized.

More frequently, myoclonias are subcontinuous but asynchronous in different muscles. In this case, their relationship with paroxysmal EEG activity is very difficult to appreciate; in this situation, the paroxysmal nature of the EEG pattern is also often difficult to recognize.

In some cases, the myoclonias are more obvious, rhythmically involving both arms and orofacial muscles. In other cases, the myoclonias are followed by a brief silent period, the result is a mixture of positive and negative phenomena. In some other cases, a negative myoclonus is predominant, which continuously fragments the voluntary movements and inhibits any fixed antigravity posturing.

Although the child is awake, the EEG is characterized by a slow activity with more or less easily recognizable paroxysmal abnormalities. These abnormalities consist of a relatively monomorphous subcontinuous, delta-theta activity (3–6 c/sec) varying in amplitude, and involving more or less asynchronously, the frontocentral regions. There are also brief sequences of rhythmic delta waves with superimposed spikes, achieving an unusual spike-and-wave, predominantly in parietooccipital regions, often elicited by eye closure (Fig. 5–1).

The ictal manifestations are characterized by brief, more or less, diffuse bursts predominating in the central regions and slow spike and waves accompanied by bilateral, more or less rhythmic, myoclonias.

When myoclonias are rhythmic and synchronous in the two sides of the body, they are strictly related to EEG diffuse paroxysms in burst, achieving an ictal pattern, similar to that of a brief myoclonic absence. In this case, the ictal discharge is also characterized by a recognizable clinical "absence" (Fig. 5–1). More frequently the myoclonias are arrhythmic and become more easy to recognize during motor arrest, for example, during absence or drowsiness when all other abnormal movements disappear.

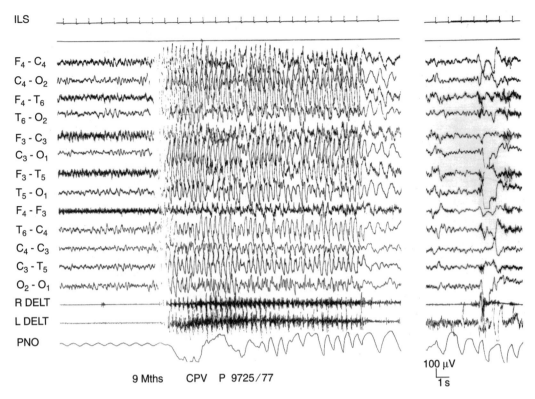

FIG. 5–1. A 9-month old girl with congenital microcephalia, bilateral frontocentral micropolygyria and callosum agenesia, massive axial hypotonia, and severe cognitive deficit presenting from the age of 5 months, with several daily brief myoclonic absences, evolving, a few months later, in long-lasting myoclonic status. See the relatively correct-for-age background activity and a myoclonic absence lasting 15 sec characterized by 3 per second diffuse spike-waves related with bilateral 3 per second rhythmic jerks inserted in a paroxysmally increased muscular tone. (R. Delt refers to right deltoid; ILS refers to intermittent light stimulation; PNO refers to pneumogram or respiration).

The electroclinical pattern of the status is often characterized by a fluctuation of the paroxysms. It is possible to observe, in fact, recurring bursts of spikes and waves or slow waves that are more or less diffuse, more or less synchronous, or asynchronous on both hemispheres. Between these bursts are inserted periods of variable duration without obvious paroxysmal discharges but with pseudorhythmic delta–theta activity of variable amplitude involving subcontinuously both central regions (Fig. 5–2).

The proof that they are not separate ictal events recurring at a more or less high frequency, but a true status, is shown by the observation that, like theta activity, positive and negative myoclonias are also subcontinuous.

In some cases, for periods of variable duration, the status is more easily recognizable because it is characterized by a continuous diffuse, but asynchronous, sequence of spike and waves of great amplitude on both hemispheres. These are related to continuous rhythmic jerks, frequently followed by negative phenomena.

During drowsiness and slow sleep, spikes and waves become continuous to the point that the spindles are not recognizable. During stages II and III of the following nocturnal cycles, the paroxysm activation is minor and spindles are clearly represented; during slow sleep, the myoclonias vanish, reappearing briefly at arousal and eventually during rapid eye movement (REM) sleep when the diffuse discharges disappear in this phase. There is a continuous rhythmic theta activity mainly involving the vertex and rolandic regions. The same theta activity,

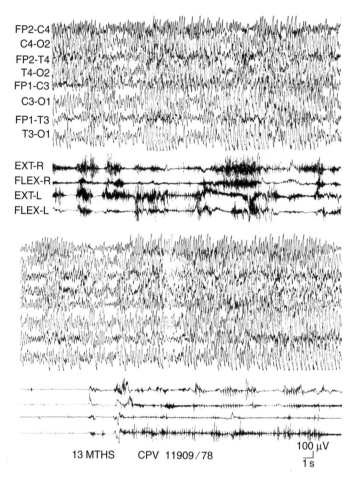

FP2-C4
C4-O2
FP2-T4
T4-O2
FP1-C3
C3-O1
FP1-T3
T3-O1

EXT-R
FLEX-R
EXT-L
FLEX-L

13 MTHS   CPV 11909/78

100 µV
1 s

FIG. 5–2. A 13-month-old girl with ataxia, jerky movements, slight acquired microcephalia, cognitive impairment, speech absence, and frequent inadequate bursts of laughter. See the subcontinuous ample delta waves fluctuating in amplitude and diffusion, mainly asynchronous on the two hemispheres, related to subcontinuous more or less rhythmic jerks partially masked by the tonic component of the other abnormal movements.

strictly related to myoclonias, is transitorily observed during waking up.

According to the electroclinical picture, three main subgroups can be recognized. The first is of subjects showing a mixed pattern of brief myoclonic absences and subcontinuous rhythmic positive jerks. These are eventually followed by a brief silent period related to a subcontinuous delta–theta activity involving the central areas, and brief sequences of rhythmic delta waves with superimposed spikes mainly involving the parietooccipital regions and often elicited by eye closure. In this first group the status is recog-

nizable just during the first year of life. They are events of variable duration, recurring sporadically in about one-half of the cases, whereas they are more "chronic" (lasting for years) in about a one-fourth of the cases. No other types of seizures are observed except for rare unilateral or generalized seizures occurring occasionally during a febrile illness.

Frequently the status results are refractory to treatment. Even benzodiazepine and corticotropin (ACTH), can have a transitory effect. In many cases, only ethosuximide, associated with valproic acid or levetiracetam, appears to induce a significant improvement. When the myoclonic status is halted or reduced by treatment, the clinical picture improves dramatically. Continuous disabling jerks and the extreme hyperactivity are reduced and some children become ambulatory.

This electroclinical picture has been mainly observed in children, with Angelman syndrome (Fig. 5–2) and with 4p- syndrome. In about one-third of these cases, the myoclonic status disappears during evolution of the disease. The intentional myoclonus can become prominent, thus achieving the picture described by Guerrini et al. (18,23) as cortical myoclonus. As we have previously outlined (12,15,28,31) and as confirmed by other authors (17,18,29), we consider this electroclinical picture as the earliest diagnostic indicator of Angelman syndrome (13).

The second subgroup include subjects which show a pattern characterized by the marked predominance of inhibitory phenomena mixed with a severe fragmented dystonic component and sudden irregular rapid lightninglike jerks. At onset, status is also often difficult to recognize because of severe mental impairment and abundance of continuous polymorphous and rough abnormal movements. The mostly erratic jerks, are therefore difficult to distinguish from the violent dyskinetic movements (Fig. 5–3). Moreover, subcontinuous multifocal slow spike-waves, predominating on the frontocentral regions, but fluctuating in amplitude and diffusion, are very difficult to correlate with the positive and negative myoclonias in the EEG (Figs. 5–3, 5–4). The result is an epileptic status characterized by a complex unregulated motor pattern inducing a peculiar "hyperkinetic complete motor inhibition."

Sometimes a long-lasting status can appear characterized by the recurrence of very ample and diffuse rhythmic slow spike-waves associated with rhythmic and generalized myoclonias

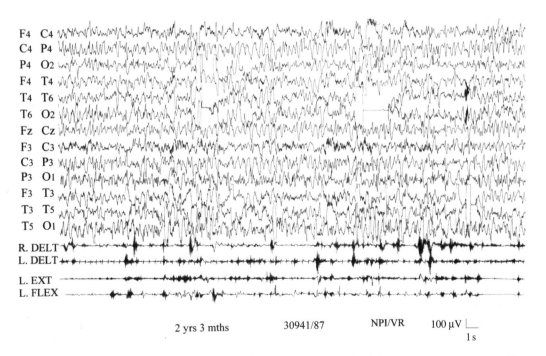

2 yrs 3 mths   30941/87   NPI/VR   100 µV |_
                                                              1 s

FIG. 5–3. A 2-year 3-month-old girl with aposturality, distonic-dyskinetic movements, severe cognitive impairment in absence of obvious neuroradiologic (MRI) abnormalities, and, showing, from the age of 7 months, long-lasting myoclonic status with subcontinuous inhibiting phenomena mixed with sudden violent dyskinetic movements. See the continuous paroxysmal motor activity related to subcontinuous frontocentral slow spike-wave mixed with unusual beta activity.

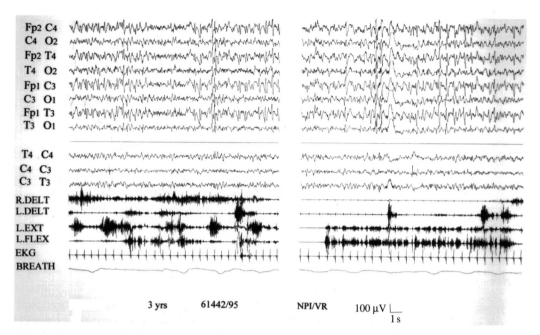

FIG. 5–4. A 3-year-old girl with microcephalia, partial callosum agenesia, vermis hypoplasia, aposturality, severe mental retardation, and distonic-dyskinetic movements, showing, from the age of 9 months, long-lasting myoclonic status. See (**left**) the multifocal paroxysms associated with erratic positive and negative myoclonus mixed with very abrupt dyskinetic movements. During the same recording (**right**), the occurrence of rhythmic inhibitory phenomena fragmenting the muscular activity, related to more rhythmic and structured paroxysmal activity on the EEG (one sister is affected by a similar disorder), were seen.

followed by an inhibitory phenomenon (Fig. 5–5) they are often resistant to intravenous benzodiazepine and requiring intensive status. Three subjects died during this status. Other types of seizures, except for brief generalized tonic-clonic seizures, sometimes in clusters, are very rare. In this subgroup, the status is always refractory to different therapies and permanent throughout the evolution with definitive aposturality and severe mental deficit. The patients showing this electroclinical picture are females affected by a nonprogressive encephalopathy of unknown etiology or sustained by a cortical malformation.

The third subgroup includes children showing only a mild neurologic impairment at onset and who suffer initially from partial motor seizures or brief myoclonic absences (Fig. 5–1). More or less rapidly and more or less subtly, a myoclonic status progressively begins, which is initially characterized by a subcontinuous sequence of generalized spike-wave-type paroxysms related to rhythmic myoclonia of face and limbs. In time, we can observe a progressive deterioration of the electrical activity morphology of EEG paroxysms are modified and become sharp theta waves with very slow pseudorhythmic continuous spikes in the central regions and vertex. At the same time, the clinical motor picture is progressively compromised and pyramidal signs and intentional tremors appear. Furthermore, continuous myoclonic inhibitory phenomena appear that sometimes can be recognized clinically and polygraphically only in the presence of an increase in the postural tone (Figs. 5–6 to 5–8). Complete motor inhibition is invariably the result.

Equally progressive, there is a severe neuropsychologic impairment, and in one-third of the cases a discrete cortical–subcortical and cerebellar atrophy is visible with MRI. A progressive pathology does not appear in any case and,

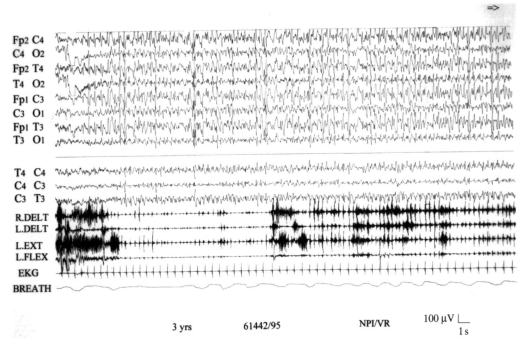

3 yrs   61442/95   NPI/VR   100 µV |⎯
                                                         1 s

FIG. 5–5. Same girl as in Fig. 5–4. Shown is a more obvious myoclonic status and a continuous recurrence of bilateral jerks related to rhythmic diffuse continuous paroxysms.

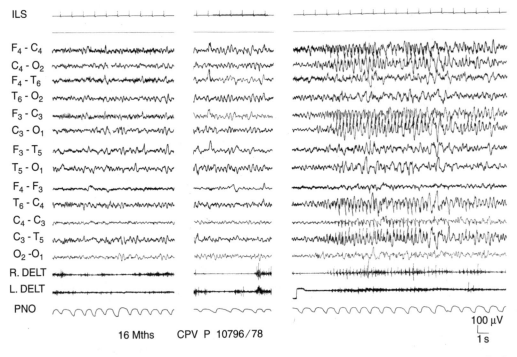

16 Mths   CPV P 10796/78   100 µV
                                      |⎯
                                       1 s

FIG. 5–6. Same girl as in Fig. 5–1. Note the appearance of long-lasting, partially modified, myoclonic status. The background activity appears slightly slowered and the ictal events are still myoclonic absences characterized, nevertheless, by a paroxysmal EEG activity involving the motor regions nearly exclusively. Motor manifestations are always obvious while attention impairment is very slight.

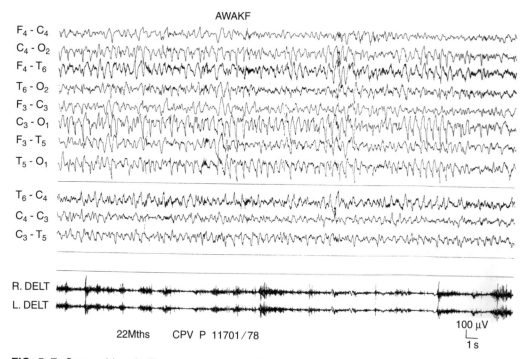

FIG. 5–7. Same girl as in Figs. 5–1 and 5–6. Clinically the neuropsychologic picture has severely worsened. The myoclonic manifestations, mixed with a subcontinuous fragmentation of muscular activity, have become subcontinuous. At the same time, any background activity organization disappears and slow spike-waves appear to be recurring subcontinuously in the centroparietal regions.

in the long term, the picture instituted remains unchanged. In one-fourth of the cases, the MRI shows the existence of a probable gyration disturbance, such as focal bilateral micropolygyria.

The electroclinical picture seems, therefore, to be one of a pharmacoresistant progressive epilepsy not sustained by a progressive disease. Partial motor seizures, predominantly tonic and only sometimes followed by generalization, are frequent, even at long term, while other types of seizures are absent.

DISCUSSION

As previously outlined, the reports in the literature describing a similar electroclinical picture are rare (11,12,16,17,27,29) and certainly do not reflect its real incidence. The main reason for this "underestimate" is probably the low frequency of using EEG polygraphic recordings for diagnosis of infantile epilepsies; on the other hand, it is probable that similar pictures have been included by some authors in other diagnostic settings such as minor motor status (1), myoclonic variant of Lennox–Gastaut syndrome (32–34), or myoclonic status in symptomatic cases of myoclonic-astatic epilepsy (35).

Some authors have, in reality, described a very similar status in cases of Angelman syndrome, but failed to recognize the prominent myoclonic character because of the absence of polygraphic recordings (19,20,25,26,36–38).

Viewing the differential diagnosis, two different conditions can present a more or less intriguing problem. Because of the significant progressive increase of neuropsychologic impairment and of the EEG paroxysmal abnormalities and the polymorphous myoclonic manifestations, the first, and often most complex step, is to rule out a progressive disease. In some cases, presenting

=>

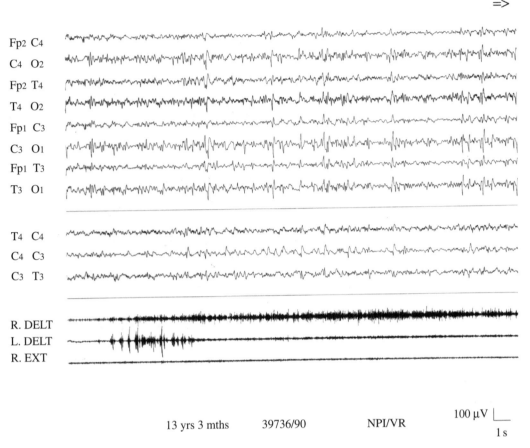

13 yrs 3 mths   39736/90   NPI/VR   100 µV

1 s

FIG. 5–8. Same girl of as in Figs. 5–1, 5–6, and 5–7. The long-term evolution is characterized by a clinical picture of tetraparetic spastic PCI with axial hypotonia and complete motor inhibition. Note the subcontinuous slow spikes and sharp waves on the centroparietal regions related to subcontinuous inhibitory phenomena fragmenting the muscular activity with insertions of bursts of positive jerks followed by an inhibitory phenomenon.

frequent atypical absences with concomitant myoclonic–atonic phenomena, the electroclinical picture can be quite similar to late infantile form of neuronal ceroid-lipofuscinosis (39–41). The absence of progressive visual impairment, normal visual-evoked potential (VEP), even when, as frequently observed, the somatosensory evoked potentials (SEP), are roughly abnormal, the absence of a paroxysmal response to intermittent light stimulation (ILS), the persistence of recognizable sleep spindles, and the more or less significant improvement of the clinical picture concomitant with a satisfactory, even if transitory, improvement of the status can help a correct diagnosis.

In the presence of the electroclinical picture of the second and third subgroups, neuropathologic and genetic molecular analyses are required to discard neuronal ceroid-lipofuscinosis. On the other hand, the differential diagnosis can be somewhat difficult with some of the cases reported in the literature as suffering from a "newborn continuous partial epilepsy" (42), "early onset progressive encephalopathy with migrant continuous myoclonus (43), or "migrating partial seizures of early infancy" (44 – 46). In fact, many of these cases can present a long-lasting status characterized by continuous discharges of diffuse spikes and waves accompanied by bilateral asynchronous myoclonias with obtundation and drooling.

CONCLUSION

As previously outlined (11,12,14,47–49), we consider that this particular type of symptomatic myoclonic epilepsy, essentially characterized by the recurrence of long-lasting atypical status, associated with an impairment of attention and continuous polymorphous jerks, mixed with other complex abnormal movements, in infants suffering from a nonprogressive encephalopathy, constitutes a peculiar syndromic entity.

Although this condition is difficult to clinically recognize (because of previous intellectual deficit and of continuous abnormal movements), it can be easily demonstrated by polygraphic recordings, which show rhythmic discharges of diffuse slow spike-waves accompanied by more or less rhythmic asynchronous myoclonias, continuous during wakefulness and, in many cases, also persisting during sleep. This status is invariably accompanied by a concomitant worsening of neuropsychologic evolution. The etiology can be various and, probably, mainly malformative and genetic; the evolution is often very poor.

We consider its recognition important because:

- It allows to exclude the hypothesis of a progressive disease evoked by the severe neuropsychologic impairment that accompanies the appearance of the status.
- Only an early recognition allows an adequate treatment avoiding or limiting neuropsychologic impairment.

Furthermore, a correct electroclinical analysis is able to distinguish three peculiar subsets having important diagnostic and prognostic significance. The first is characterized by the association of absences, subcontinuous jerks, which are at times rhythmic or arrhythmic and mainly positive, brief myoclonic absences, and hypnagogic startles. A diagnosis of Angelman syndrome or another syndromic entity sustained by a chromosomal abnormality must be considered when such a picture presents.

The second is characterized by the association of absence status and continuous rhythmic myoclonus, mainly negative, mixed with sudden uncontrolled continuous dyskinetic movements, leading to a clinical picture of hyperkinetic aposturality. This condition affects mainly females, probably with cortical malformations.

The third is characterized by continuous spike activity in rolandic regions, persisting throughout life, and accompanied by bilateral rhythmic myoclonias followed by an inhibitory phenomenon. This leads to a progressive neuromotor deterioration corresponding to a form of myoclonic progressive epilepsy in absence of progressive disease. In these cases, the etiological factor is also frequently constituted by a cortical dysplasia involving the motor area.

Finally, only a correct recognition of this electroclinical picture can help the physician to collect a greater number of cases in order to better understand the etiological features and the neurophysiologic mechanisms that sustain it.

REFERENCES

1. Brett EM. Minor epileptic status. *J Neurol Sci* 1966;3: 52–75.
2. Aicardi J, Chevrie JJ. Myoclonic epilepsies of childhood. *Neuropaediatrie* 1971;3:177–190.
3. Cavazzuti GB, Nalin A, Ferrari F, Mordini B. Encefalopatie miocloniche nel primo anno di vita. *Riv Ital EEG Neurofisiol Clin* 1979;2:253–261.
4. Pazzaglia P, Giovannardi Rossi P, Cirignotta F, et al. Nosografia delle epilessie miocloniche. *Riv Ital EEG Neurofisiol Clin* 1979;2:245–252.
5. Giovannardi Rossi P, Pazzaglia P, Cirignotta F, et al. Le epilessie miocloniche dell'infanzia. *Riv. Ital. EEG Neurofisiol Clin* 1979;2:321–328.
6. Lombroso C, Erba G. Myoclonic seizures: Considerations in taxonomy. In: Akimoto H, Kazamatsuri H, Seino M, Ward A, eds. *Advances in epileptology: The XIIIth epilepsy international symposium.* New York: Raven Press, 1982:129–134.
7. Bennett HS, Selman JE, Rapin I, et al. Nonconvulsive epileptiform activity appearing as ataxia. *Am J Dis Child* 1982;136,30–32.
8. Fejerman N. Myoclonus and epilepsies in children. *Rev Neurol* 1991;147(12):782–797.
9. Guerrini R, Parmeggiani L, Volzone A, et al. Cortical myoclonus in early childhood epilepsy. In: Majkowski J, Owczarek K, Zwolinski P, eds. *3rd European congress of epileptology.* Bologna: Monduzzi Editore, 1998:99–105.
10. Arzimanoglou A, Guerrini R, Aicardi J. Epilepsies with

predominantly myoclonic seizures. In: Arzimanoglou A, Guerrini R, Aicardi J, eds. *Aicardi's epilepsy in children.* Philadelphia: Lippincot Williams & Wilkins 2004:58–80.

11. Dalla Bernardina B, Trevisan C, Bondavalli S, et al. Une forme particulière d'épilepsies myoclonique chez des enfants porteurs d'encéphalopathie fixée. *Boll Lega It Epil* 1980;29–30:183–187.

12. Dalla Bernardina B, Fontana E, Sgrò V, et al. Myoclonic epilepsy ("myoclonic status") in nonprogressive encephalopathies. In: Roger J, Dravet C, Bureau M, Dreifuss FE, Perret A, Wolf P. eds. *Epileptic syndromes in infancy, childhood and adolescence.* 2nd ed. London: John Libbey 1992;89–96.

13. Dalla Bernardina B, Fontana E, Zullini E, et al. Angelman syndrome: electroclinical features of ten personal cases. *Gaslini* 1995;27,75–78.

14. Dalla Bernardina B, Fontana E, Darra F. Myoclonic status in nonprogressive encephalopathies. In: Gilman S, Goldstein GW, Waxman SG, eds. *Neurobase.* San Diego: Arbor Publishing. 2001.

15. Dalla Bernardina B, Fontana E, Darra F. Myoclonic status in nonprogressive encephalopathies. In: Roger J, Bureau M, Dravet C, Genton P, Tassinari CA, Wolf P, eds. *Epileptic syndromes in infancy, childhood and adolescence.* 3rd ed. London: John Libbey, 2002:137–144.

16. Chiron C, Plouin P, Dulac O, et al. Epilepsies myocloniques des encephalopathies non progressives avec etats de mal myoclonique. *Neurophysiol. Clin.* 1988;18:513–524.

17. Dulac O, Plouin P, Shewmon A. Contributors to the Royaumont Workshop. Myoclonus and epilepsy in childhood. 1996 Royaumont meeting. *Epilepsy Res.* 1998;30: 91–106.

18. Guerrini R, Bonanni P, Rothwell J, et al. Myoclonus and epilepsy. In: Guerrini R, Aicardi J, Andermann F, Hallett M, eds. *Epilepsy and movement disorders.* Cambridge: University Press 2002:165–210.

19. Matsumoto A, Kumagai T, Miura K. Epilepsy in Angelman syndrome associated with chromosome 15q deletion. *Epilepsia* 1992;33:1083.

20. Sugimoto T, Yasuhara A, Ohta T, et al. Angelman syndrome in three siblings: characteristic epileptic seizures and EEG abnormalities. *Epilepsia* 1992;33: 1078.

21. Casara GL, Vecchi M, Boniver C, et al. Electroclinical diagnosis of Angelman syndrome: A study of 7 cases. *Brain Dev* 1995;17:64–68.

22. Viani F, Romeo A, Viri M, et al. Seizure and EEG patterns in Angelman's syndrome. *J Child Neurol* 1995; 10(6):461–471.

23. Guerrini R, De Lorey TM, Bonanni P. Cortical myoclonus in Angelman syndrome. *Ann Neurol* 1996;40: 39–48.

24. Guerrini R, Carrozzo R, Rinaldi R, et al. Angelman syndrome: etiology, clinical features, diagnosis, and management of symptoms. *Pediatr Drugs* 2003;5(10):647–661.

25. Laan LA, Renier WO, Arts WF, et al. Evolution of epilepsy and EEG findings in Angelman syndrome. *Epilepsia* 1997;38(2):195–199.

26. Rubin DI, Patterson MC, Westmoreland BF, et al. Angelman's syndrome: Clinical and electroencephalographic findings. *EEG Clin Neurophysiol* 1997;102:299–302.

27. Sgrò V, Riva E, Canevini MP, et al. 4p-syndrome: A chromosomal disorder associated with a particular EEG pattern. *Epilepsia* 1995;36(12):1206–1214.

28. Dalla Bernardina B, Zullini E, Fontana E, et al. Sindrome di Angelman: Studio EEG-poligrafico di 8 casi. *Boll Lega It Epil* 1992b;79/80:257–259.

29. Mizuguchi M, Tsukamoto K, Suzuki Y, et al. Myoclonic epilepsy and a maternally derived deletion of 15pter>q13. *Clin Genet* 1994;45:44–47.

30. Engel J. A proposed diagnostic scheme for people with epileptic seizures and with epilepsy: report of the ILAE Task Force on Classification and Terminology. *Epilepsia* 2001;42(6):796–803.

31. Dalla Bernardina B, Zullini E, Fontana E, et al. Electroclinical longitudinal study of ten cases of Angelman's syndrome. *Epilepsia* 1993;34[Suppl. 2]:71.

32. Erba G, Lombroso CT. Angelman's (Happy Puppet) syndrome: Clinical, CT scan and serial electroencephalographic study. *Clin Electroenceph* 1973;20:128–140.

33. Aicardi J. Epilessie miocloniche benigne. In: Dalla Bernardina B, Tassinari CA, Beghini G. Eds. *Le epilessie infantili benigne.* Vicenza: Documenti Sigma-Tau, 1981;11–22.

34. Gastaut H. Individualisation des épilepsies dites "bénignes" ou "fonctionnelles" aux différentes ages de la vie. Appréciation des variations correspondantes de la prédisposition épileptique à ces ages. *Rev EEG Neurophysiol* 1981;11:346–366.

35. Doose H. Myoclonic astatic epilepsy of early childhood. In: Roger J, Bureau M, Dravet C, Dreifuss FE, Perret A, Wolf P, eds. *Epileptic syndromes in infancy, childhood and adolescence* London: John Libbey 1992:103–114.

36. Boyd SG, Harden A, Patton MA. The EEG in early diagnosis of the Angelman (Happy Puppet) syndrome. *Eur J Pediatr* 1988;147:508.

37. Ganji S, Duncan MC. Angelman's (Happy Puppet) syndrome: Clinical, CT scan and serial electroencephalographic study. *Clin Electroenceph* 1989;20:128–140.

38. Van Lierde A, Atza MG, Giardino D, et al. Angelman's syndrome in the first year of life. *Develop Med Child Neurol* 1990;32:1011–1021.

39. Binelli S, Canafoglia L, Panzica F, et al. Electroencephalographic features in a series of patients with neuronal ceroid lipofuscinoses. *Neurol Sci* 2000;21 [3 Suppl.]:S83–S87.

40. Veneselli E, Biancheri R, Perrone MV, et al. Neuronal ceroid lipofuscinoses: clinical and EEG findings in a large study of Italian cases. *Neurol Sci* 2000;21[Suppl 3]: S75–S81.

41. Veneselli E, Biancheri R, Buoni S, et al. Clinical and EEG findings in 18 cases of late infantile neuronal ceroid lipofuscinosis. *Brain Dev* 2001;23(5):306–311.

42. Dalla Bernardina B, Colamaria V, Capovilla V, et al. Epilessia parziale continua del lattante. *Boll Lega It Epil* 1987;58/59:101–102.

43. Gaggero R, Baglietto MP, Curia R, et al. Early-onset progressive encephalopathy with migrant, continuous myclonus. *Childs Nerv Syst* 1996;12(5):254–261.

44. Coppola G, Plouin P, Chiron C, et al. Migrating partial seizures in infancy: A malignant disorder with developmental arrest. *Epilepsia* 1995;36(10):1017–1024.

45. Gérard F, Kaminska A, Plouin P, et al. Focal seizures versus focal epilepsy in infancy : a challenging distinction. *Epil Disord* 1999;1(2):135–139.

46. Veneselli E, Perrone MV, Di Rocco M, et al. Malignant migrating partial seizures in infancy. *Epilepsy Res* 2001;46(1),22–27.
47. Dalla Bernardina B. L'EEG nelle convulsioni e nelle epilessie dei primi anni di vita. In: Canger R. ed. *Le epilessie oggi*. Milano: Masson, 1990:31–62.
48. Dalla Bernardina B, Colamaria V, Capovilla G, et al. Nosological classification of epilepsies in the first 3 years of life. In: Nisticò G, Di Perri R, *Meinardi H, eds. Epilepsy: an update on research and therapy. Progress in clinical and biological research.* New York: Liss, 1983:165–183.
49. Dalla Bernardina B, Trevisan E, Colamaria V, et al. Myoclonic epilepsy ('Myoclonic Status') in non-progressive encephalopathies. In: Roger J, Dravet C, Bureau M, Dreifuss FE, Wolf P, eds. *Epileptic syndromes in infancy, childhood and adolescence.* London: John Libbey, 1985:68–72.

6

Severe Myoclonic Epilepsy in Infancy: Dravet Syndrome

Charlotte Dravet,* Michelle Bureau,* Hirokazu Oguni,[†]
Yukio Fukuyama,[‡] and Ozlem Cokar[§]

*Centre Saint-Paul-Hôpital Henri Gastaut, Marseille, France; [†]Tokyo Women's Medical University,
Department of Pediatrics, Tokyo, Japan; [‡]Child Neurology Institute, Tokyo, Japan; [§]Haseki Research
and Education Hospital, Department of Neurology, Fatih-Istanbul, Turkey

INTRODUCTION

Severe myoclonic epilepsy in infancy (SME) was described by Dravet in 1978 (1). In 1992, there were at least 192 published cases (2). At present, it is more difficult to give a precise figure because the number of publications has greatly increased. In 2002 (3), we counted at least 253 new cases, which represent, totally, about 445 cases. It is interesting to note that most cases are reported from Japan and southern Europe, although SME has been increasingly recognized worldwide, as shown by the description of cases in the United States (4), in China (5), and in Russia (6).

According to the 1989 revised classification of the International League Against Epilepsy (7), this syndrome is characterized by febrile and afebrile generalized and unilateral clonic or tonic clonic seizures that occur in the first year of life in an otherwise normal infant and are later associated with myoclonus, atypical absences, and partial seizures. All seizure types are resistant to antiepileptic drugs. Developmental delay becomes apparent within the second year of life and is followed by definite cognitive impairment and personality disorders. It has been categorized among "epilepsies and syndromes undetermined as to whether they are focal or generalized," since the syndrome shows both generalized and localized seizure types and EEG paroxysms.

We must underline that many children have been reported by different authors with a similar picture, but without appearance of myoclonias, designated as "borderline SME" (SMEB). Most of them present with association of different seizure types (2,8–11) whereas others have only generalized tonic clonic seizures (12,13). They can have different EEG features but share the same course and the same outcome as the patients with myoclonias. Thus, they could be included in the same syndrome. This hypothesis seemed to be supported by the genetic studies performed by Doose et al. (13). For this reason, it has been proposed to change its name, first to "epilepsy with polymorphic seizures," and then to the "Dravet syndrome." In this chapter, we describe the typical syndrome according to the literature data completed by our present series (105 patients of which 60 selected on the basis of seizures recorded in video-polygraphic EEG have been exhaustively studied) and by the Tokyo Women's Medical University, Department of Child Neurology (39 patients). The Tokyo study (14) consists of a total of 84 patients, where only 39 patients have the typical form and 45 the borderline form. We shall then discuss the other forms.

GENERAL

Epidemiology

SME is a rare disorder with an incidence probably less than 1 per 40,000 (15). Almost the same figure (1/20,000 or 30,000) was reported by Yakoub et al. (10). In these studies, males are more often affected than females, in a ratio of 2:1.

Two authors calculated the percentage of SME in patients with seizure onset in the first year of life: Caraballo et al. (16) found 3% of SME in a series of 471 patients between 1992 and 1997 and Yakoub et al. (10) found 5% among 329 patients between 1980 and 1985. Two others gave a percentage related to the patients with their first seizure before the age of three: 7% (17) and 6.1% (2). In 1999, we find 8.2%. These figures show that this syndrome deserves to be recognized in infants with early convulsions.

Genetics

A large proportion of cases have a family history of epilepsy or febrile seizures (FS). The most usual percentage is about 25%, but it can be higher, up to 53% (18), 57% (15), 64.3% (19), and 71% (20).

Few authors separate FS from epilepsy in the family histories. Dravet et al. (2) mentioned 14% of FS and 18% of epilepsy. Nieto-Barrera et al. (17), in their series of 28 children, indicated 21% of FS and 32% of epilepsy within families. Among them, there were 2 families with both epilepsy and FS.

In the Tokyo study, there were 26% of FS and 13% of epilepsy. In the present Marseille series (60 cases), family antecedents are found in 22 cases (36%): FS in 10 families (16, 6%), epilepsy in 12 families (20%) of which 3 also presented with FS. Parental consanguinity is noted in three cases. The type of epilepsy found in the family is rarely indicated. In some cases, it seems to be an idiopathic generalized epilepsy. In the study by Benloumis et al. (21), patients with SME and those with FS had significantly increased incidence of FS in their relatives compared to those with absence epilepsy and to the control group. The incidence of epilepsy in relatives was higher in patients with SME and in those with absence epilepsy than in the control group, reaching a statistical significance. Epilepsy in relatives of patients with SME had the characteristics of idiopathic generalized epilepsy.

Four pairs of affected monozygotic twins (20,22,23) and one pair of dizygotic twins were reported (24). One other pair has been observed by Santucci M. (*personal communication*). In the twins published by Musumeci et al. (23), SME was associated with a Rud syndrome, which is an autosomal, recessive disease. Moreover, in two other families, the two siblings (one girl and one boy) were affected (2). In a family studied by Ogino et al. (25), one girl had a typical SME and her sister SMEB.

Recently, several publications reported SME cases in the syndrome of generalized epilepsy with febrile seizures plus (GEFS[+]) identified by Scheffer and Berkovic (26). Singh et al. (27), among eight probands with SME, found six cases with a family history of seizures. Eighteen members were affected: febrile seizures in eight, febrile seizures + in four, febrile seizures + and partial epilepsy in one, unclassified in two, SME in one, myoclonic astatic epilepsy in one, and Lennox–Gastaut syndrome in one. They conclude that in a significant number of SME cases, a genetic etiology is likely, with most family members having benign epilepsy phenotypes consistent with the GEFS[+] spectrum. Veggiotti et al. (28) reported two Italian families of GEFS[+] with two siblings affected by SME in each one.

In 2001, Claes et al. (29) found new mutations in the sodium-channel gene *SCN1A* in all the seven probands with SME that they studied. These mutations were more severe than those observed in the GEFS[+] families and occurred *de novo*. Several other studies have confirmed the finding of *SCN1A* gene mutations in most of the patients affected by SME, but not in all. The proportion varies from 85.7% (30) to 82.7% (31), 71.4% (32), 44.3% (33), 35% (34), and 33% (35). The differences between inclusion criteria are not sufficient to give a satisfactory explanation of these discrepancies. Only two patients carrying a *GABRG2* gene mutation were also reported (33,36). In a large group of 53 subjects negative for *SCN1A* mutations, the research for

GABRG2 mutation was also negative (37). More often mutations are *de novo,* but they have been detected in one of the parents of 3 patients among 28 tested parents (34), in 2 among 15 tested parents (30), and in the mother of 2 affected siblings (38). Frameshift and nonsense mutations are the most frequent, but missense and others have been reported. They have been shown in the typical as well as in the borderline forms. Correlations between phenotypes and genotypes have been studied without leading to significant differences. At the moment, these results do not allow us to have a clear understanding of the genetic background of the disease, which seems to be heterogeneous. The presence of one gene mutation in a patient supports the diagnosis, but is not yet necessary, as underlined by Scheffer (39).

Personal History

As a rule, SME occurs in normal infants. Significant antecedents were noted in 22% in our series in 1992: intrauterine growth retardation, prematurity, neonatal anoxia, and abnormal pregnancy. This data is in accordance with the literature. Only one author mentioned a percentage of 66%, in 15 patients (40). In one patient, SME was associated with a Rud syndrome (23), in one of our present series with an epidermal naevus syndrome (Solomon syndrome), and in another with a type I neurofibromatosis.

Brain Imaging

Usually, neuroimaging studies do not demonstrate brain lesions, in particular, of the malformative type. However, CT scan and MRI can show signs of slight or moderate, diffuse, cerebral atrophy, cerebellar atrophy, sometimes increased white matter signal (T2 weight) (2,18,40,41). Three times an arachnoid cyst was reported [temporal in the study by Ohki et al. (20), retrocerebellar in our present series]. In some cases, the cerebral atrophy appeared during the course of the epilepsy, while CT scan or MRI were normal at the onset.

Few authors performed interictal SPECT. Nieto-Barrera et al. (18) studied ten patients. SPECT was normal in two cases. It showed areas of hypoperfusion in eight cases, localized in one

hemisphere in five, and in both hemispheres in three. Areas of hypoperfusion were concordant with the prevalence of EEG paroxysms in two patients and discordant in two others. Lambarri San Martin et al. (42) studied four patients and found areas of hypoperfusion, temporal in three, and parietal in one.

Ferrie et al. (43) studied eight patients (of which two were considered atypical) by PET scans and MRI. They found normal MRI in all, normal PET in four, but cortical hypometabolism in four. All the latter had lateralized seizures. In one, there was a correlation between focal ictal symptoms and unilateral temporal PET abnormalities. In the three others, the correlation was unclear: asymmetric bitemporal, asymmetric bilateral posterior, marked diffuse hypometabolism.

SEMIOLOGY AT ONSET

Seizures began before 1 year in all cases. Initially, prolonged, generalized, or unilateral clonic seizures are typically triggered by fever. Several Japanese authors (8,19,22) underlined the triggering effect of a Japanese style hot water immersion, which produces a body temperature elevation (see below). These febrile seizures tend to be long (more than 20 min) [25% in our present series, 28% in the Tokyo study, 5 cases among 14 for Ohki et al. (20), and 7 among 17 for Yakoub et al. (10)] to recur in clusters in the same day (20) and to evolve into status epilepticus.

However, variations in the onset have been observed by all the authors. Afebrile seizures can occur: 28% (20), 35% in our present series, and 48% in the present Tokyo's study. In our series these afebrile seizures usually occur in the context of a vaccination or of an infectious episode, or after a bath. Later on, they are associated with febrile seizures in 80% of patients. Nieto-Barrera et al. (18) emphasized the coincidence between the first seizure and the DTP (diphtheria–tetanus–polio) vaccination.

In some patients, isolated episodes of focal myoclonic jerking are noted by parents either some weeks or some days before the appearance of the first convulsive seizure, without any fever and remain isolated, or they occur in the hours preceding the first convulsive seizure, repetitively, together with hyperthermia. Complex partial seizures can also be observed: 2 cases in our present series, at least 5 cases in the Tokyo study, and in 1 case among the 14 reported by Ohki et al. (20). Initial focal seizures are also noted by other authors (44,45).

At this stage of the disease, the EEGs are usually normal. They may display a diffuse or unilateral slowing of the background if they are recorded after a prolonged seizure. In some patients they can show generalized spike-waves elicited by the intermittent photic stimulation (IPS). This early photosensitivity was observed by Dalla Bernardina et al. (41) in 10 cases, by Renier and Renkawek (46) in 1 case, and by Dravet et al. (2) in 13 cases. Rhythmic theta activities at 4–5 Hz can be present in the centroparietal areas and the vertex (40,41).

This first seizure is often considered as a FS, few investigations are performed, and no treatment is given. However, shortly thereafter (2 weeks to 2 months, mean 6 weeks for Dulac and Arthuis, 47), other febrile seizures occur and seizures without fever also appear [2 months to 14 months, mean 5 months for Ohki et al. (20)]. Between 1 and 4 years of age, other seizure types appear, simultaneously with a slowing in the psychomotor development and the picture becomes characteristic of a steady state.

STEADY STATE

Patients with SME have multiple seizure types during the course of the disease: convulsive seizures consisting of either GTCS, generalized clonic seizures (GCS), or alternating unilateral clonic seizures, myoclonic seizures, atypical absences and obtundation status, focal seizures (simple focal motor seizures and complex partial seizures, with or without secondarily generalization), and exceptionally tonic seizures.

Convulsive Seizures

We group under this term all the seizures apparently generalized or unilateral, usually classified as tonic-clonic or clonic. They are present all over the evolution. However, the recent study

conducted in Marseille and not yet published, concerning 60 patients whose seizures have been carefully analyzed by video-polygraphic-EEG recordings, demonstrates, in many cases, peculiar clinical and EEG features of these seizures, which do not permit classification among the generalized clonic or tonic-clonic seizures. We have tried to group them by distinguishing several forms: the generalized clonic or tonic clonic seizures (9 patients), the unilateral seizures (9 patients), the "falsely generalized" seizures (10 patients), and the "unstable" seizures (11 patients). In fact, this distinction is somewhat artificial and all these seizures, except the generalized ones, seem to belong to the same category. Furthermore, they can be associated in the same patient. Most of them have been recorded during sleep, either nocturnal or diurnal, at various stages of the evolution, usually after the age of 3.

Generalized Convulsions (Nine Cases)

The generalized convulsions (nine cases) evoke the generalized tonic-clonic seizures of the idiopathic generalized epilepsies. However, they are usually shorter, with a very brief tonic phase, with few autonomic symptoms, with a transient postictal flattening quickly replaced by diffuse delta waves. These characteristics are those observed in the GTCS in childhood (Fig. 6–1). In some seizures, the initial tonic phase is almost immediately mixed with the clonic jerks, giving a vibratory aspect which is well documented in the three cases published by Ogihara et al. (48).

We did not record seizures described as clonic-tonic-clonic convulsions by Fujiwara et al. (12) and reported in 2 patients by Ohki et al. (20) and in 1 by Ohmori et al. (49), in which a short clonic phase precedes the tonic phase.

True Hemiclonic Seizures

True hemiclonic seizures, corresponding to the description by Gastaut et al. (50), become rare when patients are older. They have been recorded only in 2 young children (16 month and 3 years) in our series of 60 patients. However, there are other unilateral seizures (in seven patients) with different characteristics: shorter duration,

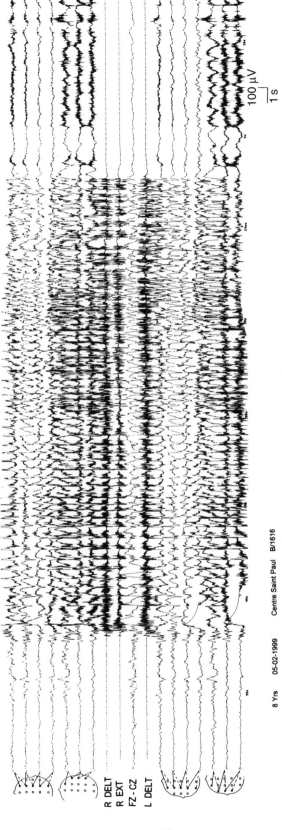

FIG. 6–1. A generalized tonic-clonic seizure in an 8-year-old boy. At onset: brief burst of fast activity (less than 1 s) progressively intermixed with slow waves. The end of the seizure is marked by a brief flattening followed by theta activity. The EMG recorded over the two deltoids shows a tonic contraction followed by sustained myoclonias that become irregular and very fast, with a vibratory aspect.

R DELT

R EXT

FZ - CZ

L DELT

100 μV

1 s

8 Yrs   05-02-1999   Centre Saint Paul   B/1616

75

association of contralateral tonus changes, ictal EEG anomalies more limited to one hemisphere. They can begin with diffuse spike-waves (49). In all the cases, there are EEG postictal asymmetric signs and, often, a postictal transitory hemiparesia. These seizures can be either on one side or on the other side in the same patient (Fig. 6–2 A, B, and C and Fig. 6–3 A and B). This pattern of alternating unilateral seizures is one of the main characteristics of the syndrome.

"Falsely Generalized Seizures" (Ten Cases)

They are characterized by a complicated semiology with some degree of discrepancy between the clinical and the EEG phenomena. The description reported by the parents seems to correspond to a generalized tonic clonic seizure. However, accurate observation through the video-polygraphic EEG recording demonstrates that they are not primarily generalized and they are different from a patient to another one. It is mainly the recording of several muscles on the two sides of the body which permits the analysis of the clinical events. They consist of a bilateral, asymmetric, tonic contraction, leading to variable postures during the seizure (extension of one limb, flexion of another). The onset can be an opening of the eyes preceding the motor phenomena, with or without deviation of the bulbs, the head, and the mouth. The patients seem to be unconscious and do not react to stimuli. Clonic jerks can start in the face or immediately involve the limbs. They are asynchronous, with an asymmetric frequency (vibratory in one side, slower in the other). They often stop on one side and persist on the other, even on a single segment. They last from 30 s to 2 min. The autonomic symptoms are slight: cyanosis, apnea, hypersalivation, and respiratory obstruction occur only at the end of the longest attacks.

The EEG discharge is always bilateral, but according to three modalities. The first consists of bilateral abnormalities from the onset, as a slow spike or a spike-wave, sometimes followed by a brief attenuation, followed by rapid activities and slow waves, still bilateral but more or less asymmetric and asynchronous. In the second, the abnormalities are initially bilateral but become and remain asymmetric during the seizure. In the third, they are bilateral but asymmetric at their very onset. The postictal EEG shows either a diffuse flattening or a diffuse slowing (Fig. 6–4). Sometimes the end of the seizure is not easy to recognize and the child continues to sleep. This asymmetry in the EEGs during the generalized tonic clonic seizures has also been described by others (11,19).

"Unstable Seizures" (11 Cases)

These seizures are characterized by the topographic changes of the ictal EEG discharge in the same seizure. The clinical manifestations are near that of the "falsely generalized" seizures with asymmetric and asynchronous tonic and clonic movements, sometimes predominant on one side or shifting from one side to the other. However, the EEG discharge involves irregularly different parts of the brain. It can start in one localized area of one hemisphere, then spread either to the entire hemisphere, either asymmetrically to the two hemispheres, or to another area of the same hemisphere or of the opposite hemisphere, then return to the first involved hemisphere. The end of the discharge can occur either in this hemisphere or contralaterally (Fig. 6–5 A and B). The ways of propagation are very variable from one seizure to another in the same patient and even in the same recording. The relationship between the clinical events and the accompanying EEG is not always clear.

All these convulsive seizures can be prolonged more than 30 min or repeated, realizing status epilepticus, requiring intravenous drug administration and, often, respiratory assistance. All the authors mention the frequency of convulsive status, mainly in the first years. Sato et al. (51) reported one patient who developed rhabdomyolisis during two febrile convulsive status epilepticus, with a complete recovery in spite of renal insufficiency and liver dysfunction.

Myoclonic Seizures

These seizures appear between the ages of 1 and 5 years, and sometimes before [with an average of 1 year 8 months in our series, 18+ or −14

(*text continues on page 85*)

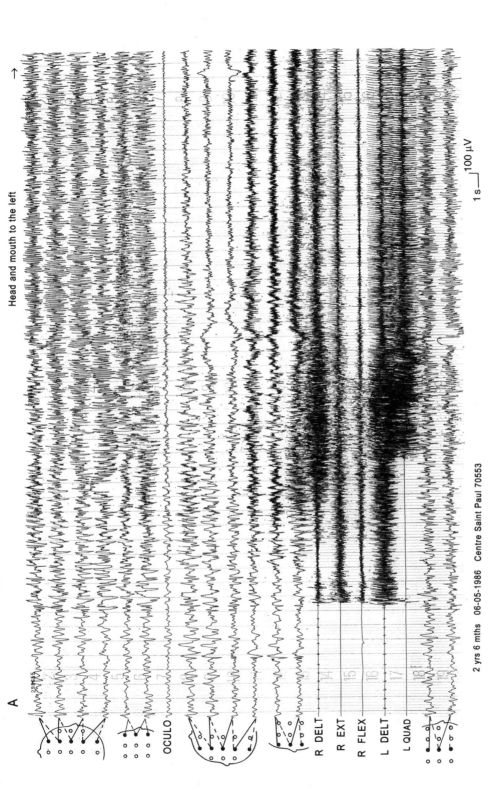

Head and mouth to the left →

A

OCULO

R DELT
R EXT
R FLEX
L DELT
L QUAD

2 yrs 6 mths   06-05-1986   Centre Saint Paul 70553

1 s $\llcorner$ 100 µV

FIG. 6–2. A left hemiclonic seizure recorded in a 2-year 6-month-old boy during a status. **A:** On the right hemisphere, spikes and slow waves during 5 s, followed by rapid, high-voltage activity; on the left hemisphere, high-voltage spikes and slow waves on the frontocentral area, followed by a low-voltage, rapid activity. Clinically, head and mouth deviation to the left. Polygraphy: diffuse tonic contraction, then vibratory phase on the left muscles.

(Continued)

77

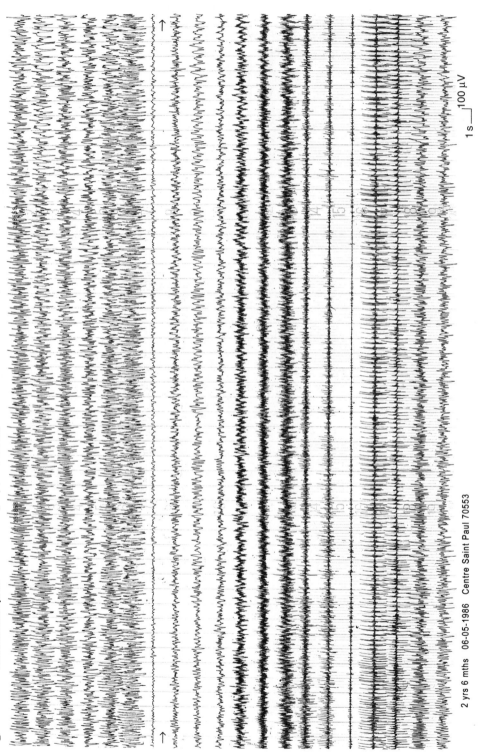

B Left hemiclonic jerks   Eyes jerks to the left

1 s ⌐ 100 µV

2 yrs 6 mths   06-05-1986   Centre Saint Paul 70553

FIG. 6–2. (*Continued*) **B:** Sustained, continuous discharge of slow waves and spikes on the right hemisphere, spreading to the left anterior region, accompanied by rhythmical clonic jerks on the left side of the body.

78

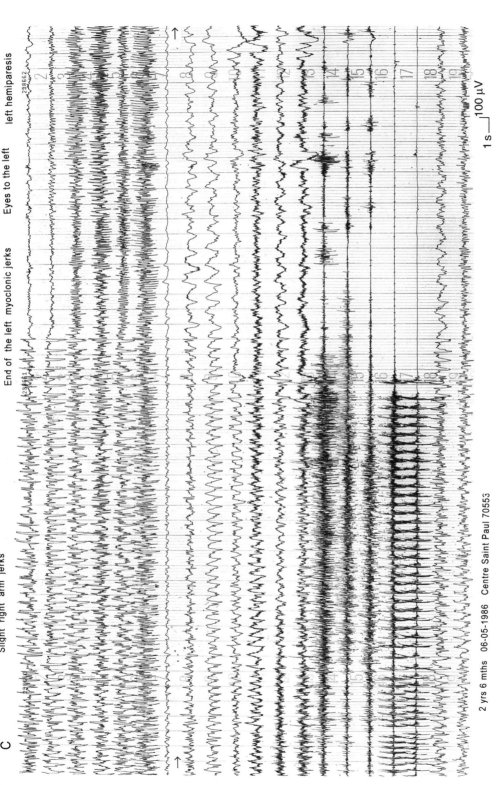

FIG. 6–2. (*Continued*) **C:** At the end, the discharge spreads to the entire left hemisphere. The postictal phase is marked by a depression on the right, associated with a left hemiparesis, immediately followed by a rapid activity, which is the onset of another seizure, whereas delta waves invade the anterior regions of the left hemisphere.

2 yrs 6 mths   06-05-1986   Centre Saint Paul 70553

79

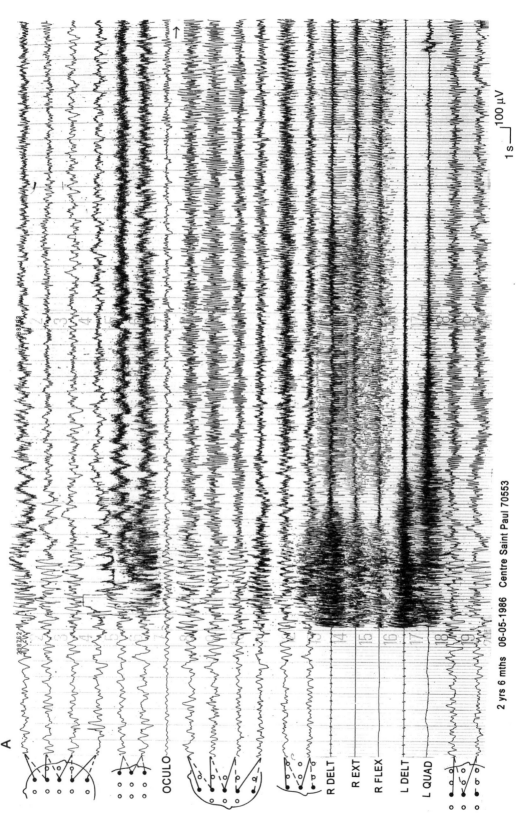

FIG. 6–3. A right hemiclonic seizure recorded in the same boy on the same day. **A** and **B:** The aspect is similar to the seizure in Fig. 6–4, but the discharge involves the left hemisphere "as a mirror".

OCULO

R DELT
R EXT
R FLEX
L DELT
L QUAD

1 s ⌐ 100 µV

2 yrs 6 mths   06-05-1986   Centre Saint Paul 70553

A

B

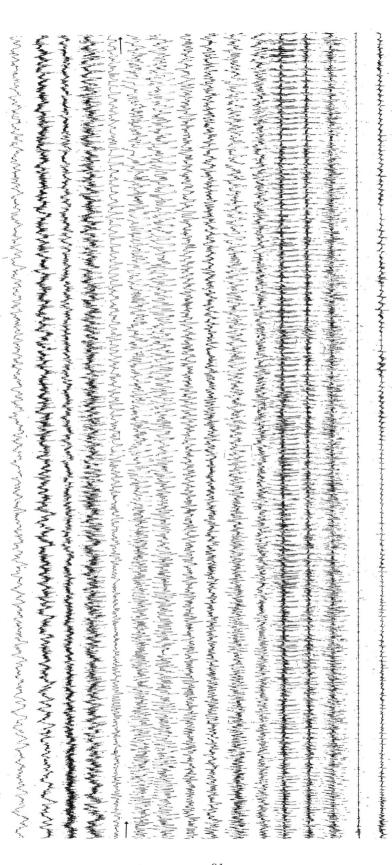

1 s — 100 µV

2 yrs 6 mths 06-05-1986 Centre Saint Paul 70553

FIG. 6–3. (*Continued*)

81

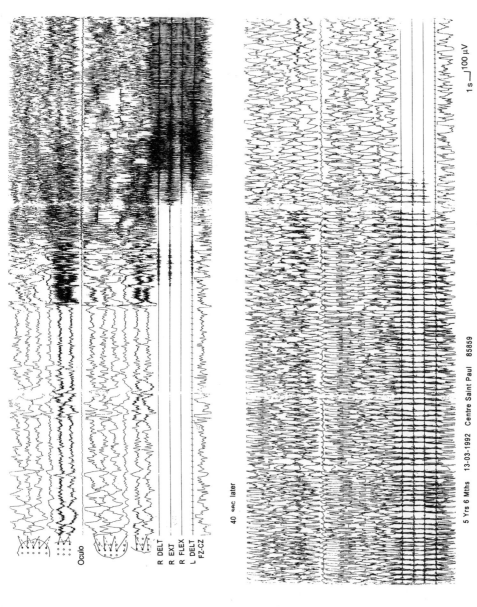

40 sec later

Oculo

R DELT
R EXT
R FLEX
L DELT
FZ-CZ

5 Yrs 6 Mths   13-03-1992   Centre Saint Paul   85859

1 s ⎤ 100 µV

FIG. 6–4. A "falsely generalized" convulsive seizure during sleep in a 5-year 6-month-old boy. **Top:** At onset a generalized slow spike followed by a low voltage theta activity, then bilateral fast activity of high voltage. Note the muscular artefacts on the EEG, which correspond to the facial onset of the clinical seizure. The EMG recording of the upper limbs shows a slight initial tonic contraction which begins 2 s after the EEG onset, remits, and then is followed by an irregular tonic contraction associated with a vibratory aspect. **Bottom:** 40 s later, diffuse spike-waves associated with bilateral myoclonias, which become progressively asynchronous and stop on the left deltoid before they stop on the right muscles. At the end of the seizure,

82

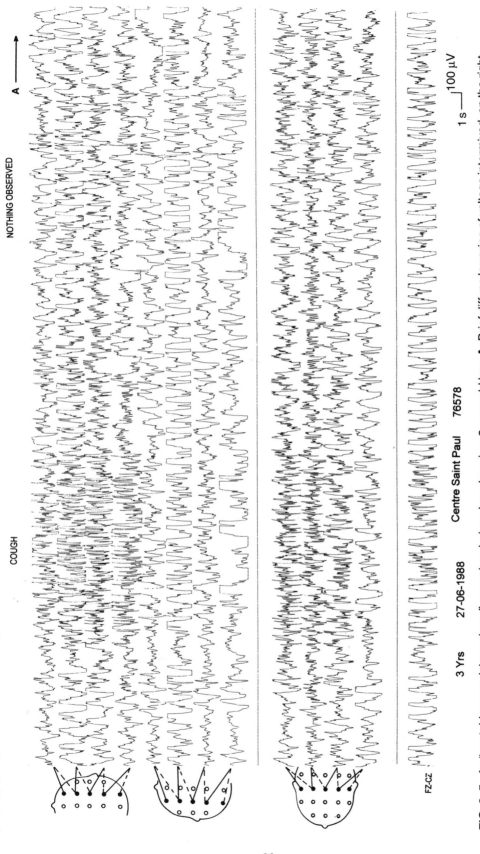

FIG. 6–5. An "unstable convulsive seizure" occurring during slow sleep in a 3-year-old boy. **A:** Brief diffuse lowering of voltage intermixed, on the right hemisphere, with rapid activity, then spikes and slow waves evident only on the right hemisphere, during 10 s, followed by a more or less rhythmic activity around 10 Hz on the right centroparietal area.

(Continued)

3 Yrs 27-06-1988 Centre Saint Paul 76578

83

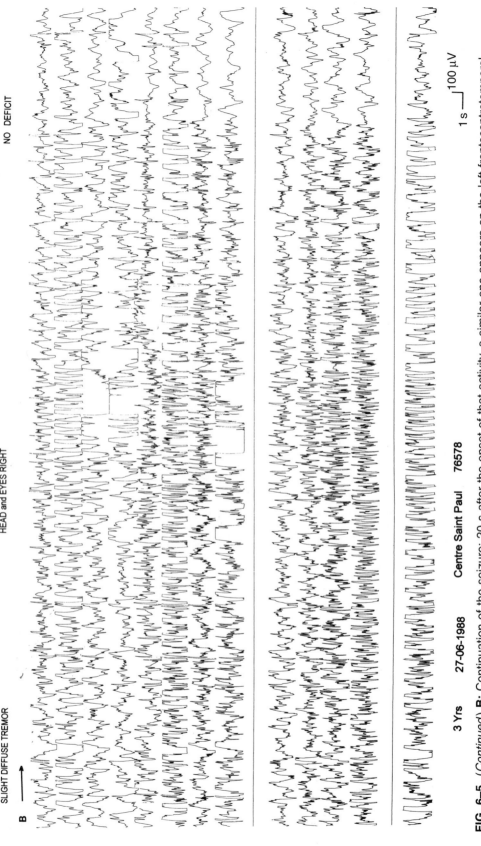

SLIGHT DIFFUSE TREMOR

B

HEAD and EYES RIGHT

NO DEFICIT

3 Yrs   27-06-1988   Centre Saint Paul   76578

1 s ⎣ 100 µV

FIG. 6–5. (*Continued*) **B:** Continuation of the seizure: 20 s after the onset of that activity, a similar one appears on the left frontocentrotemporal region, progressively associated with slow waves on the left hemisphere, becoming slower at the end of the seizure. Clinically, only a slight diffuse tremor and a head and eyes deviation to the right are observed.

84

months in the Tokyo series, and 2 years 2 months in that of Ohki et al. (20)]. They are difficult to analyze due to their variability.

They could be massive, involving whole muscles, particularly the axial ones, leading to hurling of objects held by the child and to falling. Their intensity, however, is variable, and they are sometimes barely discernible. When they are attenuated they can involve only the axial muscles (head and trunk), giving a small movement forward or backward. In some children, there is an atonic component associated with a head drop.

They can be either isolated or grouped in brief bursts, consisting of two or three jerks. They are very frequent, occurring several times a day, sometimes incessantly. In some children, they are observed only on awakening or in the minutes preceding a seizure. They persist during drowsiness and disappear during slow sleep. They can be initiated by photic stimulation, variation in light intensity, closure of the eyes, and fixation on patterns. They do not seem to be accompanied by changes in consciousness, except when they occur at very close intervals.

The polygraphic EEG recording demonstrates they are accompanied by generalized or multiple spike-waves, at 3 Hz or more, with higher voltage on the frontocentral areas and on the vertex. Their duration is usually brief (1–3 s), but it can be longer (10 s). Myoclonic electromyography (EMG) can show the postmyoclonic inhibition corresponding to the head drop (Fig. 6–6).

In the Tokyo study, the two first types, according to the intensity, the grouping, and the topography, are similar to ours. There is a third type, which consists of successive myoclonic twitching involving mostly head, eyelids, and, at times, arms, resulting in a rhythmic retropulsion of head corresponding to a burst of generalized spike-waves at 3 Hz. When they are sufficiently sustained, they appear to be atypical absence seizures with a myoclonic component (see below).

These myoclonic seizures are frequently associated with interictal segmental myoclonias: 36% of our patients in 1992 and 38% in the Tokyo study. These figures certainly are underestimated because of the variability of these myoclonias: In some patients they are rare, sometimes appearing

only before a convulsive seizure, and their diagnosis requires a special attention for this symptom. The best method of diagnosing it is the polygraphic recording. In a hyperkinetic child, one could make them evident by asking him to perform a precise activity such as drinking, piling up cubes, or holding a spoon. In the Marseille series, of 60 patients selected on the basis of seizures recorded in video-polygraphic EEG, 51 had this interictal myoclonus (85%). They involve either the limbs of the both sides, with a distal predominance, or the facial muscles, independently. They exist at rest, but are increased by voluntary movement. There is no concomitant change in the EEG. They are more frequent in the period with seizures, particularly in elder children with frequent nocturnal convulsive seizures, after awakening from attacks.

Some authors mention the occurrence of myoclonic status, sometimes lasting more than 1 day, in their patients (10,42,52). We have included them in the obtundation status.

Atypical Absence Seizures

Atypical absence seizures can appear at different ages, either between 1 and 3 years, together with the myoclonic attacks, or later on, from 5 to 12 years. In the series of Ohki et al. (20), they occurred between 4 months and 6 years. They are divided into atypical absence seizures with impaired consciousness only and those with a more or less obvious myoclonic component. Both seizure types correspond to generalized, irregular spike-waves at 2–3.5 Hz (Fig. 6–7). However, Dulac and Arthuis (47) recorded absences with rhythmical, generalized spike-waves at 3 Hz in two patients. Ohmori et al. (49) recorded atypical absences with either predominance or onset of the spike-waves in the occipital regions. Their duration varies from 3 to 10 s. In the former type, eyelid myoclonias and head fall can be observed. In the latter type, when the myoclonic component is pronounced, it is difficult to differentiate these atypical absences from the myoclonic attacks. In fact, both are probably the expression of the same epileptic process with different intensity and duration. The frequency of the atypical absences is variable in

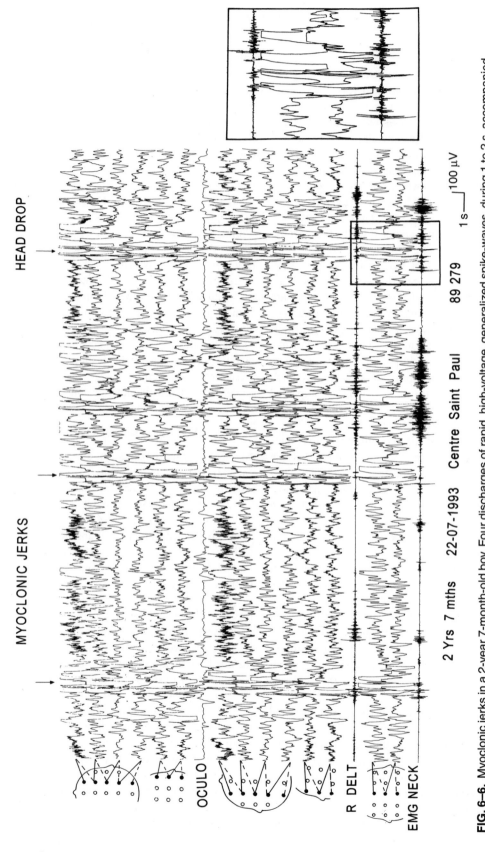

MYOCLONIC JERKS

HEAD DROP

OCULO

R DELT

EMG NECK

2 Yrs 7 mths   22-07-1993   Centre Saint Paul   89 279

1 s   100 µV

FIG. 6–6. Myoclonic jerks in a 2-year 7-month-old boy. Four discharges of rapid, high-voltage, generalized spike-waves, during 1 to 2 s, accompanied by generalized jerks recorded on the deltoid and the neck muscles. The last discharge is accompanied by a brief head drop. On the right, the enlargement of the image shows the postmyoclonic inhibition responsible for this clinical event.

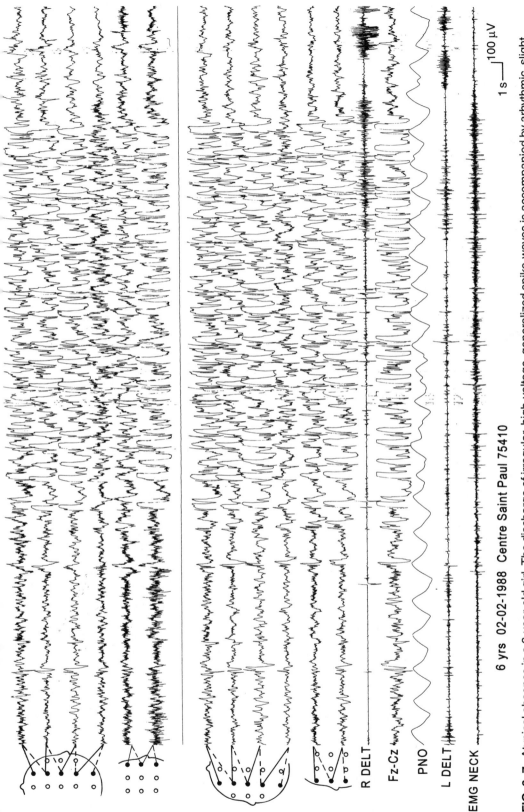

R DELT

Fz-Cz

PNO

L DELT

EMG NECK

1 s ⎣100 µV

6 yrs 02-02-1988 Centre Saint Paul 75410

FIG. 6–7. Atypical absence in a 6-year-old girl. The discharge of irregular, high-voltage, generalized spike-waves is accompanied by arrhythmic, slight myoclonic jerks, visible on the polygraphy, and by a change in the respiration.

87

the different series reported in the literature (from 40% to 93%), probably due to the overlap with the myoclonic attacks. In the Tokyo series, it is 74%; in our present series it is 95% (57/60).

Obtundation Status

Obtundation status represents a relatively characteristic symptom, reported in all the series [40% of 29 cases for Dalla Bernardina et al. (52)]. They were observed in 17 patients (43.5%) in the Tokyo study, recorded in 4, and in 18 patients in our present series (30%), recorded in 11.

In these 11 patients, we recorded 18 obtundation status, between 2 years 4 months and 19 years 9 months (mean 8 years 8 months). They consist of an impairment of consciousness, variable in intensity, the presence of fragmentary and segmental, erratic myoclonias, of low amplitude, involving the limbs and the face, sometimes associated with a slight increase of muscular tone. According to their degree of consciousness, patients can or cannot react to stimuli, have simple activities (toy manipulation and eating), interrupted by short episodes of complete loss of contact and staring. Some strong sensory stimulations can interrupt the status but never definitively. In four patients the myoclonias could realize brief synchronous fits. Convulsive seizures could either initiate, occur during, or terminate these status. These periods were prolonged for several hours, even several days, maintained by environmental light stimuli, eye closure, and the pattern fixation (dotted lines of the walls, TV screen in two recorded status). The EEG is characterized by one diffuse slow-wave dysrrhyhmia, intermixed with rare focal and diffuse spikes, sharp waves, and spike-waves, of higher voltage in the anterior regions and the vertex, without correspondence between the spikes and the myoclonias, except during the myoclonic fits (Fig. 6–8). This aspect was also described by Ohmori et al. (49). We never observed rhythmical spike-waves as in the generalized idiopathic absence status. The intravenous or rectal injection of diazepam attenuated, but did not stop these status, which we classified among the atypical absence status.

In the Tokyo study, two types of ictal EEG were documented. One type corresponded to our description (four patients), whereas the second one (one patient) corresponded to a complex partial status: Continuous posterior localized irregular slow waves or spike-waves during which the girl was unconscious with deviations of both eyes to the right. There is another case of complex partial status reported in the literature by Wakai et al. (53), with irregular spike-wave complexes over the left hemisphere, predominantly in the occipitotemporal area. In the four patients reported by Yasuda et al. (54), this status occurred every time after a GTCS, lasted from 7 to 16 min, and was accompanied by diffuse high-voltage slow waves, occasionally notched by small spikes in the frontal regions.

Focal Seizures

Simple partial seizures (SPS) of motor type or complex partial seizures (CPS), with prominent autonomic symptoms, occur in 43% to 78.6% of the patients in the largest series. They can appear early, from 4 months to 4 years (20). In our present series, they were described in 32 patients (53%), 4 with only SPS, 17 with only CPS, and 11 with both. The SPS were either versive seizures, or clonic jerks limited to a limb or a hemiface, or a combination of the two. The CPS were characterized by loss of consciousness, autonomic phenomena (pallor, cyanosis, rubefaction, respiratory changes, drooling, and sweating), oral automatisms, hypotonia, rarely stiffness, and sometimes with eyelid or distal myoclonias. When the symptomatology is mild, it is difficult to distinguish them from atypical absences without concomitant EEG. The two partial seizure types could be secondarily generalized.

Surprisingly, we have recorded them only in three patients, at 20 months, 12 years, and 27 years. The first one occurred on awakening and was a CPS, with loss of contact, right deviation of the eyes, arrhythmic myoclonias, pallor, lip cyanosis, during 1 min 45 s, accompanied by a left temporooccipital EEG discharge and a left postictal slowing. The other two occurred during a sleep recording. The first one, apparently subclinical, interested the right centrotemporal area. The second one was not well observed and interested the right temporooccipital and the vertex

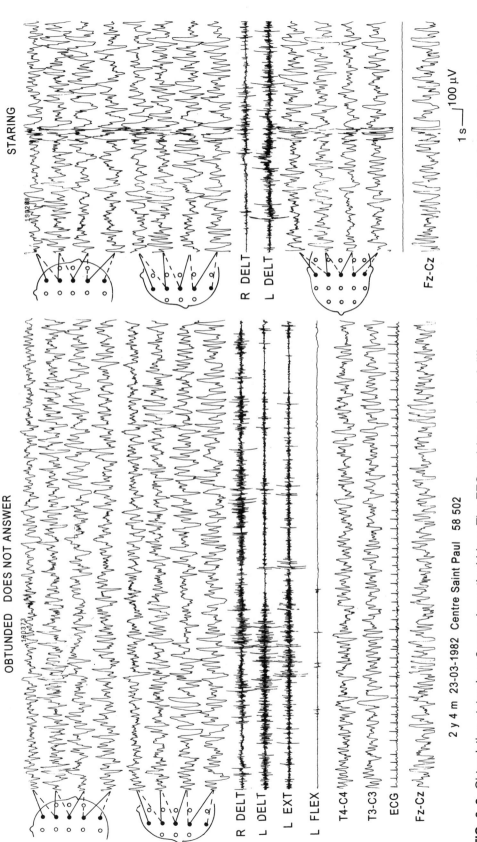

STARING

OBTUNDED DOES NOT ANSWER

R DELT
L DELT

R DELT
L DELT
L EXT
L FLEX
T4-C4
T3-C3
ECG
Fz-Cz

Fz-Cz

1 s ⌐ 100 µV

2 y 4 m 23-03-1982 Centre Saint Paul 58 502

FIG. 6–8. Obtundation status in a 2-year 4-month-old boy. The EEG activity consists of diffuse slow and sharp waves. On the right, a burst of spike-waves is accompanied by a brief staring. The polygraphy shows a slight increase in the muscular tone and arhythmical, diffuse, myoclonic jerks. When stimulated, the boy was able to walk and eat during this status, which lasted for hours, but he did not move spontaneously and did not speak.

89

areas. In the Tokyo series, SPS or CPS appeared in 23 patients (59%).

In the literature, the focal seizures reported are usually of the complex partial type with the same characteristics we have described. Ohki et al. (20) recorded 25 seizures in 8 patients with variable EEG features, beginning either in the frontal area (six records), in the temporal (nine records), or in the occipital (six records). In four patients it was not possible to determine the exact onset and in three the onset was variable from one seizure to another one. Six seizures were secondarily generalized. M. Revol (*personal communication*) also recorded four CPS in two children. Ohmori et al. (49) recorded CPS in 13 patients (occipital, temporal, and frontal). In two they were immediately preceded by a myoclonic seizure. Few authors reported SPS (5,10,40,44,55).

Tonic Seizures

Tonic seizures are exceptional in this syndrome and only four authors mentioned them in the literature (2,22,47,49). They are not mentioned in the Tokyo study's experience, but we have recorded them in nine patients, between 6 and 25 years. They are rarely described by the parents and are mainly detected by sleep EEG recordings. With variable electroclinical features, they resemble the axial tonic seizures of the Lennox–Gastaut syndrome (LGS), sometimes with a myoclonic component, but they are usually sporadic (six cases) and only in three cases were they frequently repeated during the same recording, as in the LGS. The EEG shows either a flattening or a rapid rhythm of low amplitude, followed by slow waves. Only in two cases, interictal sleep EEG is analogous to that in the LGS (rapid rhythms and multiple SWs).

Interictal Electroencephalogram

The EEGs change progressively—occurrence of generalized, focal, and multifocal abnormalities. However, we must underline the lack of specific features. Awake, the background activity is variable according to the delay after the last convulsive seizure. When the convulsive seizures are numerous, it is slow. Out of these periods it can be either normal or slow and disorganized. In some patients, a rhythmical theta activity is recorded in the central and vertex areas. The paroxysmal abnormalities are also variable and can be absent. When present, they consist of spikes, single and multiple spike-waves, generalized, symmetric or asymmetric, isolated or in brief bursts, and of localized sharp waves, slow waves, and spikes. The latter are usually seated in the central areas, bilaterally, synchronous or asynchronous, and in the vertex, and may spread to the entire hemisphere. They can be also recorded in the posterior regions, occipital or temporal. The relationship between the seat of the interictal paroxysms and the ictal discharges are not always clear. The EEGs contain more generalized paroxysms when myoclonic jerks are present. When hyperventilation is possible its effect is variable. The eye closure may facilitate the occurrence of localized and generalized abnormalities. Sleep is usually well structured with physiological patterns and cyclic organization, except when several seizures occur during the night. The paroxysmal, generalized as well as localized, activities are enhanced or appear.

Photosensitivity

It is difficult to analyze photosensitivity because it is not constant during the course of the disease. A discrepancy between the laboratory EEG and the daylife clinical photosensitivity can be observed. In our previous series (2), the EEG photosensitivity has been observed at least once in the course of the disease in 31 patients (42%), beginning between 3 months and 5 years 6 months. In eight patients it has persisted. In ten it has been observed only in one recording. In seven we were able to estimate its duration: from 3 months to 11 years 6 months. We also could observe the triggering effect of eye closure (10/63), of patterns (7/63), and of television (1/63) for myoclonus and spike-waves. Ohki et al. (20) also observed the variability of the photosensitivity in four patients.

In the Tokyo series, among 39 patients, 6 appeared to have numerous daily attacks (more than 100–200 per day), which were related to the intensity of constant light illumination, i.e., seizures became very frequent under bright conditions, while they were remarkably reduced in the dark. A strong response to IPS was also observed. Careful examination in one case showed no specific increase to intermittent low illumination light: brightness is more important. Their predominant seizure types were myoclonic seizures and atypical absence seizures with pronounced eyelid myoclonias, the latter accompanied by occasional rhythmic retropulsion of the head. They became continuous immediately after exposure to bright illumination or sunshine. Since they frequently and easily culminated into GTCS, the patients had to wear sunglasses when going outside or to remain inside. This was illustrated in a 21-month-old girl intensively studied by Morimoto et al. (56) and included in the present study. In another case, also included in this study, Miyamoto et al. (57) showed constant light sensitivity gradually decreasing around the age of 5 years and photo/pattern sensitivity at age 7. Recently, Takahashi et al. (58) showed that patients with SME have a paroxysmal response different from that observed in patients with idiopathic generalized epilepsy, dependent on the quantity of light rather than wavelength. This finding may suggest that this constant light sensitivity is at the strongest end of the photosensitive spectrum in SME patients. This group with constant light sensitivity appears to represent the most resistant type in SME, mainly when the children discover the possibility of self-stimulation. That was confirmed by Dalla Bernardina et al. (52).

Psychomotor Delay

Psychomotor delay becomes progressively evident from the second year on. Children start walking at a normal age but an unsteady gait develops for an unusually long time. About 60% of children have an ataxic gait and 20% show mild pyramidal signs.

Language also starts at the normal age, but it progresses very slowly, and often the patients do not reach the stage of constructing elementary sentences. After the age of 2 years, children become hyperkinetic, with recalcitrant behavior and major learning problems.

A neuropsychologic study was conducted in Marseille (59,60) on 20 patients aged from 11 months to 16 years 7 months, with a follow-up of over 3 years in 10 cases. Cognitive and behavioral troubles were always present, but to varying degrees. Neuropsychologic deficits concerned all skills–motor, linguistic, and visual abilities being strikingly affected. In the visuoconstructional domain, the global mode of organizing visual information was more affected than the piecemeal approach to construction. Behavior was marked by hyperactivity, psychotic type of relationships and, sometimes, autistic traits. The appearance of neuropsychologic disorders seemed to be related to the severity of the epilepsy during the first 2 years of life. Children with an initial high frequency of convulsive seizures showed earlier slowing of psychomotor development, compared to those with few such seizures in the first 2 years. Some relation was also found between the total number of convulsive seizures, their duration, and the degree of mental deterioration. Three children had a better development and their language was more preserved, even if their progresses exhibited a dysharmonic mode. This correlated with milder epilepsy, or a marked decrease in the number of convulsive seizures from the age of 6 years. One of them had an increasing number of seizures after the age of 6 years without slowing in her cognitive acquisitions nor changes in her behavior. That could be explained by a greater seizure impact on development in the first years of life. Thus, stagnation or deterioration was the rule during the first 6 years, but a positive evolution, albeit dysharmonic, was observed thereafter and some patients could attend specialized schools or sheltered work institutions.

In the literature, we did not find any other neuropsychologic study. The four main studies which considered the psychological features reported the same type of disturbances (5,10,40,52).

LONG-TERM OUTCOME

The outcome of severe myoclonic epilepsy in infancy is always unfavorable. The affected patients always have persistent seizures and all patients are cognitively impaired, often severely. In our present series, the duration of follow-up ranges from 2 years 6 months to 33 years 8 months (median: 11 years 6 months). Other series in the literature report a long follow-up: 8 to 23 years (mean 14 years 5 months) (40), 3 to 9 years (mean 6 years 2 months) (10), and 5 to 17 years (mean 11 years 1 month) (20).

Mortality Rate

The mortality rate is very high. In our previous series (2), with a mean age at follow-up of 11 years 4 months (from 3 years to 27 years) 10 patients died (15.9%). The causes were: one unknown (13 years), one seizure plus drowning (10 years), two drowning (4 and 14 years), one malignant measles under corticosteroids (3 years 4 months), one status epilepticus with hepatic failure during a respiratory infection (3 years 3 months), one accident (15 years), and two sudden unexplained deaths (7 and 13 years). In the Tokyo's series, seven patients (18%) died at a mean age of 65 ± 23 months, death being due to status epilepticus in five (between 5 and 8 years), severe infection in one (3 years 7 months), and unknown cause in one (2 years 5 months). Two other children with SME were left with residual severe neuro-logic deficits after prolonged convulsive status triggered by acute febrile illness. The age distribution of the catastrophic events suggest that careful treatment of the convulsive seizures is necessary at least until 8 years of age or more when such prolonged convulsive seizures are generally not expected.

Early death is also reported by other authors: one boy by sudden unexpected death at 17 months (46), 1/7, by drowning in a swimming pool (45), 1/20 (47), 1/10, by sudden unexpected death (9). Miyake et al. (61) found surprising data with 4/8 children dead, 3 during a status epilepticus, among a total of 128 epileptic patients who died in 14 years in a department of child neurology. We must also mention the case described by Castro-Gago et al. (62) who died at 2 years 8 months by multiorgan failure after a status, attributed to a mitochondrial cytopathy.

Treatment

Whatever their type, the seizures are extremely resistant to any kind of treatment during the first years, requiring numerous hospitalizations. Later on, partial seizures, myoclonic seizures, and atypical absences tend to disappear, but the convulsive seizures persist. They preferentially occur during the night and assume the various aspects we have described before. They can be repeated during the same night, specially in the case of fever, and then again preceded by myoclonias. In the Tokyo's series, seizure time shifted from awakefulness to sleep in only 31% of patients. The period of very active epilepsy varies from one child to another, sometimes up to the age of 12 to 13 years. As Ohki et al. (20), we did not find homogeneous data concerning the age of disappearance of the myoclonias, atypical absences, and partial seizures.

In the Tokyo series, at the final follow-up, 1 patient has been seizure-free for more than 1 year, 20 (51%) had weekly seizures, 14 (36%) monthly seizures, 3 (8%) once in 1 to 6 months, and 3 (7%) once in 6 months to 1 year. In the literature, Hurst (4) has obtained a relatively good control of seizures, but his data are not very clear, particularly concerning the follow-up duration in the patients in remission. In the study by Lambarri San Martin et al. (42), two patients are controlled by a VPA monotherapy, three by bitherapy, and six by polytherapy, but the duration of the control is not made clear. In one patient, with extremely rare seizures, the treatment was withdrawn.

Electroencephalograms

The EEGs do not have a homogeneous evolution. The background activity fluctuates, depending on the number and duration of the seizures. In our previous series (2) it remained normal in 20 patients throughout the follow-up. In 43, it has deteriorated between 5 and 10 years and showed a diffuse theta activity, sometimes associated with delta waves, still reactive. Generalized spikes and spike-waves disappeared in 19% of the cases. The localized abnormalities were variable, often recorded only during sleep. The cyclic organization of the sleep remained normal in 21 patients among 30 with several sleep recordings. The other authors also mentioned this improvement in the EEGs.

Neurologic Abnormalities

Neurologic abnormalities usually do not aggravate after the age of 4 years. The imbalance gait and the pyramidal signs tend to disappear but the patients remain clumsy, with poorly coordinated movements and often a slight action myoclonus or a tremor (63). However, in the Tokyo study's series, at the final follow-up, six patients had difficulty in walking due to severe ataxia and spastic paresis of the legs and required a wheelchair to move. In some patients of ours, we have observed a severe cyphoscoliosis and orthopedic deformation of the feet.

As mentioned before, the psychologic evolution is also more favorable in late childhood and adolescence. However, in our previous series, all the 37 patients aged more than 10 years (up to 27 years) were dependent and institutionalized. One-half were in the lowest range of deficiency (IQ lower than 50). It is important to note a change, however, in behavior, which is no more hyperkinetic and rather characterized by slowness and perseveration. Aggressiveness and acute psychiatric episodes are rare. In the other series of the literature with a long follow-up, the findings are the same (40,42,52). The mental outcome seems to be better in some cases of the series studied by Hurst (4) and by Fèrnandez-Jaén et al. (44).

Fever Sensitivity

The triggering effect of hyperthermia and infections does not disappear and febrile status epilepticus can still occur during adolescence.

In the Japanese population, all patients experienced frequent seizures triggered by fever and Japanese style hot-water immersion. Patients tended to have prolonged convulsive seizures or even status during such episodes. In the SME and SMEB patients, the epileptic seizures were always provoked by fever greater than 38°C without exception, even under intensive anticonvulsant treatments. Thus, we paid special attention to this "fever sensitivity" and also to the precipitation by hot-water immersion. It was unclear whether the infection or parainfectious change itself or merely the resulting elevation in body temperature itself was responsible for these special characteristics, because SME patients had experienced frequent episodes of hyperthermia during infancy and appeared to be susceptible to infections.

We conducted an immunological study including immunoglobulin levels, T cell function, and complement levels in 16 patients with SME and SMEB to identify the cause of susceptibility to infections. Although we found abnormal IgG, IgM, and IgA levels, it appeared to be a consequence of frequent infections rather than the cause of infection (64).

Since whole-body immersion into a bath-tub filled with hot water ranging from 39°C to 42°C for 5 to 10 min is typical as a custom in hot baths, this may be responsible for raising the body temperature. Sumi et al. (65) reported 42 children with hot-bath seizures, 27 of whom had also experienced febrile convulsions, indicating that body temperature elevation was largely responsible for the hot-bath attacks.

Thus, Awaya et al. (66,67) conducted a video–EEG study during the hot-water immersion in seven children with SME to confirm whether it could provoke attacks, and if so, to establish the guideline of safe bathing in daily life. Rectal temperature was continuously monitored during this examination. As a result, the clinical overt seizures were all provoked after 7 to 25 min of hot-water immersion, when the rectal temperature unexpectedly rose over 38°C. In addition, five of seven patients clearly showed an increase in frequency and duration of epileptic discharges, which culminated in overt clinical seizures along with elevation of the rectal temperature, i.e., atypical absence seizures, CPS, GTCS in each one, and massive myoclonic jerks developing into GTCS in two cases. They also showed no significant difference in the rate of the rectal temperature elevation during hot-water immersion between SME patients and three normal controls. This study clearly demonstrated that the epileptic seizures in SME are very sensitive to body temperature elevation itself, regardless of etiology, either due to infection, hot baths, or even physical exercise (56).

In the French patients, we did not observe the seizures provoked by the hot bath due to different practices. However, when interrogated, some parents have noted this particular sensitivity. More regularly the parents remarked on physical exercise as a seizure-triggering factor.

This fever sensitivity was most prominent during infancy and continued throughout the clinical course, although the incidences of body temperature elevation themselves dramatically decrease with age, presumably due to immunological defense, safe bathing, or maturation. Thus we strongly advocate that this unique fever sensitivity should be given more priority in the criteria of SME.

TREATMENT

Therapy is disappointing. Phenobarbital (PB), valproate (VPA), and benzodiazepines may decrease the frequency and the duration of convulsive seizures. In our experience, clonazepam (CZP) and nitrazepam are more effective than clobazam (CLB). Phenytoin (PHT) can be useful but may result in bad side effects if treatment is prolonged. Moreover, the concomitant administration of PHT and VPA increases the risk of hepatic failure. VPA, benzodiazepines, ethosuximide, and high doses of piracetam can improve the myoclonic syndrome. Clorazepate, methsuximide, acetazolamide, allopurinol, and sulthiame were used with partial results (5). Zonisamide (ZNS) was proved in SMEB with a good result when started early—around 2 years of age (68). The authors suggest that ZNS could prevent the appearance of myoclonias.

Bromide, an old-fashioned antiepileptic drug, has recently received attention for the treatment of refractory grand-mal epilepsy, including SME (69–71). In Tokyo, we conducted an add-on trial of potassium bromide (BrK) in 22 patients with SME and SMEB (72). Although it was not effective for myoclonic or absence seizures, BrK significantly improved the convulsive seizures, including GTCS, GCS, and CPS. In short-term outcomes, it brought excellent improvement in 36% and moderate improvement in 41% of the patients. It is especially worthwhile to try in children with SME or SMEB who suffer from recurrent life-threatening convulsive status. In Tokyo, the current treatment policy is to use BrK first in conjunction with VPA or CZP, ZNS, clorazepate, and to introduce a ketogenic diet if drug therapy is not sufficient.

A ketogenic diet is an option which can help some patients (16). Corticosteroids can be useful in cases of repeated status, but do not have an actual long-term efficacy. In some patients immunotherapy may give satisfactory results (personal experience).

Among the new antiepileptic drugs, the lamotrigine (LTG) experience was disappointing. An aggravating effect of this drug has been demonstrated by Guerrini et al. (73): LTG induced a worsening in 17 of 21 patients (80%), no change in three, and improvement in one. Of five patients improving in at least one seizure type, four had concomitant worsening of more invalidating seizures. This worsening appeared clearly within 3 months in most patients, but was insidious in some. Wallace (74) also mentioned this aggravating effect of LTG.

The same problem of aggravation was described in SME for carbamazepine (CBZ), but it is not so obvious. Already in 1986, Horn et al. (75) reported two patients with SME among 49 children aggravated by CBZ. However the authors have seven additional patients of whom five had adverse effects and two excellent results while treated by CBZ. In 1992, we were aware of this risk (2). Wakai et al. (53) reported a worsening effect of CBZ in at least four patients among six with SME and no effect in the two others. The authors suggest the use of CBZ in the early phase of the epilepsy as a test to confirm the diagnostic of SME when it is suspected. Wang et al. (5) used CBZ in nine patients, of whom two presented an increase in myoclonic seizures, whereas two were well controlled with VPA + CBZ, the others being in polytherapy with variable results.

Vigabatrin gave good results on convulsive and partial seizures in our older patients, when the myoclonic syndrome was attenuated. Topiramate seems to be the most promising molecule. In children and adults, as add-on therapy, it has permitted a 50% to 100% reduction of convulsive and partial seizures for more than 6 months (up to 36 months) in 23 patients out of 27 and 5 were seizure-free (76). These results are similar to those reported by other studies (77,78). We think this drug should be prescribed early in the course of the disease, but further studies with a longer follow-up, particularly in infants, are necessary to confirm its efficacy.

Another treatment type gives cause for less pessimism. The use of Stiripentol, in association with VPA and CLB was shown to be efficacious on convulsive seizures (79). In a randomized, placebo-controlled, add-on trial, 15/21 children (71%) were responders, defined as having more than 50% reduction in the seizure frequency, of whom nine were seizure free, compared to 1/20 children under placebo (5%)—none being seizure-free. These results were confirmed by a further study (80), which showed that Stiripentol is mainly efficacious on the status in the first stage of the disease.

Given the difficulties to obtain a good seizure control and the deleterious consequences of the prolonged convulsive seizures, it is necessary to avoid the status episodes by vigorous treatment and prophylaxis of infections and hyperthermia. In the case of prolonged or repeated convulsive seizures, the use of rectal diazepam can prevent the evolution into status. In case of status, the best drugs are the intravenous benzodiazepines, particularly the CZP and the midazolam (81), associated with chloral hydrate or barbiturates.

In the series reported by Dooley et al. (45), because of the inevitability of prolonged seizures and the lack of response to PB, PHT, and paraldehyde, two patients were provided with subcutaneously accessed central lines that were inserted into the external jugular vein, allowing immediate administration of intravenous medications without complications. Both children were successfully treated with pentobarbital (5 mg/kg) on multiple occasions in the emergency room.

The photo and pattern sensitivities associated with self-stimulation are extremely drug resistant and can produce long-lasting obtundation and myoclonic status in the patients. For this reason, other methods of treatment have been sought. Wearing sunglasses is usually not enough. As the monocular light stimulation fails to provoke epileptic discharges, we have obtained the complete inhibition of the self-stimulation by using glasses masking one eye, but the child did not tolerate it for long. Takahashi et al. (82) conducted a very accurate study on one child. They found that optical filters tinted with a particular color (the procion turquoise blue = MGL), were able to inhibit flickering hand movements and forced eye closure. However, the continuous use of the MGL goggles was so uncomfortable that the patient often removed them. Therefore, they designed specially adapted blue-tinted contact lenses that had transmission spectra similar to that of MGL. After a period of adjustments, the flicker hand movements disappeared completely and the contact lenses were removed after 6 months without return of the self-stimulation by hand flicker movements. Only the forced eye closure has not yet been inhibited.

DIFFERENTIAL DIAGNOSTICS

There are several diagnostic problems in SME. We envisage successively benign myoclonic epilepsy (BME), LGS, epilepsy with MAE, PME, FS, and early cryptogenic focal epilepsies.

The first two sydromes are relatively easy to eliminate. The diagnostic of BME is based on two major features: onset by brief, generalized myoclonic attacks, which represent the only ictal manifestation in a child with generalized spike-waves on the EEG without any focal abnormality (83). In the rare patients also having FS, they are always simple and infrequent. The early LGS is completely different. The occurrence of repeated FS in the first year virtually eliminates this diagnosis. The LGS starts later, in a more variable way, and often in children with preexisting brain lesions. It essentially consists of atypical absences, drop attacks, and axial tonic seizures (which are exceptional in SME), even if they are associated with myoclonias in the myoclonic variant. The EEGs always show diffuse slow spike-waves, grouped in bursts, and specific features during sleep where there is no photosensitivity (84).

More difficulties may arise in differentiating SME from MAE, a classification category in which Doose also includes those children first seen with early-onset generalized convulsive seizures triggered by fever (85). Although this onset is very similar to that of SME, the course is different, with myoclonic-astatic seizures becoming a major feature, and the absence of any focal clinical or EEG manifestation. Patients with SME do not have recurrent drop attacks. Guerrini et al. (86) clearly established the features of what can be considered now as the "true myoclonic-astatic epilepsy."

Another condition that must be ruled out is a PME. Indeed, the course of SME in its second stage could evoke a progressive disease resulting from one metabolic dysfunction, mainly the neuronal ceroid lipofuscinoses. The absence of visual disturbances, of abnormalities of the fundus, of the peculiar response to IPS in the EEGs, and the negative results of biological investigations eliminate this diagnosis. Moreover, in later childhood and adolescence there is no further deterioration and the patients present rather a picture of a static encephalopathy. A mitochondrial encephalomyopathy with ragged red fibers (MERRF) should be eliminated in the most severe cases and when there are drug-induced metabolic disturbances, by dosage of serum and cerebrospinal fluid lactate and by muscular biopsy (62).

An early cryptogenic focal epilepsy may have the same onset with FS rapidly associated to focal seizures. These patients will not present atypical absences and myoclonic jerks in the later course, but the diagnosis may remain uncertain for some months. Sarisjulis et al. (55) underlined that one focal epilepsy is improbable when the partial motor seizures affect different parts of the body and when the hemiclonic seizures are alternating.

At the very onset, the differential diagnosis is that of FS. In an infant less than 1 year, with a family history, the occurrence of long and repeated FS leads one to suspect the diagnosis of SME, mainly when the triggering fever is not high. However, it cannot be confirmed until other seizure types and myoclonic jerks occur, or one

records spike-waves resulting from photostimulation.

ATYPICAL OR BORDERLINE FORMS

The most important problem arises when the onset and the course of SME are atypical. Many authors described patients having the same characteristics as those with SME, with the exception of absence of obvious myoclonic syndrome. We also observed these patients. However, in our Marseille experience, most of the patients who do not present with myoclonic seizures have an interictal segmental myoclonus, which disturbs their motor abilities. One of them was the sister of a boy with a typical SME. In some children, the myoclonias are rare and detectable only by accurate examination and video-polygraphic recordings. In some others, myoclonic seizures can be observed and recorded only when convulsive seizures are frequent, just before they start. For this reason, we think all these patients have the same epilepsy type and we have grouped them in our series.

On the contrary, in the Tokyo series they were separated. The data above reported concerns with the group of 39 patients with typical SME. The complete study includes 45 other patients belonging to the group named "peripheral" or "borderline" SME (SMEB). Even in this group, 27% of the subjects presented massive myoclonias, with related spike-waves in the EEG, during the period of clustering seizures or hot-water immersion, and 35% had nonepileptic segmental myoclonus. However, the main characteristics of the SMEB are as follow: no atypical absences, either few EEG epileptic abnormalities, or only occasional multifocal or diffuse spike-waves during the first stage of the disease, and rare photosensitivity (2 cases/45). All the other features are similar, including the bad prognosis and the high rate of early mortality (5/45).

Other authors emphasized these two groups. Sugama et al. (8) compared the SMEB with SME and found that the EEGs were different, demonstrating no spike-waves in the SMEB, but without difference in the prognosis—always poor. Ogino et al. (25) published three cases of whom one was the brother of a child affected by a typical SME and proposed the name "polymorphous convulsive epilepsy beginning in the infant." In 1989, they added seven cases and noted that five among the ten had segmental myoclonias. In contradiction with Sugama et al. (8), they found generalized spike-waves and focal spikes in all cases.

Most of the authors in the literature do not exclude the diagnosis of SME when myoclonic seizures are absent if the children fulfill all the other criteria and they do not find differences in the long-term outcome (10,18,40,42,55).

On the other hand, in Japan, simultaneously to our SME description, Seino and Higashi (87) reported on a group of patients with refractory epilepsy in childhood characterized by predominant generalized tonic clonic seizures and Wada et al. (88) proposed to name it "high-voltage slow-wave–grand-mal syndrome (HVSW-GM)." The criteria for this syndrome are as follow: generalized and/or unilateral clonic or tonic clonic seizures in normal infants, occurring in the first year; almost no other type of seizures occur throughout the course; EEG is normal at the initial stage, then shows rather poor epileptiform discharges, such as generalized spike-waves or polyspike-waves without focal abnormalities. There is inefficiency of treatment. Psychomotor development is normal in the first stage and then slows down. Thus, the initial stage is very near that of SME. Later, Kanazawa (11,89) studied 22 patients corresponding to these criteria, aged from 3 years 3 months to 25 years at the end of the follow-up. They distinguish three groups: 12 patients with SME, 6 patients with HVSW-GM syndrome, and 4 others, considered as "variant forms." They did not find prominent differences in the outcome between these three groups—the prognosis always being poor. They conclude that these three clinical entities may be all part of one "infantile refractory grand mal syndrome," with a common physiopathological basis. Fujiwara et al. (12) found a similar result. We do not agree with this concept. A syndrome must be well-defined and the presence of multiple seizure types is one of the main features of SME, not found in the other entities. Relationship between these different forms is obvious, now supported by the results of molecular genetic studies. The

SCN1A gene mutation has been demonstrated in patients with borderline SME (33) and in patients with only refractory grand-mal seizures (30). However, as already underlined, these findings remain heterogeneous and not easy to explain and they are not sufficient to put all the cases together in the same syndrome.

Doose et al. (13) reported a series of 101 children, which met the same criteria, except an onset in the first 5 years of life: febrile or afebrile GTCS, absence of primary organic brain lesion or progressive disease, severe course with frequent febrile and/or afebrile GTCS, and failure of conventional anticonvulsive therapy. Many patients also had the characteristics of SME: onset in the first year in 74, seizures triggered by fever in 90, long duration of GTCS in 67%, "alternating hemi-grand mal" in 75%, minor seizures (myoclonic, absences, myoclonic astatic) in 55%, erratic myoclonias in 30%, and focal seizures in 35%. These features are not correlated between themselves and the authors do not seem to consider that a part of these patients could be affected by SME. However, they mention an overlap with SME, the severe type of MAE, as well as early childhood absence epilepsy with GTCS. Genetic aspects were deeply analyzed from the clinical and EEG point of view and lead to justify terming this severe form of infantile epilepsy as idiopathic epileptic encephalopathy.

The early diagnosis of SME remains a challenge and we agree with the statement by Yakoub et al. (10): this diagnosis is probable when the first seizure occurs between 2 and 9 months, in a neurologically normal baby, when the first two seizures are clonic, generalized or alternating, when they are afebrile or triggered by a moderately high temperature, and when the development is normal during the first year.

NOSOLOGIC PLACE

SME takes place in the epilepsies "undetermined whether to generalized or partial" in the international classification of the ILAE (7). Its features make it similar both to idiopathic generalized epilepsies (absence of aetiology, high familial incidence of epilepsy and FS, massive myoclonias, generalized spike-waves, and photosensitivity) and to symptomatic epilepsies (appearance of neurological signs, slowing down in the psychomotor development and further cognitive impairment, association of clinical and EEG signs of localization, and drug resistance).

In the great majority of the patients, no etiology is found. However, in the literature there are now three published patients where a mitochondrial cytopathy was suspected. Castro-Gago et al. (90) described one patient with a very severe form of SME in whom they found a high lactic acid level in cerebrospinal fluid (CFS) and urine, without metabolic acidosis or high lactacidemia. Muscle biopsy showed a slight increase in the number of mitochondria, which had a tendency toward subsarcolemmal locations, and clefts in the myofibrillar membrane that contained granular material, staining positive for oxidative enzymes, without ragged red fibers. These aspects were not specific and the quantification of the enzymatic activities was not convincing for a partial deficit of the respiratory complexes III and IV diagnosed by the authors. The same authors later published another case (62). This child had a history compatible with SME and died at 32 months, after a convulsive status, under high doses of VPA, combined with CZP, piracetam and L-carnitine, in a picture of multiorgan failure. A muscle biopsy was obtained immediately after death. Its analysis revealed a partial deficit of complex IV of the mitochondrial respiratory chain (cytochrome c oxidase 19.5 IU per IU CS). There were no point mutations at bases 8344, 8356, or 8993. The proximal cause of the death was respiratory insufficiency and generalized hypoxemia secondary to respiratory distress syndrome.

Fèrnandez-Jaén et al. (44) reported one case with the same characteristics as SME, extremely severe, in whom they found a twofold proportional rise of serum lactates (from 0.44 to 0.93 mM) 60 min after a glucose tolerance test. They performed a muscular biopsy of which the electron microscopy showed an increased number of mitochondria, some adopting a concentric and laminar structure. Enzymatic analysis showed a severe deficiency of the mitochondrial respiratory chain complex IV. Skin study revealed no alteration.

On the other hand, 14 patients were studied with complete biochemical investigations and muscular biopsy, which failed to show any obvious mitochondrial cytopathy (2,91). Thus, in rare cases, a mitochondrial dysfunction can be associated with SME, but we do not have sufficient arguments to believe that this dysfunction is at the origin of the SME which, usually, has a different course and outcome (92). These authors, in their report of eight patients with infant-onset progressive myoclonus epilepsy, found a respiratory-chain enzyme defect in three of them who did not present with the typical picture of SME. The authors give a great value to the elevation in serum or CSF lactate.

The only neuropathologic study, which has been published (46), concerned an infant dead at 19 months of age. It has shown the presence of microdysgenesis in the cerebellum, together with an irregular cortical lamination and with threefold spinal cord canals, surrounded by ectopic tissue. These abnormalities do not argue for a common specific etiology.

Presently, the recent advances in the molecular genetic studies, in spite of their complex results, let us think that SME may be due to a channelopathy related to the GEFS$^+$ syndrome with which it shares a peculiar fever sensitivity.

On the other hand, our analysis of the seizures has demonstrated that most of the convulsive seizures were not actually generalized. They probably correspond to focal seizures generated by several foci that successively fire, as shown by the "falsely generalized" and the "unstable" seizures. Our study confirms the complexity of this epilepsy was not due only to the association of multiple seizure types in the same patient, but also to these peculiar convulsive seizures. The epileptic process seems to implicate several cortical areas, either successively or alternatively, and variable from one ictal event to another one. Thus, it could be a multifocal epilepsy with an extremely rapid, sometimes simultaneous, burning of the different foci, because of a very low convulsive threshold.

The presumed topography of the epileptogenic areas involves preferentially the mesial frontal lobe, the central area, sometimes the parietal and, even, the occipital lobes. Few interictal foci are localized in the temporal area. However, some temporal seizures have been recorded by several authors. In contrast, it is surprising not to find a hippocampal sclerosis in the MRI of these patients who had prolonged and repeated severe FS.

This epilepsy cannot be considered as a primary generalized epilepsy but a predisposing genetic factor probably favors the diffuse expression of the multiple foci. This hypothesis should be stayed by other investigations, such as high-density EEG recording of the interictal paroxysms, ictal and interictal SPECT, and PET, which are difficult to perform in this type of patient. The neurophysiologic study of the myoclonus in patients with SME by Guerrini et al. (93) brings some arguments to our discussion. These authors studied the two types of myoclonus, i.e., the segmentary interictal myoclonus and the generalized ictal myoclonic jerks, by the backaveraging method, which allows detecting cortical spikes when they are not evident in the scalp EEG. For the segmentary myoclonus, time-locked EEG potentials were not detectable and C-reflex and enlarged somatosensory evoked potentials were absent. It seemed that these small jerks either are not produced in the cortex or result from discharges involving such a small number of neurons that their electrical activity is undetectable. The generalized jerks were always preceded by clearcut spike-wave discharges. Preliminary data indicated that they originate from the spread of focal cortical myoclonic activity. However, the leading hemisphere shifted from one discharge to the next, according to the muscle used as trigger, with an interside latency consistent with transcallosal spread. Thus, there is some evidence that myoclonus in SME can originate, like the other seizures, from multiple cortical areas.

Finally, it is possible to consider that several processes are concerned, associating genetic and acquired factors, and that the epileptic predisposition activates the expression of multiple epileptogenic foci.

In the new scheme proposed by the ILAE for the classification of epilepsies, the SME will be named "Dravet syndrome" because of the lack of myoclonic seizures in many patients. It will be placed among the "epileptic encephalopathies,"

defined as the conditions in which the epileptiform abnormalities themselves are believed to contribute to the progressive disturbance in cerebral function, without taking in consideration whether they are generalized or localized.

ACKNOWLEDGMENTS

We are grateful to all the authors who have kindly sent us the information we requested: Doctors Dooley and Camfield, Fèrnandez-Jaén, Fujiwara and Seino, Kanazawa, Lambarri San Martin, Nikanorova, Nieto-Barrera, Revol, Santucci, Wakai, and Wang.

REFERENCES

1. Dravet C. Les épilepsies graves de l'enfant. *Vie Méd* 1978;8:543–548.
2. Dravet C, Bureau M, Guerrini R, et al. Severe myoclonic epilepsy in infants. In: Roger J, Dravet C, Bureau M, Dreifuss FE, Perret A, Wolf P, eds. *Epileptic syndromes in infancy, childhood and adolescence.* 2nd ed. London: John Libbey, 1992:75–88.
3. Dravet C, Bureau M, Oguni H, et al. Severe myoclonic epilepsy in infancy (Dravet syndrome). In: Roger J, Bureau M, Dravet Ch, Genton P, Tassinari CA, Wolf P, eds. *Epileptic syndromes in infancy, childhood and adolescence.* 3rd ed. London: John Libbey, 2002:81–103.
4. Hurst DL. Severe myoclonic epilepsy in infancy. *Pediatr Neurol* 1987;3:269–272.
5. Wang PJ, Fan PC, Lee WT, et al. Severe myoclonic epilepsy in infancy: Evolution of electroencephalographic and clinical features. *Acta Paed Sin* 1996;37:428–432.
6. Mukhin Kiu, Nikanorova Miu, Temin PA, et al. Severe myoclonic epilepsy in infancy. *Zh Nevrol Psikiatr Im S S Korsakova* 1997;97:61–64.
7. Commission on Classification and Terminology of the International League Against Epilepsy. Proposal for revised classification of epilepsies and epileptic syndromes. *Epilepsia* 1989;30:289–299.
8. Sugama M, Oguni H, Fukuyama Y. Clinical and electroencephalographic study of severe myoclonic epilepsy in infancy (Dravet). *Jpn J Psychiat Neurol* 1987;41:463–465.
9. Ogino T, Ohtsuka Y, Yamatogi Y, et al. The epileptic syndrome sharing common characteristics during early childhood with severe myoclonic epilepsy of infancy. *Jpn J Psychiat Neurol* 1989;43:479–481.
10. Yakoub M, Dulac O, Jambaque I, et al. Early diagnosis of severe myoclonic epilepsy in infancy. *Brain Dev* 1992;14:299–303.
11. Kanazawa O. Medically intractable generalized tonic-clonic or clonic seizures in infancy. *J Epil* 1992;5:143–148.
12. Fujiwara T, Watanabe M, Takahashi Y, et al. Long-term course of childhood epilepsy with intractable Grand Mal seizures. *Jpn J Psychiatr Neurol* 1992;46:297–302.

13. Doose H, Lunau H, Castiglione E, et al. Severe idiopathic generalized epilepsy of infancy with generalized tonic-clonic seizures. *Neuropediatrics* 1998;2:229–238.

14. Oguni H, Hayashi K, Awaya Y, et al. Severe myoclonic epilepsy in infants—a review based on the Tokyo Women's medical university series of 84 cases. *Brain Develop* 2001;23:736–748.

15. Hurst DL. Epidemiology of severe myoclonic epilepsy of infancy. *Epilepsia* 1990;31:397–400.

16. Caraballo R, Tripoli J, Escobal L, et al. Ketogenic diet: Efficacy and tolerability in childhood intractable epilepsy. *Rev Neurol* (spanish) 1998;26:61–64.

17. Dalla Bernardina B, Colamaria V, Capovilla G, et al. Nosological classification of epilepsies in the first three years of life. In: Nistico G, Di Perri R, Meinardi H, eds. *Epilepsy: An update on research and therapy.* New York: Liss, 1983:165–183.

18. Nieto-Barrera M, Lillo MM, Rodriguez-Collado C, et al. Epilepsia mioclonica severa de la infancia. Estudio epidemiologico analitico. *Rev neurol* (spanish) 2000a;30:620–624.

19. Ogino T. Severe myoclonic epilepsy in infancy—a clinical and electroencephalographic study. *J Jpn Epil Soc* 1986;4:114–126.

20. Ohki T, Watanabe K, Negoro K, et al. Severe myoclonic epilepsy in infancy: Evolution of seizures. *Seizure* 1997;6:219–224.

21. Benloumis A, Nabbout R, Feingold J, et al. Genetic predisposition to severe myoclonic epilepsy in infancy. *Epilepsia* 2001;42:204–209.

22. Fujiwara T, Nakamura H, Watanabe M, et al. Clinico-electrographic concordance between monozygotic twins with severe myoclonic epilepsy in infancy. *Epilepsia* 1990;3:281–286.

23. Musumeci SA, Elia M, Ferri R, et al. Severe myoclonic epilepsy in two monozygotic subjects affected by Rud syndrome. *Boll Lega It Epil* 1992;79/80:81–82.

24. Ohtsuka Y, Maniwa S, Ogino T, et al. Severe myoclonic epilepsy in infancy: A long-term follow-up study. *Jpn J Psychiatr Neurol* 1991;4:416–418.

25. Ogino T, Ohtsuka Y, Amano R, et al. An investigation on the borderland of severe myoclonic epilepsy in infancy. *Jpn J Psychiatr Neurol* 1988;42:554–555.

26. Scheffer IE, Berkovic SF. Generalized epilepsy with febrile seizures plus: A genetic disorder with heterogeneous clinical phenotypes. *Brain* 1997;120:479–490.

27. Singh R, Scheffer IE, Whitehouse W, et al. Severe myoclonic epilepsy of infancy is part of the spectrum of generalized epilepsy with febrile seizures plus (GEFS+). *Epilepsia,* 1999;40 [Suppl. 2]:175 (abstr.).

28. Veggiotti P, Cardinali S, Montalenti E, et al. Generalized epilepsy with febrile seizures plus and severe myoclonic epilepsy in infancy: A report of two Italian families. *Epil Disord* 2001;3:29–32.

29. Claes L, Del-Favero J, Ceulemans B, et al. *De novo* mutations in the sodium-channel gene SCN1A cause severe myoclonic epilepsy of infancy. *Am J Hum Genet* 2001;68:1327–1332.

30. Fujiwara T, Sugawara T, Mazaki-Miyazaki E, et al. Mutations of sodium channel α subunit type 1 (SCN1A) in intractable childhood epilepsies with frequent generalized tonic-clonic seizures. *Brain* 2003;126:531–546.

31. Ohmori I, Ouchida M, Ohtsuka Y, et al. Significant correlation of the SCN1A mutations and severe my-oclonic epilepsy in infancy. *Biochem Biophys Res Commun* 2002;295:17–23.

32. Sugawara T, Mazaki-Miyazaki E, Fukushima K, et al. Frequent mutations of SCN1A in severe myoclonic epilepsy in infancy. *Neurology* 2002;58:1122–1124.

33. Fukuma G, Oguni H, Shirasaka Y, et al. Genetic abnormalities in core severe myoclonic epilepsy of infancy (SMEI) and borderline SMEI (SMEIB). *Epilepsia* 2003;44[Suppl 8]:50 (abstr.).

34. Nabbout R, Gennaro E, Dalla Bernardina B, et al. Spectrum of SCN1A mutations in severe myoclonic epilepsy of infancy. *Neurology* 2003;60:1961–1967.

35. Wallace RH, Hodgson BL, Grinton BE, et al. Sodium channel α1-subunit mutations in severe myoclonic epilepsy of infancy and infantile spasms. *Neurology* 2003;61:765–769.

36. Harkin LA, Bowser DN, Dibbens LM, et al. Truncation of the GABA(A)-receptor gamma2 subunit in a family with generalized epilepsy with febrile seizures plus. *Am J Hum Genet* 2002;70:530–536.

37. Madia F, Gennaro E, Cecconi M, et al. No evidence of GABRG2 mutations in severe myoclonic epilepsy of infancy. *Epilepsy Res* 2003;53:196–200.

38. Gennaro E, Veggiotti P, Malacarne M, et al. Familial severe myoclonic epilepsy of infancy: Truncation of Nav1.1 and genetic heterogeneity. *Epileptic Disord* 2003;5:21–25.

39. Scheffer IE. Severe infantile epilepsies: Molecular genetics challenge clinical classification. *Brain* 2003;126:513–514.

40. Giovanardi Rossi PR, Santucci M, Gobbi G, et al. Long-term follow-up of severe myoclonic epilepsy in infancy. In: Fukuyama Y, Kamoshita S, Ohtsuka C, Susuki Y, eds. *Modern perspectives of child neurology.* Tokyo: Asahi Daily News, 1991:205–213.

41. Dalla Bernardina B, Capovilla G, Gattoni MB. Epilepsie myoclonique grave de la première année. *Rev EEG Neurophysiol* 1982;12:21–25.

42. Lambarri San Martin I, Garaizar Axpe C, Zuazo Zamalloa E, et al. Epilepsia polimorfa de la infancia. Revision de 12 casos. *An Esp Pediatr* 1997;46:571–575.

43. Ferrie CD, Maisey M, Cox T, et al. Focal abnormalities detected by 189FDG PET in epileptic encephalopathies. *Arch Dis Child* 1996;75:102–107.

44. Fernàndez-Jaén A, Leon MC, Martinez-Granero MA, et al. Diagnostico en la epilessia mioclonica severa de la infancia: Estudio de 13 casos. *Rev neurol* (Spanish) 1998;26:759–762.

45. Dooley J, Camfield P, Gordon K. Severe polymorphic epilepsy of infancy. *J Child Neurol* 1995;10:339–340.

46. Renier WO, Renkawek K. Clinical and neuropathologic findings in a case of severe myoclonic epilepsy of infancy. *Epilepsia* 1990;3:287–291.

47. Dulac O, Arthuis M L'épilepsie myoclonique sévère de l'enfant. In: *Journées parisiennes de pédiatrie.* Paris: Flammarion, 1982:259–268.

48. Ogihara M, Hoshika A, Matsuno T, et al. EEG and polygraphical study of vibratory generalized tonic-clonic seizures (vibratory GTCS). *J Jpn Epil Soc* (Jpn) 1994;12:264–271.

49. Ohmori I, Ohtsuka Y, Murakami N, et al. Analysis of ictal EEG in severe myoclonic epilepsy in infancy. *Epilepsia* 2001;42[Suppl 6]:54 (abstr.).

50. Gastaut H, Broughton R, Tassinari CA, et al. Unilateral epileptic seizures. In: Vinken PJ, Bruyn GW, eds.

Handbook of clinical neurology: The Epilepsies, Vol. XV. Amsterdam, New York: Elsevier, 1974:235–245.

51. Sato T, Ota M, Matsuo M, et al. Recurrent reversible rhabdomyolisis associated with hyperthermia and status epilepticus. *Acta Paediatr* 1995;84:1083–1085.

52. Dalla Bernardina B, Capovilla G, Chiamenti C, et al. Cryptogenic myoclonic epilepsies of infancy and early childhood: nosological and prognostic approach. In: Wolf P, Dam M, Janz D, Dreifuss FE, eds. *Advances in epileptology,* Vol 16. New York: Raven Press, 1987:175–180.

53. Wakai S, Ikehata M, Nihira H, et al. "Obtundation status (Dravet)" caused by complex partial status epilepticus in a patient with severe myoclonic epilepsy in infancy. *Epilepsia* 1996;37:1020–1022.

54. Yasuda S, Watanabe M, Fujiwara T, et al. A peculiar state observed in 4 patients with severe myoclonic epilepsy in infancy. *Jpn J Psychiatr Neurol* 1989;43:533–535.

55. Sarisjulis N, Gamboni B, Plouin P, et al. Diagnosing idiopathic/cryptogenic epilepsy syndromes in infancy. *Arch Dis Child* 2000;82:226–230.

56. Morimoto T, Hayakawa T, Sugie H, et al. Epileptic seizures precipitated by constant light, movement in daily life, and hot water immersion. *Epilepsia* 1985;26:237–242.

57. Miyamoto A, Itoh M, Hayashi K, et al. Diurnal secretion profile of melatonin in epileptic children with or without photosensitivity and an observation of altered circadian rhythm in a case of completely under dark living condition. *No To Hattatsu (Jpn)* 1993;25:405–411.

58. Takahashi Y, Fujiwara T, Yagi K, et al. Photosensitive epilepsies and pathophysiologic mechanisms of the photoparoxysmal response. *Neurology* 1999;53:926–932.

59. Cassé Perrot C, Wolff M, Dravet C. Neuropsychological aspects of severe myoclonic epilepsy in infancy. In: Jambaqué I, Lassonde M, Dulac O, eds. *The neuropsychology of childhood epilepsy.* New York: Plenum Press/Kluwer Academic, 2001:131–140.

60. Wolff M, Cassé-Perrot C, Dravet C. Neuropsychological disorders in children with severe myoclonic epilepsy. *Epilepsia* 2001;42 [Suppl 2]:61 (abstr.).

61. Miyake S, Tanaka M, Matsui M, et al. Mortality patterns of children with epilepsies in a children's medical center. *No To Hattatsu (Jpn)* 1991;23:329–335.

62. Castro-Gago M, Martinon Sanchez JM, Rodriguez-Nunez A, et al. Severe myoclonic epilepsy and mitochondrial cytopathy. *Child's Nerv Syst* 1997;11–12:570–571.

63. Guerrini R, Dravet Ch. Severe epileptic encephalopathies of infancy, other than West syndrome. In: Engel J, Pedley. TA, eds. *Epilepsy. A comprehensive textbook,* Vol. 3. Philadelphia-New York: Lippincott-Raven, 1997:2285–2302.

64. Oguni H, Uehara T, Izumi T, et al. Immunological study of the patients with severe myoclonic epilepsy in infants (SMEI) and its variant. *Ann Rep Jpn Epil Res Found* 1994;6:195–203.

65. Sumi K, Nagaura T, Nagai T, et al. A clinical study of seizures induced by hot bathing. *Jpn J Psychiatr Neurol* 1993;47:350–351.

66. Awaya Y, Satoh F, Miyamoto M, et al. Change of rectal temperature in infants and children during and after hot water immersion. *Clin Therm (Tokyo)* 1989;9:76–82.

67. Awaya Y, Satoh F, Oguni H, et al. Study of the mechanism of seizures induced by hot bathing—ictal EEG of hot bathing induced seizures—in severe myoclonic epilepsy in infancy (SMEI). *Ann Rep Jpn Epil Res Found* (Jpn) 1990;2:103–110.

68. Kanazawa O, Shirane S. Can early zonisamide medication improve the prognosis in the core and peripheral types of severe myoclonic epilepsy in infants? *Brain Develop* 1999;21:503 (abstr.).

69. Ernst JP, Doose H, Baier WK. Bromides were effective in intractable epilepsy with generalized tonic-clonic seizures and onset in early childhood. *Brain Develop* 1988;10:385–388.

70. Tanaka J, Mimaki T, Tagawa T, et al. Efficacy of bromide for intractable epilepsy in childhood. *J Jpn Epil Soc* (Jpn) 1990;8:105–109.

71. Steinhoff B, Kruse R. Bromide treatment of pharmacoresistant epilepsies with generalized tonic clonic seizures. *Brain Develop* 1992;14:144–149.

72. Oguni H, Kitami H, Oguni M, et al. Treatment of severe myoclonic epilepsy in infants with bromide and its borderline variant. *Epilepsia* 1994;35:1140–1145.

73. Guerrini R, Dravet C, Genton P, et al. Lamotrigine and seizure aggravation in severe myoclonic epilepsy. *Epilepsia* 1998;39:508–512.

74. Wallace SJ. Myoclonus and epilepsy in childhood: A review of treatment with valproate, ethosuximide, lamotrigine and zonisamide. *Epilepsy Res* 1998;29:147–154.

75. Horn CS, Ater SB, Hurst DL. Carbamazepine-exacerbated epilepsy in children and adolescents. *Pediatr Neurol* 1986;2:340–345.

76. Villeneuve N, Portilla P, Ferrari AR, et al. Topiramate (TPM) in severe myoclonic epilepsy in infancy (SMEI): Study of 27 patients. *Epilepsia* 2002;43 [Suppl 8]:155 (abstr.).

77. Nieto-Barrera M, Candau R, Nieto-Jimenez M, et al. Topiramate in the treatment of severe myoclonic epilepsy in infancy. *Seizure* 2000;9:590–594.

78. Coppola G, Capovilla G, Montagnini A, et al. Topiramate as add-on drug in severe myoclonic epilepsy in infancy: An Italian multicenter open trial. *Epilepsy Res* 2002;49:45–48.

79. Chiron C, Marchand MC, Tran A, et al. Stiripentol in severe myoclonic epilepsy in infancy: A randomised placebo-controlled syndrome-dedicated trial. STICLO study group. *Lancet* 2000;356:1638–1642.

80. Thanh TN, Chiron C, Dellatolas G, et al. Efficacité et tolérance à long terme du stiripentol dans le traitement de l'épilepsie myoclonique sévère du nourrisson (syndrome de Dravet). *Arch Pediatr* 2002;11:1120–1127.

81. Minakawa K. Effectiveness of intravenous midazolam for the treatment of status epilepticus in a child with severe myoclonic epilepsy in infancy. *No To Hattatsu* (Jpn) 1995;27:498–500.

82. Takahashi Y, Shigematsu H, Fujiwara T, et al. Self-induced photogenic seizures in a child with severe myoclonic epilepsy in infancy: Optical investigations and treatments. *Epilepsia* 1995;36:728–732.

83. Dravet C, Bureau M. Benign myoclonic epilepsy in infancy. In: Roger J, Bureau M, Dravet Ch, Genton P, Tassinari CA, Wolf P, eds. *Epileptic syndromes in infancy, childhood and adolescence.* 3rd ed. London: John Libbey, 2002:69–79.

84. Beaumanoir A, Blume W. The Lennox–Gastaut syndrome. In: J Bureau M, Dravet Ch, Genton P, Tassinari

CA, Wolf P, eds. *Epileptic syndromes in infancy, childhood and adolescence.* 3rd ed. London: John Libbey, 2002:113–135.

85. Doose H. Myoclonic astatic epilepsy of early childhood. In: Roger J, Dravet C, Bureau M, Dreifuss FE, Perret A, Wolf P, eds. *Epileptic syndromes in infancy, childhood and adolescence.* 2nd ed. London: John Libbey, 1992:103–114.

86. Guerrini R, Dravet C, Gobbi G, et al. Idiopathic generalized epilepsies with myoclonus in infancy and childhood. In: Malafosse A, Genton P, Hirsch E, Marescaux C, Broglin D, Bernasconi R, eds. *Idiopathic generalized epilepsies.* London: John Libbey, 1994:267–280.

87. Seino M, Higashi T. The investigation on a group of secondary generalized epilepsy in childhood with onset in infancy and refractory grand mal. In: Kimura M, ed. Mental and physical disability research group sponsored by Ministry of Health and Welfare. *Report of research group of children's health and environment.* 1978:79–80.

88. Wada T, Ishida T, Watanabe Y, eds. *Epilepsy Atlas—CT and EEG.* Tokyo: Igaku Shoin, 1983.

89. Kanazawa O. Refractory grand mal seizures with onset during infancy including severe myoclonic epilepsy in infancy. *Brain Develop* 2001;23:749–756.

90. Castro-Gago M, Eiris J, Fernandez-Bustillo J, et al. Severe myoclonic epilepsy associated with mitochondrial cytopathy. *Child's Nerv Syst* 1995;11:630–633.

91. Giovanardi-Rossi P, Pini A, Santucci M, et al. Studio istologico, istochemico e biochimico muscolare nella epilessia mioclonica severa. In: Scargella M, Perniola T, eds. *Atti del XV congresso nazionale della Società Italiana di Neuropsichiatria Infantile.* Bologna: Monduzzi, 1992:279–284.

92. Harbord MG, Hwang PA, Robinson BH, et al. Infant-onset progressive myoclonus epilepsy. *J Child Neurol* 1991;6:134–142.

93. Guerrini R, Parmeggiani L, Volzone A, et al. Cortical myoclonus in early childhood epilepsy. *3rd Europe Cong of Epileptol, Warsaw, Poland.* Bologna: Monduzzi, 1998b:99–105.

7

Severe Myoclonic Epilepsy in Infancy: Clinical Analysis and Relation to *SCN1A* Mutations in a Japanese Cohort

Hirokazu Oguni,* Kitami Hayashi,* Makiko Osawa,* Yutaka Awaya,[†]
Yukio Fukuyama,[‡] Goryu Fukuma,[§] Shinichi Hirose,[§]
Akihisa Mitsudome,[§] and Sunao Kaneko[‖]

*Department of Pediatrics, Tokyo Women's Medical University, Tokyo, Japan; [†]Department of
Pediatrics, Seibo International Catholic Hospital, Tokyo, Japan; [‡]Child Neurology Institute,
Tokyo, Japan; [§]Department of Pediatrics, School of Medicine, Fukuoka University, Fukuoka, Japan;
[‖]Department of Neuropsychiatry, School of Medicine, Hirosaki University, Aomori, Japan

INTRODUCTION

After Claes et al (2001) first reported *de novo* mutations in the Na+ channel gene *SCN1A* in patients with severe myoclonic epilepsy of infancy (SME), recognition of this rare syndrome, also known as "Dravet syndrome," has accelerated around the world (1–4). However, diagnosis of SME is, at times, difficult both clinically and electroencephalographically, in part because of the wide range of clinical and EEG features that change with age and because myoclonic seizures may not be the most predominant seizure type in some patients. The latter observation made one author propose changing its name from SME to "epilepsy with polymorphic seizures" (5). According to the descriptions of Dravet and Dravet et al. (6,7), SME patients have: (1) a high incidence of family history of epilepsy or febrile convulsions; (2) normal development before onset; (3) seizures beginning during the first year of life as generalized or unilateral febrile and afebrile clonic seizures, and (4) the subsequent appearance of myoclonic and often partial seizures. EEGs in the early stage usually do not show paroxysmal discharges, but later generalized spike-waves and polyspike-waves and focal abnormalities appear. Photosensitivity may also appear early. Psychomotor development is initially normal and patients become retarded from the second year of life onward. Ataxia, pyramidal tract signs, and interictal myoclonus usually follow. All seizure types are resistant to all forms of treatment. Thus, the diagnosis of SME largely depends on the combination of clinical and electroencephalographic manifestations that change at different ages. The presence of myoclonic seizures does not appear to be most important despite its terminology.

Because of the lack of strict criteria for inclusion or exclusion, there has been some confusion as to whether patients without myoclonic seizures should be classified as SME, even if other clinical symptoms are identical to that described by Dravet and Dravet et al. (6,7). In Japan, several investigators have become aware of the existence of a distinct group of patients whose clinical findings closely resemble SME. All share most characteristic features of SME, as described by Dravet and Dravet et al. (6,7). However, they do not have myoclonic seizures, an essential diagnostic criterion for typical SME. For this group of patients, other designations have tentatively been offered (8–11), such as "SME borderline (SMEB)," a "peripheral type of SME," "infantile refractory grand-mal epilepsy," or "intractable childhood epilepsies with frequent generalized tonic-clonic seizures." Finally, the International League Against Epilepsy (ILAE) designated "Dravet syndrome" to include SME and all the SME-related or borderline groups as a part of one syndrome (12). Here, we present various phenotypic manifestations of Dravet syndrome and differences between typical and borderline groups in relation to *SCN1A* mutations.

DIFFERENT TYPES OF MYOCLONIC SEIZURES

The term "myoclonic" in SME leads to some confusion in diagnosis, because it does not specify myoclonic seizures. Instead, it is used in a broader sense to include various myoclonic phenomena (7,12,13). We evaluated patients with SME and identified four types of myoclonic attacks on video-EEG or polygraphic recordings (Fig. 7–1) (13). The first seizure type consisted of symmetrical momentary jerking or twitching of the proximal muscles and eyelids, associated with generalized 3.0–3.5 Hz spike- or polyspike-waves (typical myoclonic seizures according to ILAE classification) (Fig. 7–1A). They tended to repeat and sometimes caused the patient to fall forward or downward. The second type of myoclonic attack consisted of successive myoclonic twitching involving mostly the head and eyelids, resulting in rhythmic retropulsion of the head. In this sense, this seizure type is close to absence seizures with a strong myoclonic component or myoclonic absence seizures (Fig. 7–1B). The first and second types of myoclonic attacks occurred frequently during wakefulness, and were at times provoked by photic or pattern stimulation. The third seizure type was massive myoclonia, which was infrequent and sometimes appeared only before the onset of GTCS, i.e., GCTCS. They were frequently observed during sleep, and considered to be a fragment of GTCS, or an initial component of GTCS (Fig. 7–1C). The final type was nonepileptic segmental myoclonus, often seen during the period of frequent GTCS and later in childhood

---

FIG. 7–1. Ictal polygraph of myoclonic seizures. **A:** Myoclonic seizures. A 9-month-old girl started myoclonic seizures at the age of 5 months. Frequent episodes of myoclonic seizures occurred as single and repetitive jerks. Ictal video shows sudden elevation of both arms, extension of the trunk, and twitching of both eyelids simultaneously twice. **B:** Successive myoclonic twitching involving mostly head and eyelids. A 2-year 3-month-old girl exhibited marked photosensitivity after the age of 2 years. Attacks were characterized by twitching of eyelids and rhythmic retropulsion of the head for a few seconds. Seizures were easily triggered by photic stimulation, sunlight or a bright room. When she stayed in a dark room (under the lumination of 0 Lux), there were few generalized spike-wave discharges on the EEG (0.0625×/minutes). When she moved to a bright room (constant illumination of 100 Lux), frequent generalized spike-wave discharges were associated with myoclonic seizures (two per minute). Seizures stopped when she moved back to the dark room (constant light sensitivity). **C:** Massive bilateral myoclonia seizures were observed during all-night sleep recording in a 6-year 5-month-old girl with SME borderland (SMEB). Massive myoclonia or massive spasms (EMG discharges lasted for nearly 1 sec) were associated with diffuse sharp-slow discharge, followed by an arousal response in the EEG. During the all-night sleep recording, three independent massive spasms and one generalized tonic-clonic seizure with a preceding spasm were recorded (13). **D:** Nonepileptic segmental myoclonus. A 14-year 9-month-old boy with SMEB, developed his first seizure at the age of 3 months. He had had mainly nocturnal GTCS since the age of 6 to 7 years, occurring 6–10 times a month. He also had random and segmental myoclonus that predominantly involved distal muscles. Segmental myoclonus appeared at rest, which increased with purposeful movements. He also showed an ataxic gait. EEG showed 4–5 Hz background slowing without any epileptic abnormality. Myoclonic EMG potentials in both arms often appeared in a tremulous fashion.

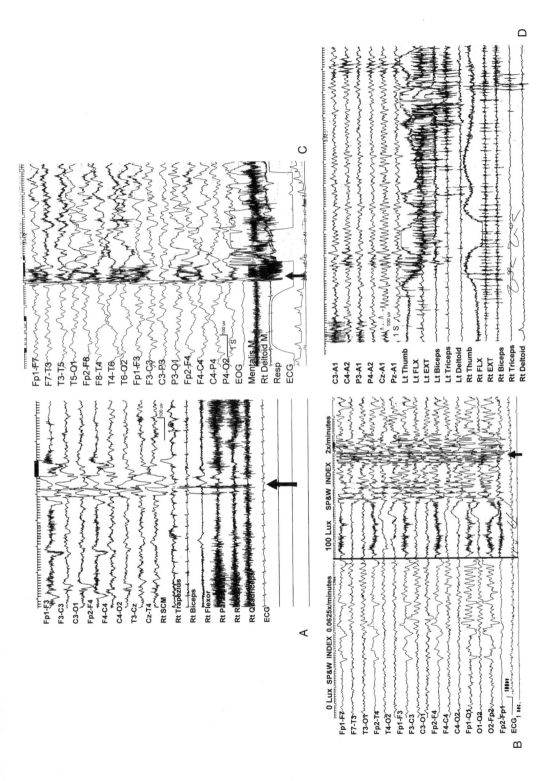

(Fig. 7–1D). This myoclonus is observed randomly and multifocally in arms and legs and most prominently when the patient is doing purposeful hand movements. Although we did not record the seizures, they appeared as focal or localized myoclonic jerks or attacks as described by other authors (14). They were probably a part of focal motor seizures or part of complex partial seizures or atypical absence seizures (or part of the obtundation status described later) rather than a part of myoclonic seizures in a strict sense.

CONVULSIVE SEIZURES MARKEDLY PRECIPITATED BY ELEVATED BODY TEMPERATURE

Among the various clinical manifestations of SME patients in Japan, special attention has been paid to the precipitation of seizures by fever and hot baths. Most authors described recurrent episodes of febrile seizures or febrile status epilepticus together with afebrile seizures during infancy and early childhood. These authors emphasized this combination of seizures as one of the characteristic features of the Dravet syndrome (14–18). In our previous study, almost 1/2 of all seizure episodes were associated with elevation of body temperature, when we included seizures during hot bath (19,20). In addition, convulsive seizures often showed polymorphic features at times starting with focal motor seizures with or without secondary generalization, unilateral or alternating unilateral clonic seizures, or other times with generalized clonic or tonic-clonic seizures.

In Japan, hot bath-induced seizures have long received attention as a special type of seizure (21). Since whole-body immersion into a bath tub filled with hot water ranging from 39°C to 42°C for 5 to 10 minutes is a typical custom in Japan, the hot bath-induced seizures were the consequence of the physiological opportunities of raising body temperature in the patients. We recorded the video–EEG during hot-water immersion of children with SME to confirm whether it could provoke attacks or not, and if it did, to establish guidelines for safe bathing (Fig. 7–2A,B) (22,23). It was surprising that clinical overt seizures were provoked in all cases

examined after 7 to 25 min of immersion in hot water, when the rectal temperature rose to over 38°. The patients clearly showed an increase in frequency and duration of epileptic discharges which culminated into overt clinical seizures. Interestingly, these seizures included atypical absences, complex partial seizures, and massive myoclonia evolving to GTCS, with elevation of the rectal temperature. Seizures were associated with diffuse irregular spike-wave discharges, culminating into diffuse ictal changes. Myoclonic seizures corresponded to brief diffuse irregular spike-wave complexes. Atypical absence seizures corresponded to longer bursts of diffuse spike-wave complexes. Complex partial seizures (CPS) were associated with more localized and longer bursts of spike-wave discharges. There was no significant difference in the rate of rectal temperature elevation during hot-water immersion between SME patients and three normal controls. Thus, we confirmed that epileptic seizures in SME are very sensitive to body temperature elevation regardless of etiology due to either infection, hot baths, or physical exercise (24).

In addition, SME patients are notoriously susceptible to infections and frequently develop hyperthermia during infancy. However, a preliminary immunological study including examination of serum immunoglobulin levels, T-cell function, and complement levels in 16 patients with SME and SMEB failed to identify any immunological abnormality as a cause of susceptibility to infections (25).

OBTUNDATION STATUS

There are a few special types of seizures observed in SME, which are difficult to classify according to the present International Classification of Seizures. Dravet et al. called them "falsely generalized seizures," "unstable seizures," and "obtundation status." Obtundation status is characterized by prolonged fluctuating disturbances of consciousness with reduced postural tone and some myoclonic jerks (7,12). We recorded the ictal video–EEG in four cases of "obtundation status." Three of these cases were reported by Fukuyama et al. (26). All cases were

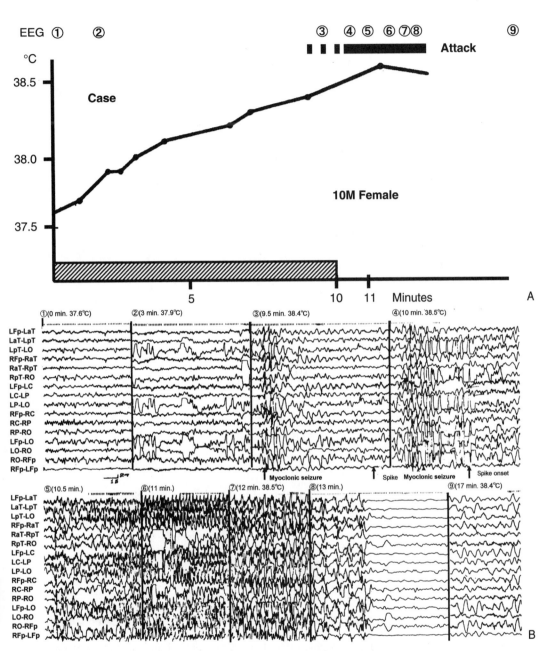

FIG. 7–2. Hot-water immersion: the relationship between rectal temperature and EEG changes in a 10-month-old girl. **A:** A 10-month-old girl, later confirmed as having SME, had recurrent febrile and afebrile unilateral seizures, partial seizures, and GTCS starting at age 5 months. Rectal temperature was 37.6°C when hot-water immersion started. Rectal temperature gradually elevated to 38.4°C 9 min later, when massive myoclonia developed, as indicated by the dotted horizontal line. Two other massive myoclonic attacks followed 30 and 60 s later, which then evolved to GTCS. **B:** This EEG was recorded during hot-water immersion. Intermittent diffuse irregular polyspike-wave discharges associated with massive myoclonias developed along with the elevation of body temperature. Massive myoclonias evolved to GTCS when rectal temperature reached 38°C. Seizure threshold seemingly decreased step-by-step as body temperature elevated. There was no difference in the speed of body temperature elevation during hot-water immersion between patients with SME and three age-matched controls. The number corresponded to that in **A.** Modified from Ref. (23)

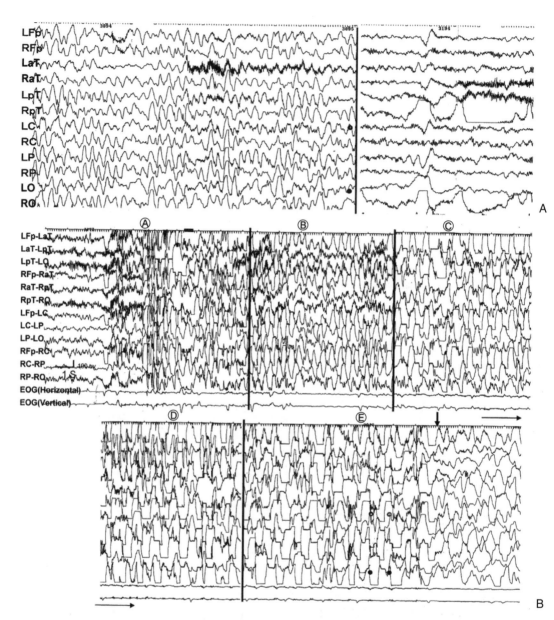

FIG. 7–3. Ictal EEG of "obtundation status." **A:** 1-year 5-month-old girl with SME "obtundation status" was observed after unilateral clonic seizures for 3 min. Ictal EEG (Lt) showed continuous diffuse high-amplitude irregular slow activity lasting more than 15 min without any change. Intravenous diazepam injection suppressed the abnormal EEG (Rt) and clinical obtundation. **B:** 2-year 3-month-old girl with SME. Generalized continuous irregular high-voltaged slow-waves at 2–2.5 Hz, mixed with some spikes. Such patterns developed suddenly and continued for 37 min with progressively slowing frequency and increasing amplitude. She appeared normal at first (**A**) then gradually became obtunded (**B**)(**C**). She became motionless (**D**) 30 min later without response. She then extended both arms (**E**) and suddenly started to move, as designated by the arrow in (**E**). This was associated with diffuse EEG slowing. She then fell asleep (13).

characterized by prolonged mild to moderate disturbances of consciousness, at times associated with cyanosis or irregular respiration and/or segmental myoclonus (Fig. 7–3A, B). "Obtundation status" has been associated with various EEG seizure patterns, which are not always identical to the original ones described by Dravet et al. (12). There are at least four EEG patterns associated with obtundation: (1) continuous diffuse dysrhythmia of slow waves, intermixed with focal and diffuse spikes, sharp waves, and spike-waves that are higher in voltage in the anterior and vertex regions (12), (2) continuous posterior localized irregular slow or spike-wave EEG discharges (13,26,28), (3) pseudorhythmic diffuse high-amplitude irregular slow waves, gradually slowing down in frequency (13), and (4) bursts of bilateral, diffuse high-voltage slow waves occasionally notched with small spikes (26,27). This heterogeneity of EEG manifestations is consistent with the polymorphous nature of the seizures in SME. This leads to difficulty in making a diagnosis of SME by diagnosing the major seizure types that characterize the syndrome.

PHOTO AND PATTERN SENSITIVITY

We identified patients who had daily numerous myoclonic and atypical absence seizures that were sensitive to constant bright light illumination (24,29). In these patients, spike discharges increased or decreased depending on the intensity of constant light illumination. Recently, Takahashi et al. (30) showed that patients with SME have a photoparoxysmal response, which depends on the quantity of light rather than on wavelength. The photoparoxysmal response in idiopathic generalized epilepsy depends on wavelength character. Patients with constant light sensitivity represent the most drug-resistant forms of SME. However, on long-term follow-up, only convulsive seizures persist. Myoclonic or absence seizures and photosensitivity disappeared with advancing age in SME.

MENTAL AND NEUROLOGIC OUTCOMES

In SME patients, psychomotor development is initially normal. Evidence of cognitive impairment start from the second year of life. Ataxia, pyramidal signs, and interictal myoclonus also follow (7,12). Neurologic deterioration depends partly on the severity of convulsive seizures. Not all patients with SME have accompanying ataxia, pyramidal signs, and interictal myoclonus, although the intellectual and seizure outcome is generally poor in most patients (13). Long-lasting repeated convulsive seizures that appear within a short interval impair brain function and intellectual ability, resulting in ataxia, pyramidal signs, and interictal myoclonus. Patients with infrequent attacks successfully treated by potassium bromide (BrK) or ketogenic diet did not show any gross neurologic signs and already impaired cognitive function did not worsen (13).

Mortality in SME patients is high due to convulsive status and sometimes due to other unexpected reasons (7,12,13,17). In our series, 12 out of 85 children with SME ($n = 7$) and SMEB ($n = 5$) died at a mean age of 65 $\pm$ 23 months (13). Seven patients died as a consequence of convulsive status and three died unexpectedly from unknown causes. Two other children with SME had residual severe neurologic deficits after prolonged convulsive status triggered by acute febrile illness. The age distribution of the catastrophic events suggests that careful treatment of convulsive seizures is critical, at least until 8 years of age, because the risk of prolonged convulsive seizures cannot be entirely eliminated until that time.

SME BORDERLINE (SMEB) GROUP

We compared clinical and EEG findings between 39 patients with SME and 45 patients with SMEB. We did not observe any difference in clinical course and ultimate prognosis that was statistically significant. However, mental outcome appeared marginally better in SMEB than SME (13). SMEB, regardless of whether it is referred to as "high-voltage slow waves grand mal," "refractory grand-mal epilepsy in infancy," "fever sensitive grand mal," or "severe idiopathic generalized epilepsy of infancy," is essentially part of the clinical spectrum of SME (8–11). This clinical continuum extends from SMEB, as the mildest end, to SME, as the most severe end, with constant light sensitivity and intermediates of frequent or infrequent myoclonic and absence seizures in-between. This concept has been consolidated by recent reports that SMEB patients have the same molecular pathology as SME, namely, *SCN1A* mutations (31). This spectrum concept could explain the various clinical manifestations of SME and SMEB during early childhood.

PHENOTYPE–GENOTYPE IN RELATION TO *SCN1A* MUTATIONS

We studied the clinical and EEG differences between Dravet syndrome (SME + SMEB) patients who had mutations in the gene encoding the alpha 1 subunit of the Na^+ channel, *SCN1A*, and patients who did not have mutations in *SCN1A*.

Are *SCN1A* mutations truly responsible for this epilepsy syndrome (32)? We studied 12 patients with SME and 17 patients with SMEB. We analyzed *SCN1A*, *SCN1B*, *SCN2A*, *SCN2B*, and *GABRG2* genes using methods which were previously described (32).

Among 29 patients, we identified 14 *SCN1A* mutations in 14 patients (48%) that included 8 missense mutations, 2 deletions, 2 nonsense, and 2 frame-shift mutations (Fig. 7–4). SME patients had more frequent mutations than SMEB patients, although there were no significant differences in the ratio of *SCN1A* mutations {[SME = 8/12 (67%) vs. SMEB = 6/17 (35%) ($P > 0.05$)} (Table 7–1). The types of mutation (nonsense, deletions, and frame-shift mutations vs. missense mutations) did not appear to correlate with intellectual and seizure outcomes.

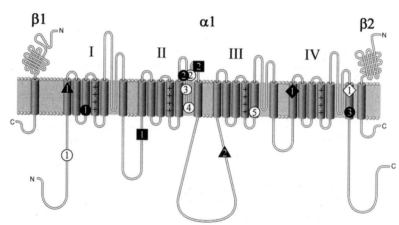

FIG. 7–4. Site of the Na^+ channel mutations in 14 patients with Dravet syndrome. Neuronal voltage-gated Na^+ channels are composed of three subunits: an α subunit and two auxiliary β subunits, $\beta1$ and $\beta2$. The α subunit is a large pore-forming, bell-shaped molecule whose expression alone is sufficient to function as a Na^+ channel. The α subunit has four homologous domains (I–IV), each of which is comprised of six membrane-spanning segments. The fourth segment of each domain functions as a voltage sensor. The ion pore is formed between the fifth and sixth segments (45). Identified mutations in SME are depicted with solid symbols: ●, ■, ▲, and ♦ indicating missense, nonsense, and frameshift mutations resulting in a premature stop, respectively. Mutations identified in SMEB are depicted with open symbols: ○ and ◊ indicate missense mutations and an in-frame deletion mutation, respectively. Mutations in SME consist of missense (numbers on ●): (1) c.568T>C: W190R, (2) c.2772G>C: M924I, and (3) c.5312A>G: Y1771C; nonsense (numbers on ■): (1) c.2101C>T: R701X and (2) c.2825G>A: W942X; frameshift (numbers on ▲): (1) c.429-30delGT: V143fsX148 and (2) c.3494-5delTT: L1165fsX1172; in-frame (♦1): c.4641-3delAAT:M1549del. Mutations in SMEB consist of missense (numbers on ○): (1) c.302G>A: R101Q, (2) c.2772G>A: M924I, (3) c.2801T>C: V934A, (4) c.2807G>A: R936H, and (5) c.4034T>C: L1345P; in-frame (◊1): c.5266-8delTTT: F1756del.
*The nucleotide and amino acid numbers were based on the mRNA of human *SCN1A* registered as NCBINM-006920. Nomenclature for mutations is based on the recommendations by Dunnen and Antonarakis (46).

TABLE 7–1. *Comparisons of the various clinical and EEG features between the two groups*

	Positive *SCN1A* mutations	Negative *SCN1A* mutations	P value
N	14	15	
Age at the study (m)	165 ± 92	215 ± 106	0.143
Follow-up period (m)	103 ± 75	132 ± 91	0.179
Gender (F/M)	12/2	13/2	>.9999
Age onset of epilepsy (m)	6.5 ± 2.5	5.9 ± 278	0.259
FH of convulsive disorders	9	10	>.9999
FC	8	6	
Epi	1	4	
SME/SMEB	8/6	4/11	0.139
Status epilepticus	10	13	0.390
Photopattern sensitivity	3	5	0.682
Intellectual outcomes			0.422
> = Mild	2	4	
Moderate	8	5	
Severe	4	6	
Seizure outcomes			0.202
Daily	3	0	
Weekly	5	4	
Monthly	2	3	
Yearly	4	8	

SMEB = SME borderland, Mild = 50 < IQ < 70, Moderate = 35 < IQ < 50, Severe = IQ < 35.

However, there were more patients with SME among nonsense, deletions, and frameshift mutations. Seizure and intellectual outcomes did not appear to be different between SME patients with *SCN1A* mutations patients without *SCN1A* mutations. Taking into account the general mutation rate of GEFS+ (5.6%) (33) and our present results, we consider SME, SMEB, and GEFS+ as part of a clinical spectrum caused by *SCN1A* mutations with SME as the most severe, GEFS+ as the mildest, and SMEB in-between. This agrees with the original suggestion of Singh et al. (34) (Fig. 7–5). Thus, the spectrum concept to explain clinical variabilities of SME is appropriately supported by both clinical and genetic findings.

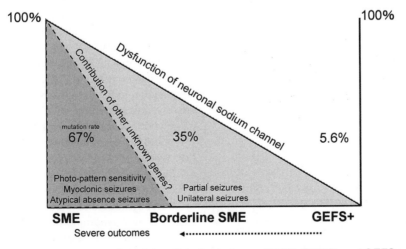

FIG. 7–5. Schematic representation of the clinical spectrum of SME, SMEB, and GEFS+ in relation to *SCN1A* mutations.

TREATMENT

SME is one of the most malignant and catastrophic epilepsies. In contrast to Lennox–Gastaut syndrome (LGS) and West syndrome, both of which are believed to be comparable catastrophic epilepsies, patients with SME suffer from frequent prolonged convulsive seizures, sometimes culminating in life-threatening convulsive status, which require pentobarbital anesthesia (13). Although they also have myoclonic seizures and atypical absence seizures, the most striking seizures are convulsive attacks that occur spontaneously or are provoked by body-temperature elevation. Myoclonic or absence seizures can be partially controlled by ACTH, clonazepam, and combinations of valproate and ethosuximide. Convulsive seizures are most resistant to all available antiepileptic drugs (35). In addition, carbamazepine sometimes aggravates preexisting seizures (7,12,35). Potassium bromide (BrK), an old-fashioned antiepileptic drug, was recently reevaluated for the treatment of SME (36–39). The authors retrospectively analyzed the short-term and long-term efficacy of BrK in 33 patients with SME and SMEB (Table 7–2). After 3 months of trial in 33 patients, results were excellent in 11 patients and moderate in another 11 patients. Results showing poor response were seen in the remaining 11 patients. After 12 months of trial in the 31 patients, results were excellent in 9, moderate in 6, and poor in 16 of the 31 patients. Seven children without response to BrK were placed on ketogenic diet and two of them showed excellent result. Although it was not effective for myoclonic or absence seizures, BrK is particularly useful in treating children with SME or SMEB who demonstrate recurrent life-threatening status convulsivus, often triggered by fever (37). After introduction of BrK, episodes of status convulsivus were entirely eliminated in all patients with SME, although recurrence of brief GTCS was difficult to control. Ketogenic diet is effective not only for GTCS, but also for myoclonic and absence seizures when successfully introduced (35). Continuous infusion of midazolam was reported to successfully suppress status epilepticus that were resistant to intravenous diazepam, phenytoin, and lidocaine (40). In Europe, a new drug stiripentol has recently been shown to be effective for convulsive seizures in patients with SME, although it is not commercially available in most countries (41). The prognosis of patients with SME depends mostly on the control of these catastrophic seizures. Development of new anticonvulsant drugs, which work specifically on the protein product of *SCN1A*, is urgent.

ETIOLOGY AND NOSOLOGIC SITUATION

Despite vigorous administration of conventional AEDs, hyperthermia-sensitive seizures in Dravet syndrome are almost never prevented, and persist from onset to later in life. Based on our results, we strongly advocate that fever sensitivity or seizures very sensitive to body-temperature elevation be given special priority in the diagnostic criteria of SME. Fever sensitivity was most prominent during infancy, and persisted throughout the clinical course. The incidence of seizures induced by body-temperature elevation dramatically decreased with age, presumably due to immunological defense, safe bathing, or maturation. *SCN1A* mutations in this syndrome may explain why seizures are unusually sensitive to hyperthermia. Na$^+$ channels have been known to be thermosensitive, as shown in paramyotonia congenita (*SCN4A* mutation), Brugada syndrome (*SCN5A* mutation) induced by fever, and temperature-sensitive paralytic mutation in *Drosophilia* (*Drosophilia* sodium channel a subunit dysfunction) (42–44).

There are still many questions about the causes of Dravet syndrome that are unanswered. What causes Dravet syndrome in those 20% to 65% of cases with SME who do not have *SCN1A* mutations? Other disease-causing genes may be responsible. Hence, we also analyzed *SCN1A*,

TABLE 7–2. *Effect of BrK for GTCS*

Trial period	3M ($n = 33$)	12M ($n = 31$)
• Excellent (75%<)	11(3/8)*(33%)	9 (3/6)(29%)
• Moderate (50–75%)	11 (6/5)	6 (3/3)(19%)
• No effect (50%>)	11 (6/5)	16 (9/7)(52%)

SCN1B, SCN2A, SCN2B, and *GABRG2.* In 52% of patients, we did not observe any mutations in *SCN1A, SCN1B, SCN2A, SCN2B,* and *GABRG2* genes. It is true that SME patients had more frequent mutations than SMEB. Although identification of *SCN1A* mutations in patients with Dravet syndrome has marked a new era in the basic understanding of this catastrophic epilepsy, there should exist other disease-causing genes associated with SME, modifier genes affecting *SCN1A,* or some *SCN1A* mutations that have not been detected by the present methodology.

CASE EXAMPLES OF SME PATIENTS WITH AND WITHOUT *SCN1A* MUTATIONS

Case 1

The patient is a 14-year-old female. She was born uneventfully at 39 weeks of gestation and weighed 3620 g. There is no family history of seizure disorders. She developed her first seizure at the age of 6 months. Later she experienced prolonged GTCS and unilateral seizures, often triggered by fever and hot baths. Myoclonic seizures were first recognized at 1 year of age.

At 1 year 6 months of age, we identified strong photo- and pattern-sensitive myoclonic seizures. When she was looking at vertical stripes and checkered patterns, myoclonic seizures appeared with diffuse spike-wave discharges (Fig. 7–6). Myoclonic attacks were also provoked when the pattern was flushed in a dark room. She also experienced recurrent so-called "obtundation status" characterized by fluctuating levels of consciousness and flaccid posture associated with continuous irregular large spike-wave discharges, which predominated over both posterior head regions. Intravenous diazepam terminated the spike-wave discharges and she regained consciousness. Recurrent *status epilepticus* triggered by fever prompted several visits to the emergency clinic. Myoclonic seizures successively occurred, which looked like myoclonic absence seizures, at times evolving to GTCS. At 2 years 2 months of age, treatment-resistant status epilepticus, triggered by high fever, left her with quadriplegia and severe mental retardation (Fig. 7–7). After recovery from status epilepticus, she had fewer severe convulsive seizures and only occasional pattern-sensitive attacks. She had GTCS once every 6 months and pattern-sensitive versive seizures once a month. A

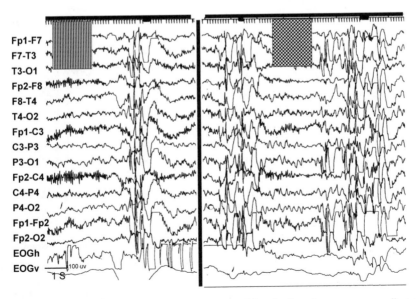

FIG. 7–6. Pattern-sensitive myoclonic seizures in case 1. Myoclonic seizures were easily precipitated by pattern stimulation at the age of 1 year 7 months.

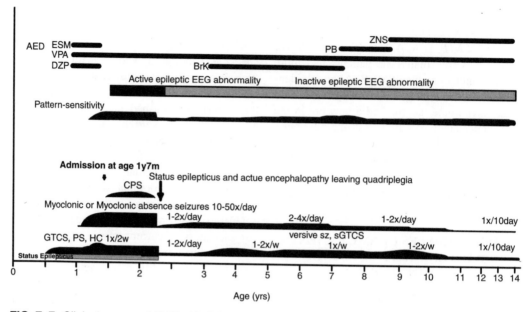

FIG. 7–7. Clinical course of SME with *SCN1A* mutations (14 year 4-month-old girl).

non-sense mutation of *SCN1A* (1 in Fig. 7–4) was identified at 14 years of age.

Case 2

The patient is a 13-year 5-month-old boy with SME. His mother experienced febrile convulsions twice during infancy. He was born uneventfully at 40 weeks of gestation and weighed 3320 g. His development was normal until 7 months of age, when he developed febrile GTCS lasting for 45 min. Since then, he experienced recurrent febrile and afebrile GTCS often lasting more than 15 min. In addition, hot baths provoked GTCS. Myoclonic seizures started at 1 year of age. Complex partial seizures characterized by cloudiness of consciousness with eye deviation followed later. He also had focal motor seizures that evolved to unilateral seizures or GTCS. At 2 years 2 months of age, video-EEG examinations recorded spontaneous myoclonic seizures that occurred 10–20 times per day. Photic and pattern stimulations easily provoked attacks that often evolved to GTCS (Fig. 7–8). Photo and pattern sensitivity persisted until the age of 8 years and disappeared. GTCS

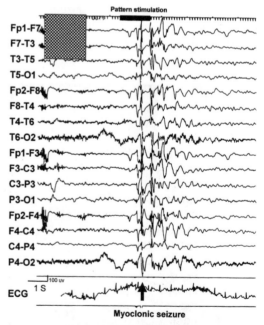

FIG. 7–8. Pattern-sensitive myoclonic seizures in case 2. Myoclonic seizures were easily precipitated by pattern stimulation and at times progressed to secondarily generalized seizures at the age of 2 years 3 months.

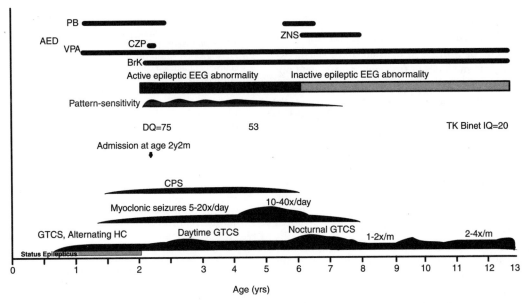

FIG. 7–9. Clinical course of SME without *SCN1A* mutations (13-year 4-month-old boy).

occurred exclusively during wakefulness until 8 years of age, when they began to gradually develop during sleep. Now he has had GTCS once a week. No myoclonic seizures were found (Fig. 7–9). EEG showed generalized spike-wave discharges and moderate slowing of background activity. At 8 years of age, epileptic EEG abnormalities gradually disappeared, even during IPS. He was now moderately retarded without apparent ataxia or pyramidal signs. No mutation of *SCN1A, SCN1B, SCN2A, SCN2B,* and *GABRG2* gene was identified.

CONCLUSION

SME in infants is one of the most malignant epileptic syndromes recognized in the latest classification of epileptic syndromes. Diagnosis of SME depends largely on the combination of clinical and electroencephalographic manifestations at different ages, of which the most important are myoclonic seizures. However, different types of myoclonic attacks and the lack of strict criteria for diagnosing SME has caused some confusion as to whether patients without myoclonic seizures or myoclonus should be classified as SME, despite other identical clinical symptoms

[SME borderlands (SMEB) group]. Among the various clinical manifestations of SME in Japan, special attention has been paid to the easy precipitation of seizures by fever and hot baths. We have demonstrated that seizures in these patients are very sensitive to elevation of body temperature regardless of etiology. Using simultaneous EEG and rectal temperature monitoring during hot-water immersion, we showed that epileptic discharges increased in frequency and eventually developed into seizures at temperatures over 38°. We believe that the unique fever sensitivity observed in SME is similar to, but more intense, than that of febrile convulsions. We have also identified a group of patients who had countless daily myoclonic and atypical absences, which were sensitive to constant bright light illumination. In these cases, spike discharges increased or decreased depending on the intensity of constant light illumination. Although these cases form the most drug-resistant SME, they gradually lost the constant-light sensitivity at the age of 5 or more years, leaving only fever-sensitive grand-mal seizures. In the long run, only convulsive seizures continue, while myoclonic or absence seizures and photosensitivity disappear with advancing age. It is conceivable that SMEB constitutes a basic epileptic condition underlying SME. There is a clinical continuum, which extends from the mildest end of SMEB to the severest end of SME with constant-light sensitivity, with intermediates of frequent or infrequent myoclonic and absence seizures in-between. This "spectrum concept" appropriately explains the clinical variabilities between SME and SMEB during early childhood. Our etiologic speculation has been confirmed by analysis of *SCN1A* mutation in both groups of patients. SME patients had more frequent mutations than SMEB patients, although there were no significant differences in the ratio of *SCN1A* mutations. Taking into account the general mutation rate of GEFS$^+$ (5.6%) and the present result, SME, SMEB, and GEFS$^+$ probably represent a clinical spectrum caused by *SCN1A* mutations. The "clinical spectrum" ranges from SME at the most severe end to GEFS$^+$ at the mildest end, and SMEB in-between. Thus, the "spectrum concept" to explain the variety of clinical manifestations of SME is appropriately supported by both clinical and genetic findings.

REFERENCES

1. Claes L, Del-Favero J, Ceulemans B, et al. De novo mutations in the sodium-channel gene SCN1A cause severe myoclonic epilepsy of infancy. *Am J Hum Genet* 2001;68(6):1327–1332.
2. Sugawara T, Mazaki-Miyazaki E, Fukushima K, et al. Frequent mutations of SCN1A in severe myoclonic epilepsy in infancy. *Neurology* 2002;9;58(7):1122–1124.
3. Ohmori I, Ouchida M, Ohtsuka Y, et al. Significant correlation of the *SCN1A* mutations and severe myoclonic epilepsy in infancy. *Biochem Biophys Res Commun* 2002;5;295(1):17–23.
4. Nabbout R, Gennaro E, Dalla Bernardina B, et al. Spectrum of SCN1A mutations in severe myoclonic epilepsy of infancy. *Neurology* 2003;24;60(12):1961–1967.
5. Ogino T, Ohtsuka Y, Amano R, Yamatogi Y, Ohtahara S. An investigation on the borderland of severe myoclonic epilepsy in infancy. *Jpn J Psychiatr Neurol* 1988;42:554–555.
6. Dravet C. Les epilepsies graves de l'enfant. *Vie Med* 1978;8:543–548.
7. Dravet C, Bureau M, Roger J. Severe myoclonic epilepsy in infants. In: Roger J, Bureau M, Dravet C, Dreifuss FE, Perret A, Wolf P. eds. *Epileptic syndromes in infancy, childhood and adolescence.* 2nd ed. London: John Libbey, 1992:75–88.
8. Sugama M, Oguni H, Fukuyama Y. Clinical and electroencephalographic study of severe myoclonic epilepsy in infancy (Dravet). *Jpn J Psychiatr Neurol* 1987;41:463–465.
9. Ogino T, Ohtsuka Y, Yamatogi Y, et al. The epileptic syndrome sharing common characteristics during early childhood with severe myoclonic epilepsy in infancy. *Jpn J Psychiatr Neurol* 1989;43:479–481.
10. Fujiwara T, Watanabe M, Takahashi Y, et al. Long-term course of childhood epilepsy with intractable grand mal seizures. *Jpn J Psychiatr Neurol* 1992;46:297–302.
11. Kanazawa O. Medically intractable generalized tonic-clonic or clonic seizures in infancy. *J Epil* 1992;5:143–148.
12. Dravet C, Bureau M, Oguni H, et al. Severe myoclonic epilepsy in infants (Dravet syndrome). In: Roger J, Bureau M, Dravet C, Genton P, Tassinari CA, Wolf P. eds. *Epileptic syndromes in infancy, childhood and adolescence.* 3rd ed. London: John Libbey, 2002:81–103.
13. Oguni H, Hayashi K, Awaya Y, et al. Severe myoclonic epilepsy in infants—A review based on the Tokyo Women's Medical University series of 84 cases. *Brain Develop.* 2001;23(7):736–748.
14. Ogino T. Severe myoclonic epilepsy in infancy—A clinical and electroencephalographic study *Tenkan Kenkyu (in Jpn) (Tokyo)* 1986;4:114–126.
15. Fujiwara T, Yagi K, Watanabe M, Terauchi N, et al. A clinico-electrical study of 32 patients with severe myoclonic epilepsy in infancy (Dravet). In: Seino M, ed. *The 1986 annual report of the research committee on prevention and treatment of intractable epilepsy.* Supported by the Ministry of Health and Welfare. (*Jpn*) Shizuoka, 1987:129–139.
16. Ohtsuka Y, Maniwa S, Ogino T, et al. Severe myoclonic epilepsy in infancy: a long-term follow-up study. *Jpn J Psychiatr Neurol* 1991;45:416–418.
17. Maniwa S. Severe myoclonic epilepsy in infancy: a longitudinal study. *Tenkan Kenkyu (Jpn) (Tokyo)* 1993;11:226–235.
18. Ohki T, Watanabe K, Negoro K, et al. Severe myoclonic epilepsy in infancy: Evolution of seizures. *Seizure* 1997;6:219–224.
19. Hayashi K, Oguni H, Osawa M, et al. Clinical study of childhood epilepsies with onset in the first year of life: A new international classification of epilepsies and epileptic syndromes. *J Tokyo Wom Med Coll (Jpn)* 1995;65:38–47.
20. Hayashi K, Oguni H, Osawa M, et al. Clinical study of childhood epilepsies with onset in the first year of life: Clinical features of epilepsies with fever sensitive seizure. *J Tokyo Wom Med Coll (Jpn)* 1995;65:48–57.
21. Sumi K, Nagaura T, Nagai T, et al. A clinical study of seizures induced by hot bathing. *Jpn J Psychiatr Neurol* 1993;47:350–351.
22. Awaya Y, Satoh F, Miyamoto M, et al. Change of rectal temperature in infants and children during and after hot water immersion. *Rinsyo Taion (Tokyo) (Jpn)* 1989;9:76–82.
23. Awaya Y, Satoh F, Oguni H, et al. Study of the mechanism of seizures induced by hot bathing—Ictal EEG of hot bathing induced seizures in severe myoclonic epilepsy in infancy (SMEI). *1990 Ann Rep Jpn Epil Res Found (Osaka) (Jpn)* 1990;2:103–110.
24. Morimoto T, Hayakawa T, Sugie H, et al. Epileptic seizures precipitated by constant light, movement in daily life, and hot water immersion. *Epilepsia* 1985;26:237–242.
25. Oguni H, Uehara T, Izumi T. Immunogenetic study of the patients with severe myoclonic epilepsy in infants

(SMEI) and its variant. *1994 Ann Rep Jpn Epil Res Found (Osaka) (Jpn)* 1994;6:195–203.

26. Fukuyama Y, Hayashi K, Izumi T, et al. Clinical study of SMEI: A peculiar paroxysmal state of prolonged consciousness disturbance. In: Seino M, ed. *The annual report of the research committee on cause and therapy of intractable epilepsies.* Supported by the Ministry of Health & Welfare. Shizuoka. 1989:147–153.

27. Yasuda S, Watanabe M, Fujiwara T, et al. A peculiar state observed in 4 patients with severe myoclonic epilepsy in infancy. *Jpn J Psychiatr Neurol* 1989;43:533–535.

28. Wakai S, Ikehata M, Nihira H, et al. "Obtundation Status (Dravet)" caused by complex partial status epilepticus in a patient with severe myoclonic epilepsy in infancy. *Epilepsia* 1996;37:1020–1022.

29. Miyamoto A, Itoh M, Hayashi K, et al. Diurnal secretion profile of melatonin in epileptic children with or without photosensitivity and an observation of altered circadian rhythm in a case under completely dark living conditions. *No To Hattatsu (Tokyo) (Jpn)* 1993;25:405–511.

30. Takahashi Y, Fujiwara T, Yagi K. Photosensitive epilepsies and pathophysiologic mechanisms of the photoparoxysmal response. *Neurology* 1999;22:926–932.

31. Fujiwara T, Sugawara T, Mazaki-Miyazaki E, et al. Mutations of sodium channel alpha subunit type 1 (*SCN1A*) in intractable childhood epilepsies with frequent generalized tonic-clonic seizures. *Brain* 2003;126(Pt 3):531–546.

32. Oguni H, Awaya Y, Osawa M, et al. How *SCN1A* mutations contribute to Dravet syndrome—A comparison of clinical and EEG features between Dravet syndrome with and without *SCN1A* mutations: *Program&Abstracts, The 4th Asian and Oceanian Epilepsy Congress, Karuizawa Nagano, Japan,* 2002;Sept 11–14:262.

33. Wallace RH, Scheffer IE, Barnett S, et al. Neuronal sodium-channel alpha1-subunit mutations in generalized epilepsy with febrile seizures plus. *Am J Hum Genet.* 2001;68(4):859–865.

34. Singh R, Scheffer IE, Whitehouse W, et al. Severe myoclonic epilepsy in infancy is part of the spectrum of generalized epilepsy with febrile seizure plus (GEFS$^+$). *Epilepsia* 1999;40[Suppl 2]:175.

35. Okada N, Miyamoto A, Hayashi K, et al. Severe myoclonic epilepsy in infancy. A reevaluation of various therapeutic trials at our department. *J Jpn Pediatr Soc (Jpn)* 1990;94:1409–1413.

36. Ernst JP, Doose H, Baier WK. Bromides were effective in intractable epilepsy with generalized tonic clonic seizures and onset in early childhood. *Brain Develop* 1988;10:385–388.

37. Tanaka J, Mimaki T, Tagawa T, et al. Efficacy of bromide for intractable epilepsy in childhood. *J Jpn Epil Soc (Jpn)* 1990;8:105–109.

38. Steinhoff B, Kruse R. Bromide treatment of pharmaco-resistant epilepsies with generalized tonic-clonic seizures. *Brain Develop* 1992;14:144–149.

39. Oguni H, Hayashi K, Oguni M, et al. Treatment of severe myoclonic epilepsy in infants with bromide and its borderline variant. *Epilepsia* 1994;35:1140–1145.

40. Minakawa K. Effectiveness of intravenous midazolam for the treatment of status epilepticus in a child with severe myoclonic epilepsy in infancy. *No To Hattatsu (Tokyo) (Jpn)* 1995;27:498–500.

41. Chiron C, Marchand MC, Tran A, et al. Stiripentol in severe myoclonic epilepsy in infancy: A randomised placebo-controlled syndrome-dedicated trial. STICLO study group. *Lancet* 2000;356(9242):1638–1642.

42. Sugiura Y, Aoki T, Sugiyama Y, Hida C, et al. Temperature-sensitive sodium channelopathy with heat-induced myotonia and cold-induced paralysis. *Neurology.* 2000;13;54(11):2179–2181.

43. Hodges DD, Lee D, Preston CF, tipE regulates Na$^+$-dependent repetitive firing in Drosophila neurons. *Mol Cell Neurosci* 2002;19(3):402–416.

44. Mok NS, Priori SG, Napolitano C, et al. A newly characterized SCN5A mutation underlying Brugada syndrome unmasked by hyperthermia. *J Cardiovasc Electrophysiol.* 2003;14(4):407–411.

45. Hirose S, Okada M, Yamakawa K, et al. Genetics abnormalities underlying familial epilepsy syndromes. *Brain Develop* 2002;24:211–222

46. Dunnen J, Antonarakis S. Nomenclature for the description of human sequence variations. *Hum Genet* 2001;109:121–124.

8

Myoclonic Seizures in the Context of Generalized Epilepsy with Febrile Seizures Plus (GEFS⁺)

Michel Baulac*,§, Isabelle Gourfinkel-An*,†, Stephanie Baulac†, and Eric Leguern†,‡

*Neurology/Epilepsy Department and Paris VI University, Hôpital Pitie-Salpetriere, Paris, France; †INSERM U 289, Hôpital Pitie-Salpetriere, Paris, France; ‡Département de Génétique, Cytogénétique et Embryologie, Hôpital Pitie-Salpetriere, Paris, France

INTRODUCTION

The GEFS⁺ Familial Condition

Generalized epilepsy with febrile seizures plus (GEFS⁺) is a recently described familial condition [1] in which febrile seizures (FS) and epilepsy coexist in affected families. Indeed, in this heterogeneous familial context, some affected members have febrile seizures which are particular, called febrile seizures plus (FS⁺), because they persist beyond the classical limit of 6 years of age. They are often multiple in a given individual. On the other hand, some other family members may have typical FS, disappearing before the age of 6. Moreover, variable types of afebrile seizures are observed in affected individuals, most often generalized seizures, tonic-clonic (GTCS), absence, atonic, tonic seizures, including myoclonias and myoclonic seizures as well. Hemiconvulsives, temporal, and frontal lobe seizures have been also reported, extending the GEFS⁺ spectrum to partial seizures [1,2]. These afebrile seizures may begin in childhood in association with the FS, this continuum between febrile and afebrile seizures being very characteristic (Fig. 8–1). However, afebrile seizures may also appear after a variable seizure-free period, or in subject without known previous history of FS.

Several types of seizures, including myoclonic seizures, can coexist in a given patient with more or less typical electroclinical features of idiopathic generalized epilepsies (Fig. 8–2). In some instances, they may constitute myoclono-astatic epilepsy (MAE) or severe myoclonic epilepsy in infancy (SMEI), although this latter syndrome has, thus far, been very rarely reported in the GEFS⁺ pedigrees. Finally, some electroclinical patterns that do not correspond to any of the well-established syndromes of the international classification can be encountered.

PLACE OF MYOCLONIC SEIZURES IN THE GEFS⁺ SPECTRUM

In the GEFS⁺ familial context, the spectrum of individual phenotypes includes all the generalized seizure types. Myoclonic seizures have been reported in patients with FS or FS⁺.

In one of their families, Singh et al. [3] describe two individuals: one had two FS at the age of 1.5 years and a brief period of frequent myoclonic seizures at the age of 2 during an intercurrent infection. He then became seizure-free

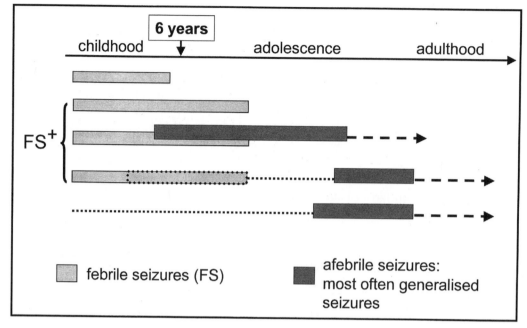

FIG. 8–1. Familial GEFS+ context. Temporal sequence of clinical expression of febrile seizures and afebrile seizures.

off treatment at the age of 4. The other individual, evaluated at the age of 5, had FS, afebrile GTCS, and myoclonic seizures starting at the age of 1.

In another family, consistent with the GEFS+ phenotype (2), one individual only, aged 18 at the time of the study, presented myoclonic seizures.

He had several FS, starting at the age of 1, including an episode of prolonged FS, and then, without free interval, he started to have GTCS accompanied by other seizure types. Myoclonic jerks were sporadic. Absence seizures were consistent with the description usually made in GEFS+, with rare

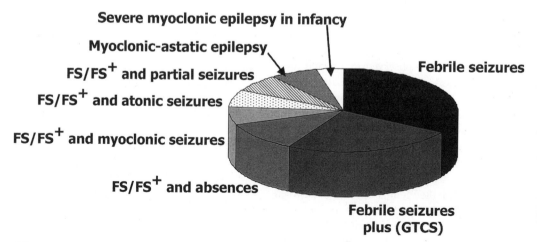

FIG. 8–2. GEFS+ phenotypic variability. Diversity of seizure types. (Adapted from Scheffer and Berkovic, *Brain* 1997.)

episodes lasting longer than the typical absences. He became pharmacoresistant and had moderate intellectual impairment. EEG recordings showed a slow background and generalized spike-waves. Myoclonic jerks were not directly observed and polyspike waves were not recorded, however.

In spite of their well-established presence in the GEFS+ spectrum, myoclonic seizures account for a small proportion of the diverse seizure types. In a survey of ten families consistent with the GEFS+ phenotype, including 94 affected individuals, typical FS were reported in 35%, FS+ in 25%, FS or FS+ and absences in 7.5%, while FS or FS+ and myoclonic seizures were reported in only 3% of the patients (3).

Myoclonic seizures are also present as one of the seizure types of the syndromes that can be observed in GEFS+ families. MAE is the most frequent of these syndromes and ten of them are reported in a meta-analysis of ten families (3). However, eight out of these ten cases were observed in each of the eight small families included in this survey. The mean age of seizure onset was 1.5 years, all but one with fever. Four had explosive onset of multiple seizure types and developed a combination of myoclonic, absence, and GTCS seizures, myoclonic seizures occurring singly or in clusters.

SMEI, which is usually a sporadic condition, is a relatively rare phenotype in GEFS+ pedigrees and very few affected members have, thus far, been reported (4). Some studies, however, lead to the observation that FS and FS+ could be encountered more frequently than expected in SMEI relatives. Among 39 affected relatives of 12 SMEI probands, 14 relatives with FS, 7 with FS+, 2 with partial epilepsies, and single individuals with SMEI, MAE or Lennox–Gastaut syndrome (LGS) were identified (5). These findings suggested that SMEI could be the most severe condition of an extended GEFS+ spectrum.

Finally, juvenile myoclonic epilepsy (JME) seems to be a rare condition in GEFS+. One case was reported in the original pedigree leading to the initial delineation and description of the GEFS+ condition, but at the stage of molecular analysis it was found that this patient did not have the mutation that was present in most of the other affected members (6). Another very probable case is reported as the proband for a family consistent with the classification of GEFS+. He had myoclonic seizures without preceding FS, with a polyspike wave pattern (7).

The conclusion seems to be that myoclonic jerks are not a very frequent phenotype in GEFS+ families, although a few individuals have the characteristic sequence FS or FS+ and myoclonic seizures. The interest in myoclonias occurring in GEFS+ families, however, lies in all the genetic findings that have been made in this context and which may, to some extent, contribute to the pathophysiology of myoclonic seizures.

GENETICS FINDINGS IN GEFS+

GEFS+ is inherited as an autosomal dominant trait with incomplete penetrance (70–80%); it is genetically heterogeneous. The first locus was mapped to the chromosome 19q13.1 and a mutation (Cys121Trp) in the *SCN1B* gene, encoding the $\beta1$ subunit of the neuronal voltage-gated sodium channel, was identified in an Australian family (8). This mutation altered the tertiary structure of the protein by disrupting a disulfuric bridge in the extracellular immunoglobulin-like domain of the auxiliary $\beta1$ subunit of the voltage-gated sodium channel. Using electrophysiological recordings from mammalian cell lines, Meadows et al. (9) reported that Cys121Trp mutation causes subtle effects on channel function and subcellular distribution that bias neurons toward hyperexcitability and epileptogenesis. A few years later, only two other mutations in SCN1B were identified in GEFS+ families (10) and this gene has been excluded in the vast majority of families with GEFS+.

A second disease locus mapping to region 2q21-q33 has been reported (2,11). In the two French families studied, two different mutations (Arg1648His and Thr875Met) have been identified in the *SCN1A* gene. This gene encodes the $\alpha1$ subunit of the neuronal voltage-gated sodium channel, which forms the pore of the channel (12). These two mutations are located in the transmembrane segment S4 of II and IV domains that are responsible for channel activation in response to the potential. Mutations in the *SCN1A* gene seem to be more frequently implicated in GEFS[+] families as additional numerous point mutations in this gene have been later described (6,7,13,14). Mutations in *SCN1A* were also reported in patients (isolated cases or familial cases) with febrile seizures and partial epilepsy (15,16). The *SCN2A* gene, also located in 2q21-q33 and encoding the α2 subunit of the voltage-gated sodium channel, may be also implicated (17).

Electrophysiologic studies have demonstrated that mutations in the β1, α1, and α2 subunits interfere with the functional properties of the sodium channel (8,18–22).

The neuronal voltage-gated sodium channel is not the only channel to be implicated in GEFS[+]. Indeed, by performing a genome scan in a large French family with GEFS[+], Baulac et al. (22) localized a new gene on chromosome 5q34 (GEFS[+]2), where the cluster of genes, *GABRA1, GABRA6, GABRB2,* and *GABRG2,* encoding the α1, α6, β2, and γ2 subunits of the GABA$_A$ receptor, respectively, was located. The Lys289Met mutation was identified in the second transmembrane domain of the γ2 subunit of GABA$_A$ receptor.

Electrophysiologic studies in *Xenopus* oocytes showed that this mutation led to a drastic decrease in chloride GABA-induced currents, but that the sensibility to benzodiazepines was conserved. Concomitantly, Wallace et al. (23) described the Arg43Gln mutation in the same subunit of the GABA$_A$ receptor in a family comprising patients with FS and childhood absence epilepsy (CAE). This mutation was located in the binding site of benzodiazepines. Electrophysiologic studies in HEK cells showed an absence of potentiation by diazepam. Additional mutations in GABRG2 were recently associated with either the GEFS[+](4) or FS/CAE phenotype (25).

MYOCLONIC SEIZURES AND THE GENETIC HETEROGENEITY OF GEFS[+]

The GEFS[+] condition is genetically heterogeneous in the ways that multiple genes have been found. Yet, many families, consistent with the GEFS[+] description, are not carrying mutations in any of these four genes thus far discovered. Two ion channel genes, however, *GABRG2* and

SCN1A, have been implicated in several GEFS[+] families and, more importantly, may contribute to the phenotype. This leads us to ask the following questions: Do the phenotypes associated with a *GABRG2* mutation differ, to some extent, from the phenotypes associated with a *SCN1A* mutation? Does one of these two genes contribute to myoclonic seizures in a different way from the other?

The four families harboring *GABRG2* mutations and who presented a GEFS[+]-compatible familial phenotype can be pooled altogether. This analysis includes the family described under the phenotype childhood absence and FS (23), because several of its affected individuals had FS[+], while many others had FS followed or not by afebrile seizures. The small family reported by Kananura et al. (24) is also included on the grounds that all the three affected individuals had FS followed by other seizure types, absence and/or GTCS.

This pooled analysis considers three levels: (a) distribution of FS, FS[+], and afebrile seizures, (b) prevalence of the different seizure types regardless the syndrome, if any, and (c) occurrence of well-defined syndromes (Table 8–1). The same analysis was done with four of the GEFS[+] families carrying *SCN1A* mutations (1;2;6;7;11;12;14;25) and is presented in Table 8–2.

In terms of distribution of FS, FS[+], and afebrile seizures, it appears that many more individuals had pure FS in association with *GABRG2* (48%) than with *SCN1A* (17%), whereas many more had FS[+] with *SCN1A* (57%) than with *GABRG2* (13%). The continuum between FS and afebrile seizures, very typical of GEFS[+], was more frequent with the sodium channel gene mutations. In terms of seizure types, GTCS were twice as frequently observed with *SCN1A* as compared to *GABRG2*—absence seizures and atonic seizures being not very different. Typical CAE was not reported in the presence of *SCN1A* mutations, whereas it represented 20% of the patients carrying a *GABRG2* mutation. The large family combining CAE and FS, who contributes both to the GEFS[+] and CAE phenotypes is accounting for a large proportion, with 7 out of a total of 9 patients. The pedigree of this family

TABLE 8–1. Analysis of the four families with the phenotype or traits of GEFS+ harboring a GABRG2 mutation

GABRG2 mutation	K289M (Ref. 22)	R43Q (Refs. 23,26)	Q351X (Ref. 4)	IVS6 (Ref. 24)	All	%
Phenotype(s)	GEFS+	CAE/FS	GEFS+	CAE/FS		
N affected and mutation	13	25	3	3	44	100
Total FS	11	21	3	3	38	86
FS only	8	10	2	1	21	48
FS and epilepsy	3	11	1	2	17	38
FS+	2	3	1		6	13
Total epilepsy	5	15	1	2	23	52
Epilepsy only	2	4	0	0	6	13
Absence seizures	1	9	1	2	13	29
GTC seizures	2	10	1	2	15	34
Myoclonic seizures		2	1		3	7
Atonic seizures		1	1		2	4
CAE		7		2	9	20
MAE		2			2	4
SMEI		0	1		1	2
Partial seizures/epilepsy	1	1			2	4
Unclassified	2	1			3	3

Distribution of febrile seizures (FS), febrile seizures plus (FS+) and afebrile seizures, prevalence of seizure types (GTC for generalized tonic clonic), and occurrence of syndromes (CAE for childhood absence epilepsy and SMEI for severe myoclonic epilepsy in infancy).

was particular, bilineal, and a second gene underlying the CAE phenotype was hypothesized, but not found (26). However, the contribution of GABRG2 to the CAE phenotype was also observed in the small family of three affected individuals, two of them with typical CAE (24).

Regarding myoclonic seizures, they accounted for 9% of the seizure types with SCN1A and 7% with GABRG2. In terms of well-defined epilepsy syndromes, including myoclonic seizures among their seizure types, MAE seems more frequent with SCN1A (9% versus 4%). Only one JME

TABLE 8–2. Analysis of four of the GEFS+ families associated with a SCN1A mutation

SCN1A mutation	R1648H (Refs. 2,12)	T875M (Refs. 11,12)	W1204R (Ref. 7)	D188V (Refs. 1,6,25)	All	%
Phenotype(s)	GEFS+	GEFS+	GEFS+	GEFS+		
N affected and mutation	13	11	5	13	42	100
Total with FS	9	11	4	11	35	83
FS only	2	3	1	1	7	17
FS and epilepsy	7	8	3	10	28	67
FS+	6	7	2	9	24	57
Total with epilepsy	11	8	4	12	35	83
Epilepsy only	4		1	2	7	17
Absence seizures	2	3	1	4	9	21
GTC seizures	10	4	3	10	27	64
Myoclonic seizures	1		2	1	4	9
Atonic seizures		2	1	2	5	12
CAE and JAE						0
MAE	0	2	1	1	4	9
SMEI						0
JME			1			2
Partial seizures/epilepsy	1	1			3	7
Unclassified			1	2	3	7

Same legend as in Table 8–1. JME, juvenile myoclonic epilepsy.

case was reported in association with a *SCN1A* mutation (7). SMEI was not observed in the typical GEFS$^+$ families associated with *SCN1A* mutations, which contrasts with the findings made in *de novo* cases where a high frequency of *de novo SCN1A* mutations is found (27), often leading to truncated proteins. Interestingly, some mutations are not *de novo*, but transmitted by asymptomatic or mildly affected parents (28). Moreover, these mutations do not always lead to truncated proteins. These findings are consistent with the notion that SMEI may be part of an extended GEFS$^+$ spectrum (5). In families carrying a *GABRG2* mutation, only one individual had this severe myoclonic epilepsy phenotype (4). Regarding *de novo* patients, the implication of the *GABRG2* gene was found in one single individual in a series of 22 (29), with a nonsense mutation, and in none of another series of 53 subjects whose results were negative for *SCN1A* mutations (30).

In conclusion, myoclonic seizures were observed in approximately 8% of the patients from the GEFS$^+$ families harboring a *SCN1A* or *GABRG2* mutation, including patients with FS or FS$^+$ and myoclonic seizures, as well as patients presenting a well-defined syndrome like MAE or SMEI. These figures are consistent with the prevalence of myoclonic seizures in GEFS$^+$ families, in general, regardless of their genetic background, another gene, such as *SCN1B*, or the absence of any of the genes identified so far. This percentage may not be, in fact, very different from the prevalence of myoclonic seizures in the general population with epilepsy. Taking into account, however, the fact that GEFS$^+$, in spite of the presence of partial epilepsy phenotypes (1;2;16), remains predominantly a context of generalized seizures or syndromes, a relative higher prevalence of myoclonic seizures would be expected. Therefore, the gene mutations found in the typical GEFS$^+$ pedigrees so far do not seem to contribute strongly to the specific generation of myoclonic seizures.

REFERENCES

1. Scheffer IE, Berkovic SF. Generalized epilepsy with febrile seizures plus: a genetic disorder with heterogeneous clinical phenotypes. *Brain* 1997;120:479–490.

2. Baulac S, Gourfinkel-An I, Picard F, et al. A second locus for familial generalized epilepsy with febrile seizures plus maps to chromosome 2q21-q23. *Am J Hum Genet* 1999;65:1078–1085.

3. Singh R, Scheffer IE, Crossland K, et al. Generalized epilepsy with febrile seizures plus: a common childhood-onset genetic epilepsy syndrome. *Ann Neurol* 1999;45:75–81.

4. Harkin LA, Bowser DN, Dibbens LM, et al. Truncation of the GABAA-receptor gamma2 subunit in a family with generalized epilepsy with febrile seizures plus. *Am J Hum Genet* 2001;17:70.

5. Singh R, Andermann E, Whitehouse WPA, et al. Severe myoclonic epilepsy of infancy: Extended spectrum of GEFS$^+$? *Epilepsia* 2001;42:837–844.

6. Wallace RH, Scheffer IE, Barnett S, et al. Neuronal sodium-channel alpha1-subunit mutations in generalized epilepsy with febrile seizures plus. *Am J Hum Genet* 2001;68:859–865.

7. Escayg A, Heils A, MacDonald BT, et al. A novel SCN1A mutation associated with generalized epilepsy with febrile seizures plus- and prevalence of variants in patients with epilepsy. *Am J Hum Genet* 2001;68:866–873.

8. Wallace RH, Wang DW, Singh R, et al. Febrile seizures and generalized epilepsy associated with a mutation in the Na$^+$-channel beta1 subunit gene SCN1B. *Nature Genet* 1998;19:366–370.

9. Meadows LS, Malhotra J, Loukas A, et al. Functional and biochemical analysis of a sodium channel beta1 subunit mutation responsible for generalized epilepsy with febrile seizures plus type 1. *J Neurosci* 2002;22:10699–10709.

10. Wallace RH, Scheffer IE, Parasivam G, et al. Generalized epilepsy with febrile seizures plus: Mutation of the sodium channel subunit SCN1B. *Neurology* 2002;58:1426–1429.

11. Moulard B, Guipponi M, Chaigne D, et al. Identification of a new locus for generalized epilepsy with febrile seizures plus (GEFS$^+$) on chromosome 2q24-q33. *Am J Hum Genet* 1999;65:1396–1400.

12. Escayg A, MacDonald BT, Meisler MH, et al. Mutations of SCN1A, encoding a neuronal sodium channel, in two families with GEFS$^+$2. *Nature Genet* 2000;24:343–345.

13. Ito M, Nagafuji H, Okazawa H, et al. Autosomal dominant epilepsy with febrile seizures plus with missense mutations of the sodium-channel alpha 1 subunit gene, SCN1A. *Epilepsy Res* 2002;48:15–23.

14. Cossette P, Loukas A, Lafreniere RG, et al. Functional characterization of the D188V mutation in neuronal voltage-gated sodium channel causing generalized epilepsy with febrile seizures plus (GEFS). *Epilepsy Res* 2003;53:107–117.

15. Sugawara T, Mazaki-Miyazaki E, Ito M, et al. Nav1.1 mutations cause febrile seizures associated with afebrile partial seizures. *Neurology* 2001;28:703–705.

16. Abou-Khalil B, Ge Q, Desai R, et al. Partial and generalized epilepsy with febrile seizures plus and a novel SCN1A mutation. *Neurology* 2001;57:2265–2272.

17. Sugawara T, Tsurubuchi Y, Agarwala KL, et al. A missense mutation of the Na$^+$ channel alpha II subunit gene Na(v)1.2 in a patient with febrile and afebrile seizures causes channel dysfunction. *Proc Natl Acad Sci USA* 2001;98:10515.

18. Tammaro P, Conti F, Moran O. Modulation of sodium current in mammalian cells by an epilepsy-correlated beta-1 subunit mutation. *Biochem Biophys Res Commun* 2002;291:1095–1101.

19. Alekov A, Rahman MM, Mitrovic N, et al. A sodium channel mutation causing epilepsy in man exhibits subtle defects in fast inactivation and activation in vitro. *J Physiol* 2000;3:533–539.

20. Alekow AK, Rahman MM, Mitrovic N, et al. Enhanced inactivation and acceleration of activation of the sodium channel associated with epilepsy in man. *Eur J Neurosci* 2001;13:2171–2176.

21. Spampanato J, Escayg A, Meisler MH, et al. Functional effects of two voltage-gated sodium channel mutations that cause generalized epilepsy with febrile seizures plus type 2. *J Neurosci* 2001;21:7481–7490.

22. Baulac S, Huberfeld G, Gourfinkel-An I, et al. First genetic evidence of GABAA receptor dysfunction in epilepsy: A mutation in the gamma2 subunit gene. *Nat Genet* 2001;28:46–48.

23. Wallace RH, Marini C, Petrou S, et al. Mutant GABAA receptor gamma2-subunit in childhood absence epilepsy and febrile seizures. *Nat Genet* 2001;28:49–52.

24. Kananura C, Haug K, Sander T, et al. A splice-site mutation in *GABRG2* associated with childhood absence epilepsy and febrile convulsions. *Arch Neurol* 2002;59:1137–1141.

25. Lopes-Cendes I, Scheffer IE, Berkovic SF, et al. A new locus for generalized epilepsy with febrile seizures plus maps to chromosome 2. *Am J Hum Genet* 2000;66:698–701.

26. Marini C, Harkin LA, Wallace RH, et al. Childhood absence epilepsy and febrile seizures: a family with a GABA(A) receptor mutation. *Brain* 2003;126:230–240.

27. Sugawara T, Mazaki-Miyazaki E, Fukushima K, et al. Frequent mutations of SCN1A in severe myoclonic epilepsy in infancy. *Neurology* 2002;58:1122–1124.

28. Nabbout R, Gennaro E, Dalla Bernardina B, et al. Spectrum of SCN1A mutations in severe myoclonic epilepsy of infancy. *Neurology* 2003;60(12):1961–1967.

29. Fukuma G, Oguni H, Shirasaka Y, et al. Genetic abnormalities in core severe myoclonic epilepsy of infancy (SMEI) and borderline SMEI (SMEB). *Epilepsia* 2003;44 [Suppl 8]:50 (abstr.).

30. Madia F, Gennaro E, Cecconi M, et al. No evidence of GABRG2 mutations in severe myoclonic epilepsy of infancy. *Epilepsy Res* 2003;53:196–200.

9

Benign Myoclonic Epilepsy in Infancy

Charlotte Dravet* and Michelle Bureau*

*Centre Saint-Paul-Hôpital Henri Gastaut, Marseille, France

INTRODUCTION

The syndrome of benign myoclonic epilepsy in infancy (BMEI) was not clearly identified before the first description in seven infants in 1981 (1). In this article, it was defined as the occurrence of myoclonic seizures (MS) without other seizure types, except rare simple febrile seizures (FS), in the first 3 years of life in normal infants. These MS were easily controlled by a simple treatment and remitted during childhood. The psychomotor development remained normal and no severe psychologic consequences were observed. Many other cases have been published since. BMEI was classified among the generalized idiopathic epilepsies in the 1989 international classification (2). Several authors have described cases with reflex MS, triggered by noise or contact, and have proposed distinguishing two separate entities, the second one being named *Reflex myoclonic epilepsy in infancy* (3). We do not think this distinction is necessary, and we will describe all the cases as BMEI.

To our knowledge, there are, at present, 115 cases published in the literature, of which 95 correspond to the classic description (4–21) and 20 were reported as *reflex* BMEI (3,22–28). We now have five new cases, of which four have associated spontaneous and reflex seizures, making a total of 120. One also must mention that in the first description, the onset was before 3 years of age, whereas in the following reports some cases have a later onset, up to 4 years 8 months (15). That means the same type of epilepsy may appear at different ages, but tends to be more frequent in some periods (29).

GENERAL BACKGROUND

Epidemiology

According to the few available epidemiological data, BMEI seems to represent less than 1% of all the epilepsies (30 and unpublished data from the Centre Saint-Paul, 1999), 2% of all idiopathic generalized epilepsies (unpublished data from the Centre Saint-Paul, 1997), 1.3%, and 1.72% of epilepsies, which begin in the first year of life (14,19), around 2% of epilepsies, which begin in the first 3 years of life (4), and 0.39% of epilepsies which begin in the first 6 years of life (12).

Sex

When the sex is mentioned, it appears that boys outnumber girls: 62 vs. 34.

Genetics

Genetics of BMEI are unknown. Cases are rare and no family cases of BMEI have been described. A family history of epilepsy or febrile seizures (FS) was present in 44% of 88 cases. In 78 cases, the rate of FS in the family was 17% and the rate of epilepsy 27%. The epilepsy type found in relatives is difficult to assess. In ten cases, it was probably an idiopathic epilepsy. In the case described by Arzimanoglou et al. (13) the proband was the second of two brothers and the oldest was affected by a typical epilepsy with myoclonic-astatic seizures (EMAS, Doose syndrome). In the family of the patient described by Biondi et al. (8), other members had dubious epilepsy. Sleep EEGs were obtained for the father and his two sisters and demonstrated brief bursts of generalized spike-waves. In one of our patients (unpublished case), the maternal aunt suffered from myoclonic jerks at adolescence, but the diagnosis of juvenile myoclonic epilepsy was not established.

Personal History

Most patients do not have any pathologic history prior to the onset of the MS. Only two (1.9%) had an associated disease: Down's syndrome (10) and hyperinsulinic diabetes (5). One bleeding during pregnancy (15) and one cesarean birth (22) were mentioned, and Badinand-Hubert et al. (7), indicated that three patients presented with "neurological or neuropsychological syndromes" without precision.

However, the occurrence of FS is not uncommon: 20 patients among 81 (25%). They were always simple, usually rare (one or two), and were observed before the onset of the myoclonias and before initiation of treatment (15 cases). One single study (17) reported the description by the parents of infrequent, generalized afebrile seizures, at the early onset or during drug withdrawal, never observed by professionals. The authors believed they were repeated MS.

CLINICAL AND ELECTROENCEPHALOGRAM MANIFESTATIONS

The age at onset is usually between 4 months and 3 years. An earlier onset is uncommon. A later onset was reported, at 4 years 9 months (15) and at 3 years 9 months (17).

Initially, the MS are brief, often rare, involving the upper limbs and the head, and rarely the lower limbs. In babies, they may be barely noticeable and the parents sometimes have difficulty in determining their exact onset and their frequency. They often speak of "spasms" or "head nodding." Later on, their frequency increases.

Video-EEG and polygraphic recordings have enabled us to make a precise analysis of these seizures. They are more or less massive myoclonic jerks, involving the axis of the body and the limbs, provoking a head drop and an upward-outward movement of the upper limbs, with flexion of the lower limbs, and, sometimes, a rolling of the eyeballs. Their intensity varies from one child to the other and from one attack to another in the same child. The most severe forms cause a sudden projection of the objects held in the hands, and, sometimes, a fall. The mildest forms provoke only brief forward movement of the head, or, even, a simple closure of the eyes. As a rule, the seizures are very brief (1–3 s), although they may be longer, especially in older children, consisting of pseudorhythmically repeated jerks lasting no more than 5 to 10 s. They occur several times a day at irregular and unpredictable times. Unlike infantile spasms, they do not occur in long series. They are not favored by awakening, but rather by drowsiness. In some patients, they can be triggered by intermittent photic stimulation (IPS). In the patients with reflex BMEI, they are triggered by a sudden noise or a sudden contact. The state of consciousness is difficult to assess in isolated seizures. Only when they are repeated is there a slight impairment of consciousness without interruption of activity. The patient reported by Zafeiriou et al. (28) presented reflex myoclonic seizures of a longer duration (up to 5 s) with eyelid myoclonias and an absence component. This seizure type was also reported by Prats-Vinas et al. (21) in three of their eight patients. We never observed the sudden brief vocalization reported by Lin et al. (17), ascribed by the authors to the involvement of the diaphragm and/or the abdominal muscles producing an expiratory noise. In reflex BMEI, the myoclonus is elicitable both in wakefulness and in sleep, with a threshold lower in stage I and increasing gradually during the slower stages (3). No REM sleep was recorded and tested in patients with reflex MS.

As the development continues normally, parents and pediatricians tend not to consider these movements as pathologic events.

When an EEG is performed, it can be normal on awakening if no myoclonic fit is recorded. However, myoclonias are always associated with an EEG discharge. Polygraphic recordings demonstrate that the myoclonias are accompanied by a discharge of fast generalized spike-waves or polyspike-waves at more than 3 Hz, lasting the same time as the myoclonias (Fig. 9–1). This discharge is more or less regular and can start in the two anterior areas and the vertex. Myoclonias are brief (1–3 s) and usually isolated. The myoclonic jerk may be followed by a brief atonia, sometimes, after the attack. There is a voluntary movement, visible as a normal muscular contraction. In only one patient did we observe the association of myoclonias in the deltoid muscle with a pure atonia in the neck muscles. During drowsiness, there is an enhancement of the myoclonias; they usually, but not always, disappear during slow sleep. The MS triggered by tactile and acoustic stimuli have the same characteristics. Ricci et al. (3) noted that the initial manifestation generally, but not always, consisted of a blink, followed 40–80 msec later by the first myoclonic arm jerk. After a myoclonic attack there was a refractory period, lasting 20 to 30 s to 1 to 2 min, during which sudden stimuli did not provoke attacks, even when the startle reaction was easily elicited. IPS can also provoke MS (10,11,15,17,21).

The interictal EEG is normal for the child's age. Spontaneous spike-wave discharges are rare; some slow waves may be found over the central areas. Surprisingly, the patient with reflex BMEI reported by Kurian and King (27) had an awake EEG with numerous discharges of spike-waves and polyspike-waves without clinical correlate. IPS does not provoke spike-waves without concomitant myoclonia at the onset. Nap sleep recordings have shown a normal organization of sleep; generalized spike-wave discharges may occur during rapid eye movement (REM) sleep (Fig. 9–1).

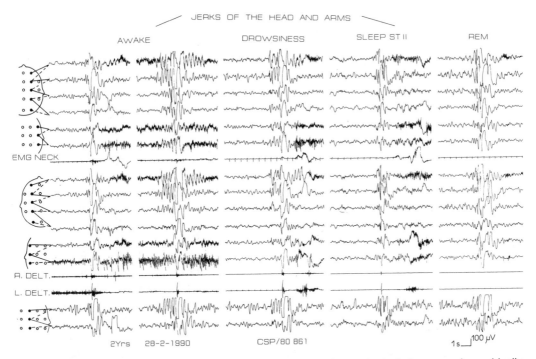

FIG. 9–1. In a 2-year-old girl, before any treatment, several myoclonic jerks are polygraphically recorded when awake, persisting during drowsiness, and attenuated during sleep, stage II. They are accompanied by generalized spike-wave, sometimes preceded by spike-wave localized in the anterior regions. The same type of generalized discharge appears during REM without concomitant clinical event. R DELT: right deltoid muscle; L DELT: left deltoid muscle. (From Dravet C, Bureau M, Roger J. Benign myoclonic epilepsy in infants. In: Roger J, Bureau M, Dravet C, Dreifuss FE, Perret A, Wolf P, eds. *Epileptic syndromes in infancy, childhood and adolescence, 2nd ed.* London, Paris: John Libbey, 1992:67–74. With permission.)

EVOLUTION AND TREATMENT

No other type of seizure is observed in children with BMEI, even if they are left untreated (for up to 8.5 years in one of our patients), particularly no absence or tonic seizure. Clinical examination is normal. Interictal myoclonus was described only by one author (15) in six patients. By reviewing our own patients, we found a mild interictal myoclonus in two, revealed by polygraphic recordings.

Many patients were not investigated, but when CT scan and MRI were performed they were normal (43 patients).

The outcome seems to depend on an early diagnosis and treatment. Myoclonias are easily controlled by Valproate (VPA) alone and the child may then develop regularly, according to the normal milestones. If left untreated, the patient continues to experience myoclonic attacks and this may lead to impaired psychomotor development and behavior disturbances.

The therapeutic modalities are known more or less precisely in 91 patients. It consisted of a monotherapy in 81 patients, polytherapy in 7, and no therapy in 3. Monotherapies were with VPA in 76, with phenobarbital (PB) in 2, with clobazam (CLB) in 2, and with nitrazepam (NTZ) in 1. Seventy one (88%) became seizure-free (67 with VPA, 2 with PB, and 2 with CLB). Nine patients with VPA had a seizure reduction, of which four became seizure-free after addition of PB, clonazepam (CZP) or CLB (15). We do not know the evolution for the five others. One patient with NTZ also had a seizure reduction, followed by a complete control after addition of VPA. Six patients (11) received bitherapy with primidone (PRM), and ethosuximide (ESM), of which only one became seizure-free. In the other five, the addition of VPA followed by VPA monotherapy allowed complete control. Only in one patient did myoclonic seizures persist, in spite of various polytherapies and even a ketogenic diet (21). Finally, three patients presenting with reflex seizures did not receive any treatment and became seizure-free spontaneously (3). On the whole, 85 patients (93%) became seizure free.

These data confirm that VPA is the drug of first choice in BMEI. However, the treatment must be monitored using plasma-level assessments because an irregular intake can lead to a relapse and falsely mimic a drug-resistant epilepsy. Lin et al. (17) gave a very detailed study of the treatment in their patients. They also underlined the necessity of this monitoring and of the use of high doses at the onset (30–40 mg/k) to obtain levels more than 100 mg/l, 3 hours after the morning intake, in some patients. The daily dose was reduced to usual therapeutic plasma levels (50–100 mg/l) after seizures were controlled.

LONG-TERM OUTCOME
AND PROGNOSIS

The length of follow-up is known in 72 cases, lasting from 6 months to 28 years, equal to or more than five years in 57. The age at follow-up is shown in Fig. 9–2.

In all these cases, MS disappeared. Their duration is known in 62 cases (Fig. 9–3). In most patients they lasted less than 1 year. The longest duration (from 4 years 10 months to 6 years 4 months) was observed only in the first publication, before the recognition of the syndrome and its treatment (10). Progressively, while the duration of follow-up is longer, the number of patients who have other seizure types after the end of the myoclonic seizures increases. Presently they are 13 to be reported among the 72 cases with a known follow-up (18%). The occurrence of rare generalized tonic-clonic seizures (GTCS) was reported in 11 patients, without associated MS. Three of them had GTCS during drug withdrawal, between 11 and 15 years, again controlled by VPA: we do not have other information in one case (15); in the second, VPA was definitively withdrawn later (15). In the third case, VPA was continued because of persisting sensitivity to IPS and eye closure (10). In another patient (17), VPA was tentatively withdrawn very early, at 4 years 9 months. A new control was obtained and VPA again stopped without relapse. For the other seven patients, GTCS occurred between 9 and 16 years, but we do not have further details (11,18,21). Two other patients, after the drug withdrawal and a free interval, presented absences, respectively, at 10 and 11 years (21). They were described as "petit mal" for the first patient

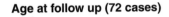

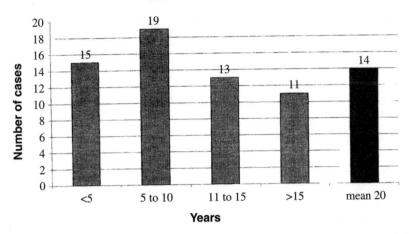

FIG. 9–2. Age at the follow-up. (From Dravet C, Bureau M. Benign myoclonic epilepsy in infancy. In: Roger J, Bureau M, Dravet Ch, Genton P, Tassinari CA, Wolf P. eds. *Epileptic syndromes in infancy, childhood and adolescence.* London: John Libbey, 2002:69–79. With permission.)

and as absences with marked eyelid myoclonia for the second one. The latter were completely controlled by ESM. Due to a photomyoclonic response on the EEG, ESM was substituted at 12 years by VPA and was stopped at 17 years, without relapse, during the following 3 years.

Among the 91 patients whose treatment is known, it was stopped in 35 patients aged more than 6 years and in one aged 4. It is still present in six patients more than 6 years, because of a persisting photosensitivity in two (10), of one GTCS during withdrawal in one (15), and for an unknown reason in three (15). It is still present in 16 patients aged less than 6 years. Three patients aged less than 6 years remained without treatment (3). In 30 patients, we have no information.

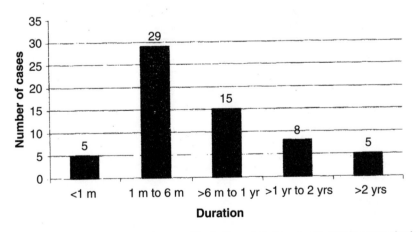

FIG. 9–3. Duration of the myoclonic seizures. (From Dravet C, Bureau M. Benign myoclonic epilepsy in infancy. In: Roger J, Bureau M, Dravet Ch, Genton P, Tassinari CA, Wolf P. eds. *Epileptic syndromes in infancy, childhood and adolescence.* London: John Libbey, 2002:69–79. With permission.)

TABLE 9–1. *EEG at follow-up (55 Cases)*

Authors and number of cases	Normal	Spontaneous generalized spike-wave	Photosensitivity	Focal abnormalities awake	Sleep abnormalities
Salas Puig et al. (1 case)	1	/	/	/	None
Todt and Müller (14 cases)	8	6	/	/	?
Giovanardi Rossi et al. (11 cases)	2[a]	7	2	2	?
Deonna and Despland (1 case)	1[a]	/	/	/	?
Revol et al. (1 case)	1	/	/	/	None
Cuvelier et al. (1 case)	1[b]	/	/	/	?
Lin et al. (10 cases)	8	/	2	/	?
Dravet et al. (5 cases)	5[c]	/	1	1	5 (Focal)
Ribacoba and Salas Puig (1 case)	/	/	1	/	1 (Generalized)
Total	27	13	6	3	6

From Dravet C, Bureau M. Benign myoclonic epilepsy in infancy. In: Roger J, Bureau M, Dravet Ch, Genton P, Tassinari CA, Wolf P. eds. *Epileptic syndromes in infancy, childhood and adolescence.* London: John Libbey, 2002:69–79. With permission.
[a] Follow-up less than 3 years in 1 patient.
[b] Follow-up less than 3 years.
[c] Follow-up less than 3 years in 2 patients.

The EEG outcome is known for 55 patients (Table 9–1). It is interesting to note that the photosensitivity can appear after the disappearance of the MS, as reported by different authors (15–17) and can persist for many years (11), even up to the adult age, after MS stops (Dravet, *unpublished cases*). At this age, it is only an EEG response without clinical correlate. Another finding is the association of focal abnormalities. They were recorded during waking in five patients (15, 17, and Dravet, *unpublished cases*). Usually they were spike-waves located in the two frontocentral and the vertex area, but they could be fron-

toparietal and frontotemporal. They disappeared during the evolution. Conversely, in other patients, they appeared during the evolution and during sleep (15) (Dravet, *unpublished cases*). They were still present, only during sleep, at the end of the follow-up in five of our patients.

On the whole, the psychological outcome is favorable and most of the patients are normal. In the 17 recently published cases (21,26–28), 14 patients (82%) are normal but no details are provided and some are still very young. The psychologic outcome is precisely known in 69 cases (Table 9–2). Fifty-seven (83%) were normal, of

TABLE 9–2. *Psychological outcome (69 Cases)*

Author, number of cases	Normal	Mild mental retardation	Mental retardation personality disorders
Salas Puig et al. (1 case)	1	\	\
Todt and Müller (14 cases)	11	3	\
Colamaria et al. (1 case)	\	1	\
Arzimanoglou et al (1 case)	1	\	\
Giovanardi et al. (11 cases)	9	2	\
Deonna and Despland (1 case)	1	\	\
Revol et al. (1 case)	1	\	\
Ricci et al. (6 cases)	6	\	\
Cuvellier et al. (1 case)	1	\	\
Lin et al. (10 cases)	9	1	\
Sarisjulis et al. (6 cases)	6	\	\
Dravet et al. (16 cases)	11	3	2
Total	57	10	2

From Dravet C, Bureau M. Benign myoclonic epilepsy in infancy. In: Roger J, Bureau M, Dravet Ch, Genton P, Tassinari CA, Wolf P. eds. *Epileptic syndromes in infancy, childhood and adolescence.* London: John Libbey, 2002:69–79. With permission.

whom 38 were aged 5 years or more. Ten (14%) presented with a mild retardation and attended a specialized school, but none were institutionalized. Among them, the patient reported by Colamaria et al. (5) had several hypoglycemic convulsions and motor disturbances in the first weeks of life. One of our patients is less than 2 years and can still improve, as observed in another case (31). Two others had MS until the ages of 6 and 8 years without treatment. We do not have details about the others. Two patients (3%) had a cognitive deficit and personality disturbances. The first had a Down syndrome and a strong photosensitivity. The second had MS until 5 years, with a sensitivity to IPS and to eye closure. The psychotic disturbance appeared around 10 years of age and progressively worsened. Prats-Vinas et al. (21) reported one patient who suffered from an acute mania, perhaps related to a prolonged VPA administration.

This psychologic outcome partly depends on an early diagnostic permitting appropriate treatment and reassurance of the family about the future. The early occurrence of epilepsy often generates great anxiety and leads to incorrect educational attitudes. However, there are also other factors related to an associated pathology or to an abnormal family structure and a disturbed mother–infant relationship. However, in some cases, the etiology of the mental retardation is unclear and could be due to the neurobiologic process responsible for epilepsy.

These findings confirm the usual good prognosis of BMEI. Attacks provoked by noise or contact were more easily controlled than spontaneous ones. Patients with reflex BMEI always had a normal psychomotor evolution, but their follow-up is relatively short. Conversely, photosensitivity was more difficult to control and persisted several years after the end of seizures.

DIFFERENTIAL DIAGNOSIS

When myoclonias start in the first year of life, the other diagnosis that comes to mind is that of *cryptogenic infantile spasms (IS)*. IS are clinically different from benign myoclonias: they are more intense, involving a strong flexion (or extension) of the whole body, which is never observed in

BMEI; isolated, sporadic spasms are always associated with serial spasms in the same infant; long serial spasms are favored by awakening. Polygraphic recordings of IS show a typical pattern of a brief tonic contraction, well-described by Fusco and Vigevano (32), rarely a prolonged myoclonia. The ictal EEG is not a fast generalized polyspike-waves. It is variable: sudden interruption of hypsarrhythmia by a flattening with or without superimposed fast rhythms, large slow wave followed by a flattening, or even no visible change. The occurrence of IS is associated with behavioral changes, poor quality of contact, and a slowing down of psychomotor acquisitions leading to arrest and regression. The interictal EEGs are always abnormal, demonstrating either a true hypsarrhythmia or a modified hypsarrhythmia or focal abnormalities; they never show the isolated or brief bursts of bilateral synchronous spike-waves as in BMEI.

When both the psychomotor development and the EEG remain normal after several examinations performed during awake and sleep, seizures resembling IS must suggest the diagnosis of *benign nonepileptic myoclonus* (33). In these patients, even the ictal EEG is normal (34,35).

In the first year of life, *severe myoclonic epilepsy of infancy* (SMEI) could be evoked, but it always begins with long and repeated febrile convulsive seizures. Exceptionally, they can be immediately preceded by myoclonic attacks, more often focal. They are drug-resistant and associated with other seizure types. The psychomotor development becomes retarded during the second year of life (36).

When myoclonias begin after the end of the first year of life, the diagnosis of a *cryptogenic Lennox–Gastaut syndrome* (LGS) may come to mind. In LGS (37), seizures are mainly not myoclonic, but myoclonic-atonic, or purely atonic, or more often tonic, leading to sudden falls and injuries. Their polygraphic expression is heterogeneous and the ictal EEG is either a recruiting rhythm or a flattening, or a high slow wave, followed by runs of low-voltage rapid rhythms. Interictal EEGs can be normal at the very onset and the typical diffuse slow spike-wave discharges may appear progressively. The typical electroclinical features during sleep can be delayed in time. The diagnosis is based upon the rapid association of different types of seizures, such as atypical absences and axial tonic seizures, the constant impairment of behavior and learning, and the lack of efficacy of antiepileptic drugs.

If myoclonic seizures remain isolated or are associated with GTCS, the diagnosis of *myoclonic-astatic epilepsy of early childhood* (EMAS) must be entertained, although the onset of myoclonic-astatic seizures in this syndrome is rare before the age of 3 years (38). There are two essential differences: (a) the first is the clinical aspect of the seizures, which always consist of falls in EMAS, while falls are rare in BMEI, and which are combined with other types of seizures, particularly status of minor seizures with stupor, which are never observed in BMEI (29); and (b) the EEG features are also different: spike-waves and polyspike-waves are more numerous, grouped in long bursts, and associated with a typical theta rhythm over the centroparietal areas. However, some cases, included by Doose, should probably be classified as BMEI. In the same way, the group studied by Delgado-Escueta et al. (39) under the name of early childhood myoclonic epilepsy (ECME) seems to include both cases of EMAS and of BMEI.

One recent study (21) emphasizes the relationship between BMEI and the *syndrome of eyelid myoclonias with absence* (40), because the authors observed eyelid myoclonias during the myoclonic seizures in three children and one of them, later on, at 10 years, had this seizure type. This evolution was not observed by other authors.

Finally, one should consider other epilepsies beginning in the first 3 years of life in which myoclonias are the main type of seizures and which have a variable prognosis. They are heterogeneous: combination of other types of seizures, constant presence of EEG focal abnormalities, previous delayed psychomotor development, and poor response to drugs. Their prognosis is uncertain (9,41).

DIAGNOSTIC WORK UP

The diagnosis work up is simple, requiring a good clinical description and repeated polygraphic video-EEG recordings in order to demonstrate the presence of MS with generalized spike-wave discharges, either spontaneous or facilitated by drowsiness, by noise, by contact, or by IPS. A sleep recording shows slight activation of discharges, without change in morphology, without appearance of rapid rhythms and focal abnormalities. Neuroimaging can be useful to confirm the absence of brain lesions, but is not mandatory when the symptomatology is typical. Neuropsychologic assessment is more useful to check the good psychomotor development and to follow the evolution. Biologic investigations can be necessary in case of associated symptoms evoking another disease.

MANAGEMENT

The first intention treatment is VPA in monotherapy, which must be applied as soon as possible. The use of solution is preferable to that of syrup to avoid rejection by the infant. Plasma levels must be monitored carefully. A daily dose of 30 mg/kg t.i.d. is usually sufficient, but higher doses are necessary in some patients (17). VPA is also effective against possible febrile seizures. If myoclonias are not completely controlled by VPA, the addition of either a benzodiazepine (CLB or NTZ) or ESM can be proposed and the diagnostic must be reviewed. The treatment should be maintained for 3 or 4 years, after the onset, if it is well tolerated. In the cases of purely reflex seizures, drug therapy may be avoided. When it is applied it can be stopped early, but not in cases of photosensitivity. The occurrence of a generalized tonic clonic seizure at adolescence can require a new brief period of treatment at this age. The medical treatment must be associated with psychologic help to the family.

NOSOLOGIC PLACE

Before our princeps publication (1), cases similar to those reported here were described by several authors within the confusing frame of "myoclonic epilepsies" (42–46). In their taxometric classification, Loiseau et al. (47) identified a "group C" corresponding to the Aicardi "cryptogenic myoclonic epilepsy." Jeavons (48) gave the name "myoclonic epilepsy of childhood" to a similar type of epilepsy, beginning at a later age (3 years). Gastaut (49) confirmed our description. In 1989, the International League Against Epilepsy (ILAE) included this name in the idiopathic generalized epilepsies (2). However, in a study of 40 cases, Aicardi and Levy-Gomez (50) did not recognize a group with a constant favorable outcome and Lombroso (51) indicated that he found no fundamental difference between BMEI and severe myoclonic epilepsy. From 1989, all the series concerning childhood epilepsies now include the BMEI syndrome (30), which means that the syndrome is well recognizable. We must also mention the report of a *familial infantile myoclonic epilepsy* in a large kindred with autosomal recessive inheritance (52). The affected patients present with clinical and EEG characteristics that could evoke those observed in BMEI, as well as in SMEI, but are different from them. In this family, the locus was mapped to chromosome 16p13 (53). The authors discuss the possible relationship between the various forms of idiopathic epilepsies with myoclonias in children and suggest investigating a linkage to chromosome 16 in familial cases of infantile myoclonic epilepsies, including BMEI.

In practice, the diagnosis of BMEI must be restricted to those patients fulfilling the following criteria:

- brief MS, spontaneous or provoked by noise or contact,
- onset between 4 months and 3 years,
- in a previously normal child,
- not associated to other seizure types, except rare simple FS,
- in the EEGs: generalized fast spike-wave and polyspike-wave during MS, rare interictal spike-wave when awake, and
  spike-wave enhanced by drowsiness and slow sleep, sometimes by IPS, normal background, and absence of focal discharges
- good response to VPA monotherapy.

Faced with this typical picture, if treatment is given without delay, the clinician may predict a good clinical outcome for seizures and for cognitive functions. In cases with less typical features, particularly in the presence of focal EEG discharges, the diagnosis remains dubious until a long remission is observed (19). When the onset is later than 3 years, the diagnosis may be the same (29).

We do not believe it is legitimate to separate a syndrome with reflex seizures. Considering all the cases reported, we found that the MS triggered by noise and/or contact were isolated in 14 patients, among the 24 in whom this data was available. In the other ten patients they were associated with spontaneous MS. (In one of our patients, the reflex MS were observed only during a short period at the very beginning). They had the same semiology as the spontaneous MS. The EEGs were not different, except for the absence of photosensitivity. In one case (28), the EEG showed numerous interictal spike-waves and polyspike-waves. Treatment could not always be avoided and seizure control was not obtained easily in all patients (22) (Dravet, *unpublished cases*). However, overall, it is probably the most benign form. As Ricci et al. (3) and Caraballo et al. (26), we found a higher rate of family history in our reflex BMEI: 57 vs. 39% in the whole group. Here, we want to report a peculiar case. A girl started at 6 months with MS occurring both as she drank from her bottle and spontaneously. We recorded her EEG with videopolygraphy at 1 year 6 months. During the bottle drinking, the EEG showed long bursts of spike-waves localized in the vertex and the two central areas, culminating in MS with generalized spike-waves. The MS were only controlled by high doses of VPA. She is now seizure-free and completely normal at 5 years 6 months. Deonna (54), in his review of the literature on reflex myoclonic seizures, only wonders what their relationships to BMEI are. Caraballo et al. (26) conclude that reflex BMEI may be considered either as an idiopathic stimulosensible syndrome or as a variant of the BMEI. We hypothesize that these two subgroups have a common genetic background, with modifying factors explaining their slight differences.

Obviously this syndrome belongs to the group of the idiopathic generalized epilepsies (2). It seems to be the infantile equivalent of *juvenile myoclonic epilepsy* (JME), but the two syndromes have never been observed successively in the same patient. We only know of one unpublished case in the Centre Saint-Paul population who probably started at 3 years in what has been considered as a JME later on. However, we have few data concerning the onset and it is not included in our present series. Delgado-Escueta et al. (39) did not find cases of JME in their study of 24 affected family members of early childhood myoclonic epilepsy (ECME), whereas they found 76% of other types of idiopathic generalized epilepsies. The relationship with EMAS should be investigated as suggested by the case reported by Arzimanoglou et al. (13). Moreover, Doose (38) mentioned the case of a patient with a previous EMAS who had two children. The first was affected by EMAS, but the second by a BMEI.

The last problem is that of the denomination of this syndrome. In 1981, it was legitimate to name it "benign" because of the constant disappearance of seizures and the usually good psychologic outcome. In 2001, this benignity becomes questionable when the definition given by the ILAE Commission report (55) is considered: "a benign epilepsy syndrome is a syndrome characterized by epileptic seizures that are easily treated, or require no treatment, and remit without sequelae." However, whether the cognitive and personality disorders described in rare patients are the sequelae of those with epilepsy or not is difficult to establish, given the early age of onset. In some patients the syndrome can be associated with another pathology, as it is accepted in other idiopathic and benign epilepsies, such as the benign epilepsy with centrotemporal spikes (56).

REFERENCES

1. Dravet C, Bureau M. L'épilepsie myoclonique bénigne du nourrisson. *Rev EEG Neurophysiol* 1981;11:438–444.
2. Commission on Classification and Terminology of the International League Against Epilepsy: proposal for revised classification of epilepsies and epileptic syndromes. *Epilepsia* 1989;30:389–399.
3. Ricci S, Cusmai R, Fusco L, et al. Reflex myoclonic epilepsy: A new age-dependent idiopathic epileptic syndrome related to startle reaction. *Epilepsia* 1995;36:342–348.
4. Dalla Bernardina B, Colamaria V, Capovilla G, et al. Nosological classification of epilepsies in the first three years of life. In: Nistico G, Di Perri R, Meinardi H, eds. *Epilepsy: An update on research and therapy.* New York: Liss, 1983:165–183.
5. Colamaria V, Andrighetto G, Pinelli L, et al. Iperinsulinismo, ipoglicemia ed epilessia mioclonica benigna del lattante. *Boll Lega It Epil* 1987;58/59:231–233.
6. Salas-Puig J, Ramos Polo E, Macarron Vincente J, et al. Benign myoclonic epilepsy of infancy. Case report. *Acta Paediatr Scand* 1990;79:1128–1130.
7. Badinand-Hubert N, Revol M, Isnard H, et al. About 9 observations of benign myoclonic epilepsy of infancy. *Abstracts book VII Riunione congiunta delle Leghe Italiana-Francese-Portughese e Spagnola contro l'Epilessia* 1990;Taormina 12-15 maggio:106.
8. Biondi R, Sofia V, Tarascone M, et al. Epilessia mioclonica benigna dell'infanzia: contibuto clinico. *Boll Lega It Epil* 1991;74:93–94.
9. Dravet C. Les épilepsies myocloniques bénignes du nourrisson. *Epilepsies* 1990;2:95–101.
10. Dravet C, Bureau M, Roger J. Benign myoclonic epilepsy in infants. In: Roger J, Bureau M, Dravet C, Dreifuss FE, Perret A, Wolf P. eds. *Epileptic syndromes in infancy, childhood and adolescence.* 2nd ed. London, Paris: John Libbey, 1992:67–74.
11. Todt H, Müller D. The therapy of benign myoclonic epilepsy in infants. In: Degen R, Dreifuss FE, eds. *Epilepsy Research, Suppl 6. The benign localized and generalized epilepsies in early childhood.* Amsterdam: Elsevier Science, 1992:137–139.
12. Ohtsuka Y, Ohno S, Oka E, et al. Classification of epilepsies and epileptic syndromes of childhood according to the 1989 ILAE classification. *J Epil* 1993;6:272–276.
13. Arzimanoglou A, Prudent M, Salefranque F. Epilepsie myoclono-astatique et épilepsie myoclonique bénigne du nourrisson dans une même famille: quelques réflexions sur la classification des épilepsies. *Epilepsies* 1996; 8:307–315.
14. Caraballo R, Cersósimo R, Galicchio S, et al. Epilepsies during the first year of life. *Rev Neurol* (Spanish) 1997; 25:1521–1524.
15. Giovanardi Rossi P, Parmeggiani A, Posar A, et al. Benign myoclonic epilepsy: long-term follow-up of 11 new cases. *Brain Develop* 1997;19:473–479.
16. Ribacoba Montero R, Salas Puig J. Benign myoclonic epilepsy in childhood. A case report. *Rev Neurol* (in Spanish) 1997;25:1210–1212.
17. Lin YP, Itomi K, Takada H, et al. Benign myoclonic epilepsy in infants: video-EEG features and long-term follow-up. *Neuropediatrics* 1998;29:268–271.
18. Mukhim KI, Petrukhin AS, Pylaeva OA, et al. Benign myoclonic epilepsy in infancy. *Zh Nevrol Psikiatr Im SS Korsakova (Russ)* 1999;99:4–8.
19. Sarisjulis N, Gamboni B, Plouin P, et al. Diagnosing idiopathic/cryptogenic epilepsy syndromes in infancy. *Arch Dis Child* 2000;82:226–230.
20. Dravet C, Bureau M. Benign myoclonic epilepsy of infancy. In: Meinardi H, ed. *Handbook of clinical neurology 73: The epilepsies. Part II.* Amsterdam: Elsevier Science, 2000:137–142.
21. Prats-Vinas JM, Garaizar C, Ruiz-Espinoza C. Benign myoclonic epilepsy in infant. *Rev Neurol* (Spanish) 2002;34:201–204.
22. Revol M, Isnard H, Beaumanoir A, et al. Touch evoked myoclonic seizures in infancy. In: Beaumanoir A, Naquet R, Gastaut H, eds. *Reflex seizures and reflex epilepsies.* Genève: Médecine et Hygiène, 1989:103–105.
23. Deonna T, Despland PA. Sensory-evoked (touch) idiopathic myoclonic epilepsy of infancy. In:

Beaumanoir A, Naquet R, Gastaut H, eds. *Reflex seizures and reflex epilepsies*. Genève: Médecine et Hygiène, 1989:99–102.

24. Cuvellier JC, Lamblin MD, Vallée L, et al. Epilepsie myoclonique bénigne réflexe du nourrisson. *Arch Pediatr* 1997;8:755–758.

25. Fernandez Lorente J, Pastor J, Carbonell J, et al. Reflex benign myoclonic epilepsy of childhood. A propos of a new case. *Rev Neurol* (Spanish) 1999;29:39–42.

26. Caraballo R, Cassar L, Monges S, et al. Reflex myoclonic epilepsy in infancy: a new reflex epilepsy syndrome or a variant of benign myoclonic epilepsy in infancy. *Rev Neurol* (Spanish) 2003;36:429–432.

27. Kurian MA, King MD. An unusual case of benign reflex myoclonic epilepsy of infancy. *Neuropediatrics* 2003;34:152–155.

28. Zafeiriou D, Vargiami E, Kontopoulos E. Reflex myoclonic epilepsy in infancy: A benign age-dependent idiopathic startle epilepsy. *Epileptic Disord* 2003;5:121–122.

29. Guerrini R, Dravet Ch, Gobbi G, et al. Idiopathic generalized epilepsies with myoclonus in infancy and childhood . In: Malafosse A, Genton P, Hirsch E, Marescaux C, Broglin D, Bernasconi R, eds. *Idiopathic generalized epilepsies: clinical, experimental, and genetic aspects*. London, Paris: John Libbey, 1994:267–280.

30. Loiseau P, Duché B, Loiseau J. Classification of epilepsies and epileptic syndromes in two different samples of patients. *Epilepsia* 1991;32:303–309.

31. Cassé-Perrot C, Dravet C, Genton P. Epilepsie myoclonique sévère, épilepsie myoclonique bénigne, épilepsie myoclono-astatique (Doose): étude neuropsychologique (résultats préliminaires). *Epilepsies* 1997;9:191–194.

32. Fusco L, Vigevano F. Ictal clinical and electroencephalographic findings of spasms in West syndrome. *Epilepsia* 1993;34:671–678.

33. Lombroso CT, Fejerman N. Benign myoclonus of early infancy. *Ann Neurol* 1977;1:138–143.

34. Dravet C, Giraud N, Bureau M, et al. Benign myoclonus of early infancy or benign non-epileptic spasms. *Neuropediatrics* 1986;17:33–38.

35. Pachatz C, Fusco L, Vigevano F. Benign myoclonus of early infancy. *Epileptic Disorders* 1999;1:57–61.

36. Dravet C, Bureau M, Oguni H, et al. Severe myoclonic epilepsy in infancy (Dravet syndrome). In: Roger J, Bureau M, Dravet Ch, Genton P, Tassinari CA, Wolf P. eds. *Epileptic syndromes in infancy, childhood and adolescence*. London: John Libbey, 2002:81–103.

37. Beaumanoir A, Dravet Ch. The Lennox-Gastaut syndrome. In: Roger J, Bureau M, Dravet C, Dreifuss FE, Perret A, Wolf P. eds. *Epileptic syndromes in infancy, childhood and adolescence*. 2nd ed. London, Paris: John Libbey, 1992:115–132.

38. Doose H. Myoclonic astatic epilepsy of early childhood. In: Roger J, Bureau M, Dravet C, Dreifuss FE, Perret A, Wolf P. eds. *Epileptic syndromes in infancy, childhood and adolescence,* 2nd ed. London, Paris: John Libbey, 1992:103–114.

39. Delgado-Escueta AV, Greenberg D, Weissbecker A, et al. Gene mapping in the idiopathic generalized epilepsies: Juvenile myoclonic epilepsy, childhood absence epilepsy, epilepsy with grand mal seizures, and early childhood myoclonic epilepsy. *Epilepsia* 1990;31[Suppl 3]:S19–S29.

40. Panayiotopoulos CP. Absence epilepsies. In: Engel J, Pedley TA eds. *Epilepsy. A comprehensive textbook*. Philadelphia: Lippincott-Raven, 1997:2327–2346.

41. Dravet C, Bureau M, Genton P. Benign myoclonic epilepsy of infancy: electroclinical symptomatology and differential diagnosis from the other types of generalized epilepsy in infancy. In: Degen R, Dreifuss FE, eds. *Epilepsy Research, Suppl. 6. The benign localized and generalized epilepsies in early childhood*. Amsterdam: Elsevier Science, 1992:131–135.

42. Harper JR. True myoclonic epilepsy in childhood. *Arch Dis Child* 1968;43:28–35.

43. Doose H, Gerken H, Leonardt R, Volzke E, Voltz C. Centrencephalic myoclonic astatic Petit Mal. *Neuropediatrie* 1970;2:59–78.

44. Aicardi J, Chevrie JJ. Myoclonic epilepsies of childhood. *Neuropediatrie* 1971;3:177–190.

45. Kruse R. Epilepsien des Kindesalters. In: Matthes A, Kruse R, eds. *Neuropediatrie*. Stuttgart: Georg Thieme Verlag, 1973:354–425.

46. Aicardi J. Course and prognosis of certain childhood epilepsies with predominantly myoclonic seizures. In: Wada JA, Penry JK, eds. *Advances in epileptology: The Xth Epilepsy International Symposium*. New York: Raven Press, 1980:159–163.

47. Loiseau P, Legroux M, Grimond P, et al. Taxometric classification of myoclonic epilepsies. *Epilepsia* 1974;15:1–11.

48. Jeavons PM. Nosological problems of myoclonic epilepsies in childhood and adolescence. *Develop Med Child Neurol* 1977;19:3–8.

49. Gastaut H. Individualisation des épilepsies dites "bénignes" ou "fonctionnelles" aux différents âges de la vie. *Rev EEG Neurophysiol* 1981;11:346–366.

50. Aicardi J, Levy-Gomez A. The myoclonic epilepsies of childhood. *Cleve Clin J Med* 1989;56 [Suppl. 1]:S34–S39.

51. Lombroso CT. Early myoclonic encephalopathy, early infantile epileptic encephalopathy, and benign and severe infantile myoclonic epilepsies: A critical review and personal contributions. *J Clin Neurophysiol* 1990;7:380–408.

52. De Falco FA, Majello L, Santangelo R, et al. Familial infantile myoclonic epilepsy: Clinical features in a large kindred with autosomal recessive inheritance. *Epilepsia* 2000;42:1541–1548.

53. Zara F, Gennaro E, Stabile M, et al. Mapping of a locus for a familial autosomal recessive idiopathic myoclonic epilepsy of infancy to chromosome 16p13. *Am J Hum Genet* 2000;66:1552–1557.

54. Deonna T. Reflex seizures with somatosensory precipitation. Clinical and electroencephalographic patterns and differential diagnosis, with emphasis on reflex myoclonic epilepsy of infancy. In: Zifkin BG, Andermann F, Beaumanoir A, Rowan AJ. eds. *Reflex epilepsies and reflex seizures. Advances in Neurology*, Vol 75. Philadelphia: Lippincott-Raven, 1998:193–206.

55. Engel J, Jr. A proposed diagnostic scheme for people with epileptic seizures and with epilepsy: report of the ILAE Task Force on Classification and Terminology. *Epilepsia* 2001;42:1–8.

56. Gelisse P, Genton P, Raybaud C, et al. Benign childhood epilepsy with centro-temporal spikes and hippocampal atrophy. *Epilepsia* 1999;40:1312–1315.

10

Autosomal Recessive Benign Myoclonic Epilepsy of Infancy

Federico Zara* and Fabrizio A De Falco[†]

*Laboratory of Neurogenetics, Department of Neuroscience and Rehabilitation, Institute G. Gaslini, Genova, Italy; [†]Department of Neurology, Loreto Nuovo Hospital, Napoli, Italy.

INTRODUCTION

The nosologic classification of epilepsies with myoclonic manifestations occurring in infancy and early childhood has always been difficult (1–8). In fact, myoclonic events may be non-specific manifestations occurring in a variety of epileptic disorders.

Epileptic syndromes of infancy and early childhood presenting with myoclonic manifestations include complex phenotypes characterized by different type of seizures, variable neurologic symptoms, and often a poor prognosis, such as early myoclonic encephalopathy, West syndrome, Lennox–Gastaut syndrome (LGS), severe myoclonic epilepsy of infancy (SMEI), myoclonic-astatic epilepsy (MAE), and phenotypes in which myoclonic seizures are the prominent clinical feature with absence of other types of seizures or neurologic signs, such as the benign myoclonic epilepsy of infancy (BMEI) (9).

This heterogeneous group of disorders includes symptomatic forms characterized by pre-existent brain damage, usually acquired in the prenatal or neonatal periods or in infancy and forms without evidence of brain pathology before the onset of the seizures, likely of genetic origin. Except for the SMEI, the mode of inheritance and the genetic etiology of these forms are largely unknown.

However, the clinical heterogeneity and the sporadic nature of these disorders have compli-cated their classification into homogenous syndromic entities and many cases of myoclonic epilepsy with onset in infancy remain unclassified.

Among these disorders, familial myoclonic epilepsy with onset in infancy (FIME) is a peculiar form characterized by autosomal recessive inheritance, myoclonic seizures associated to generalized tonic-clonic seizures persisting into adulthood if not controlled by an appropriate treatment, normal psychomotor development, and benign outcome (10,11) (Table 10–1).

CLINICAL FEATURES

FIME was observed in eight patients belonging to a large Italian family (Fig. 10–1). Clinical features are homogeneous among patients with slight differences in the clinical onset and occurrence of febrile seizures.

Clinical Onset

The disease could begin with afebrile generalized tonic-clonic seizures between the 4th and the 7th months of age (patients III-2 to III-5) or with myoclonic seizures between the 12th and 18th months (patients III-8, III-9, and III-10). In one patient, it began with febrile seizures at the age of 3 years (patient III-6).

TABLE 10–1. *Clinical features of eight FIME patients*

| ID | Sex | Clinical onset | | Seizures | | | EEG | Psychomotor development |
		Age (mo)	Type of seizure	MS (age)	GTCS (age)	FS (age)		
III-2	F	4	GTCS	5	4	4	Normal	Normal
III-3	F	7	GTCS	9	7	12	Polyspikes in IPS	Normal
III-4	M	5	GTCS	7	5	8	Normal	Normal
III-5	M	5	GTCS	8	5	12	Normal	Normal
III-6	F	36	FS	36	36	36	Normal	Normal
III-8	M	16	MS	16	18	—	Normal	Normal
III-9	M	12	MS	12	18	—	Left temporal abnormalities	Normal
III-10	M	12	MS	12	48	—	Polyspikes in IPS	Normal

Seizures

- Febrile seizures occurred between 5 and 36 months of age, in five affected individuals, all in branch I from the first offspring (patients III-2 to III-6).
- Myoclonic seizures (MS) represented the dominant seizure type and were present in all the affected subjects from both branches of offspring, showing the same clinical features. They appeared between 5 and 36 months of age and persisted to adulthood in all patients. Clinical features varied with age. In childhood, MS were spontaneous and could be erratic, bilateral or massive. They occurred isolated or in clusters, several times a day, and could last for many hours (sporadic myoclonic status epilepticus), with preserved consciousness, sometimes preceding a convulsive seizure. Dur-

ing adolescence, MS occurred several times a week, sometimes lasting 30 min or longer, or persisting until the appearance of generalized tonic–clonic seizures (GTCS), which marked the end of the myoclonic status. During youth, myoclonic attacks more often had a localized pattern. They were spontaneous and facilitated by fatigue or drowsiness, or induced by intense and persistent stimulation (acoustic stimuli or variations in light intensity) or by repetitive movements. MS could have onset from the hands while peeling potatoes or from the legs after long walks. One subject reported the onset of myoclonic jerks in the legs culminating in a GTCS after standing up in back of a truck while riding over rough terrain during military service. After persistent light stimulus, patients complained of involuntary rapid eyelid and eyeball movement and almost none

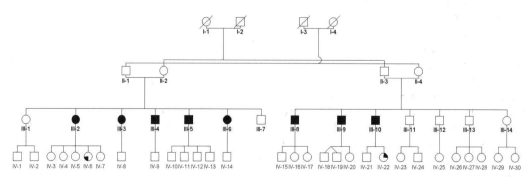

FIG. 10–1. Pedigree of the family affected by familial infantile myoclonic epilepsy of infancy. Solid symbols, affected subjects. Patient IV had idiopathic generalized epilepsy with onset in adolescence. Patient IV-22 had febrile seizures.

of the subjects tolerated intense green and thus, could not take a walk through the woods. All the subjects had learned to avoid situations triggering myoclonic jerks and recognize those attacks that preceded a generalized seizure. The trigger stimuli in our patients were unlike those of the reflex myoclonic epilepsy of infancy described by Ricci et al. (12) in 1995, where surprise appeared fundamental in triggering attacks, regardless of the type of stimulus used. In all types of reflex epilepsy the unexpected nature of the stimulus is the main factor in precipitation (13), while in our family the MS was induced by persisting trigger stimuli.

GTCS occurred in all affected subjects, with onset in early infancy in branch I (patients III-2 to III-6) and between 4 and 8 years in branch II (patients III-8 to III-10). They were spontaneous or followed a prolonged myoclonic status. GTCS were more frequent in infancy and in adolescence, but persisted even into adulthood, except for patient III-4, who presented his last GTCS at 19 years of age. A patient (III-6) presented a true status convulsivus after appendectomy and repeated GTCS at delivery.

Other Clinical Features

The neurologic examination was normal in all affected individuals and neuroradiologic investigations (cranial C T and/or MRI), carried out on five patients were unremarkable. All subjects had normal psychomotor development and had no signs of cognitive deterioration. All were married with children.

CLINICAL COURSE AND THERAPY

In the affected subjects myoclonic attacks showed the maximal incidence between the ages of 4 and 12 years and GTCS between 12 and 16 years. Both lessened during adulthood. Drug treatment with valproate (CVPA) was effective on GTCS, but its suspension is followed by new attacks. Patient III-2 began treatment with VPA in 1997 after a further generalized seizure, achieving total control of GTCS. In the five treated patients, MS are reduced but still persist on therapy. Three patients, not receiving therapy,

still present MS provoked by repetitive movements or fatigue and sporadic GTCS every 2 to 3 years.

ELECTROENCEPHALOGRAM FEATURES

An ictal EEG recording was not obtained in any of the patients. It was impossible to precipitate MS by repetitive movements in the EEG laboratory, also because many of the patients were on antiepileptic drugs. The interictal recording was generally normal or showed mild left temporal abnormalities that were not specific for epilepsy (patient III-9). In two patients IPS induced a pathologic response. A 40-year-old woman (patient III-3, first branch of the pedigree) showed a diffuse abnormal background activity, with slow and irregular occipital alpha rhythm mixed to diffuse theta activity and sporadic isolated bilateral sharp waves over the occipital regions (Fig. 10–2A). In this patient IPS induced moderate voltage irregular spike and slow wave complexes and paroxysmal bursts of high-voltage polyspikes more evident over the occipital region (Fig. 10–2B and C). A 44-year-old man (patient III-10, second branch) had a normal background activity, but prolonged IPS first induced a normal driving response (Fig. 10–3A), then synchronous eyelid myoclonias (Fig. 10–3B), and, finally, a burst of high-voltage polyspike and slow wave complexes with maximal expression over the occipital regions (Fig. 10–3C): the patient asked to stop the examination because "he felt the seizure coming."

GENETIC FEATURES

FIME shows a clear autosomal recessive pattern of inheritance. The eight patients descend from two asymptomatic intermarried sib pairs. One parent (subject II–2) showed mild aspecific paroxysmal abnormalities on the EEG. None of their 20 offsprings was affected by FIME. One subject (IV–7) had two generalized tonic-clonic seizures when she was 18 years old and no epileptic manifestations during infancy or childhood. A 12-year-old girl (subject IV–22) had febrile seizures when she was 7 months old and 3 years old and no additional seizures.

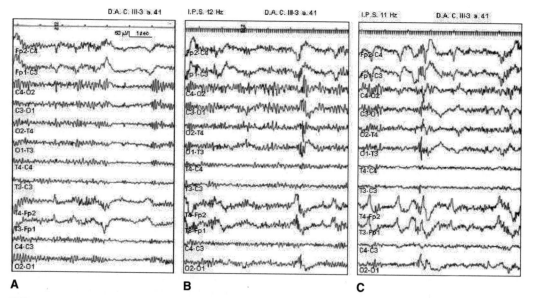

FIG. 10–2. Patient III-3 is a 42-year-old affected woman. The EEG examination showed a diffuse abnormal background activity, with sporadic isolated bilateral sharp waves over the occipital regions (**A**). IPS induced the appearance of moderate voltage irregular spike and slow wave complexes and paroxysmal bursts of high-voltage polyspikes with maximal expression over the occipital regions (**B** and **C**). From de Falco et al., ref. 10.

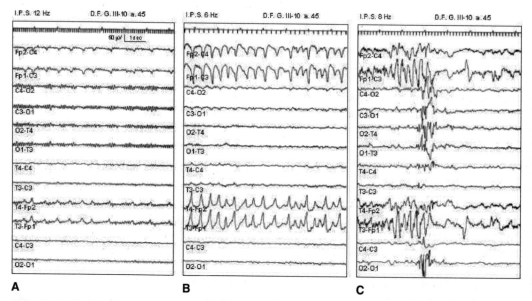

FIG. 10–3. Patient III-10, a 46-year-old affected man. The EEG examination showed normal background activity with a normal driving response to IPS (**A**). Prolonged IPS induced synchronous eyelid myoclonias (**B**) and, finally, a burst of high-voltage polyspike and slow wave complexes over the occipital regions (**C**). From de Falco et al., ref. 10.

Linkage analysis led to the identification of the FIME locus on a 2-Mb segment of chromosome 16p13.3. Two different disease haplotypes were identified in the affected subjects despite the typing of densely spaced markers, indicating that the two mutations arose from different ancestors. Thus far the gene involved is not known. The core of symptoms in FIME was very homogenous, although we observed slight clinical differences in the onset of the disease between the two branches of the family. In the first branch, the onset is characterized by a convulsive type of seizure and in the second branch by myoclonic seizures. This finding might indicate that the phenotype may be influenced by other genetic factors.

DIFFERENTIAL DIAGNOSIS AND NOSOLOGIC CLASSIFICATION

The clinical features of FIME place it in the broad spectrum of the myoclonic epilepsies of infancy. The classification of myoclonic epilepsies of infancy has always been controversial. In fact, in the clinical practice, several patients developing myoclonic epilepsy with onset in infancy or early childhood do not fit any specific epilepsy syndrome, even if they share important clinical features. Thus, for instance, it has been proposed to extend the clinical spectrum of the SMEI including similar phenotypes with a minor myoclonic component (Dravet syndrome).

Myoclonic seizures occurring in the first year of age may be suspected as the initial manifestation of West syndrome. Infantile spasms (IS), however, are brief tonic contractions, only rarely prolonged, and are associated with psychomotor retardation and often with neurologic abnormalities. The interictal EEGs in the West syndrome is always abnormal, with typical hypsarrhythmia and, sometimes, with focal abnormalities.

In FIME, clinical onset is frequently an afebrile GTCS that can also be the initial symptom of SMEI. However, SMEI patients develop a drug-resistant epilepsy with different type of seizures, such as unilateral motor seizures, and constantly show psychomotor retardation (14).

The LGS and MAE have a later onset and different clinical manifestations, including myoclonic-atonic, atonic, and tonic seizures for the first and myoclonic astatic seizures and minor seizures for the latter.

FIME has a peculiar phenotype and does not match any previously described myoclonic epilepsy. However, it shares some important clinical features with benign myoclonic epilepsy of infancy: FIME is a generalized idiopathic epilepsy of infancy characterized by myoclonic seizures with negative personal history, absence of psychomotor or neurologic impairment, and good response to VPA treatment. Like in BMEI the interictal EEG of patients was normal or with mild abnormalities, but frequently with paroxysmal features of intermittent photic stimulation (IPS). However, in BMEI, febrile seizures are infrequent and GTCS, before or after the onset of MS, sometimes following therapy withdrawal (15–19), are rare. Conversely, the frequent occurrence of febrile convulsions, the constant presence of GTCS and their persistence in adulthood in all patients, the frequency and duration of the MS, sometimes continuous, particularly preceding a convulsive seizure, are characteristic of FIME.

Prolonged myoclonic attacks (true myoclonic status epilepticus), lasting hours, and sometimes preceding a GTCS, have been described in children with benign form by Dulac (20) and in his series of "infantile myoclonic epilepsy following febrile convulsions" by Lombroso (21). We cannot exclude that some of these patients could be FIME patients.

Different authors observed that benign and severe forms could not be sharply separated due to the presence of intermediate forms and grouped them within the same heading of cryptogenic myoclonic epilepsy of infancy. This cryptogenic myoclonic epilepsy closely resembles the early childhood myoclonic epilepsy (ECME), as defined by Delgado–Escueta (22).

A peculiar feature of FIME is the autosomal recessive mode of inheritance. It is known that genetic factors play an important role in the etiology of myoclonic epilepsies. Recently, a mutation in the gene encoding the alpha1 subunit of the GABA$_A$ receptor—*GABRA1*—and α1 subunit of the neuronal voltage-gated sodium channel—*SCN1A*—have been identified in a family affected by autosomal dominant juvenile myoclonic epilepsy and in subjects affected by the SMEI, respectively (23,24). Moreover, different loci have been mapped for benign adult familial myoclonic epilepsy and mendelian subsets of juvenile myoclonic epilepsy (JME) (25–27). A high frequency of positive family history was also found in different myoclonic epilepsies such as in the cryptogenic myoclonic epilepsy reported by Fejerman (7), in ECME (22), and in BMEI (28).

Autosomal recessive inheritance in myoclonic epilepsy was only reported by Panayiotopoulos and Obeid in families affected by JME (29).

More, in general, however, autosomal recessive inheritance is a very rare event in human idiopathic epilepsy.

Neubauer and colleagues proposed autosomal recessive (AR) inheritance for benign epilepsy with centrotemporal spikes and reported evidence of linkage on chromosome 15q (30) in a cohort of nuclear families. AR inheritance has been demonstrated in an inbred family affected by rolandic epilepsy, paroxysmal exercise-induced dystonia, and writer's cramp (31).

Conversely, idiopathic epilepsy is often transmitted as AR trait in other mammals (dogs, 32; rats, 33; mice, 34–36) and in more distant species such as chickens (37) and *Drosophila* (38). It is possible that the occurrence of AR epileptic traits in animals is due to the high inbreeding rate of specific populations or to a bias in the evaluation of more severe AR phenotypes compared to milder autosomal dominant (AD) forms.

On the other hand, AR traits may be underestimated in humans because of the low clustering of affected cases in families segregating AR traits and phenotypic variability of epilepsies. Thus, several AR epileptic traits may be present in the general population as clinically and genetically distinct sporadic phenotypes.

The peculiar genealogical structure of the family affected by FIME suggests that it may be an isolated condition. However, most mendelian epilepsies were initially described in sporadic pedigrees and then reported worldwide. It is possible that sporadic cases affected by FIME are present within the heterogeneous group of myoclonic epilepsy of infancy, not included in known epileptic syndromes.

The identification of the mutant gene will provide an important tool to verify the role of FIME in the general populations and to better elucidate the pathogenesis of myoclonic epilepsies.

REFERENCES

1. Aicardi J, Chevrie JJ. Myoclonic epilepsies of childhood. *Neuropediatrie* 1971;3:177–190.
2. Jeavons PM. Nosological problems of myoclonic epilepsies in childhood and adolescence. *Develop Med Child Neurol* 1977;19:3–8.
3. Dravet C, Roger J, Bureau M, et al. Myoclonic epilepsies in childhood. In: Akimoto H, Kazamatsuri H, Seino M, Ward A. eds. *Advances in epileptology: XIIIth epilepsy international symposium*. New York: Raven Press, 1982:135–140.
4. Lombroso CT, Erba G. Myoclonic seizures: considerations in taxonomy. In: Akimoto H, Kazamatsuri H, Seino M, Ward A, eds. *Advances in epileptology: XIIIth epilepsy international symposium*. New York: Raven Press, 1982:129–134.
5. Roger J, Dravet C, Bureau M, Dreifuss FE, Perret A, Wolf P. eds. *Epileptic syndromes in infancy, childhood and adolescence*. London: John Libbey, 1992.
6. Aicardi J. Myoclonic epilepsies of infancy and childhood. *Adv Neurol* 1986;43:11–31.
7. Fejerman N. Myoclonies et épilepsies chez l'enfant. *Rev Neurol (Paris)* 1991;147:782–797.
8. Aicardi J. Myoclonic epilepsies of infancy and early childhood. In: Aicardi J. ed. *Epilepsy in children*. 2nd ed. New York: Raven Press, 1994:67–79.
9. Commission on Classification and Terminology of the International League Against Epilepsy: Proposal for Revised Classification of Epilepsies and Epileptic Syndromes. *Epilepsia* 1989;30:389–399.
10. de Falco FA, Majello L, Santangelo R, et al. Familial infantile myoclonic epilepsy: Clinical features in a large kindred with autosomal recessive inheritance. *Epilepsia* 2001;42:1541–1548.
11. Zara F, Gennaro E, Stabile M, et al. Mapping of a locus for a familial autosomal recessive idiopathic myoclonic epilepsy of infancy to chromosome 16p13. *Am J Hum Genet* 2000;66:1552–1557.
12. Ricci S, Cusmai R, Fusco L, et al. Reflex myoclonic epilepsy in infancy: a new age-dependent idiopathic epileptic syndrome related to startle reaction. *Epilepsia* 1995;36:341–348.
13. Deonna T. Reflex seizures with somatosensory precipitation. Clinical and electroencephalographic patterns and differential diagnosis, with emphasis on reflex myoclonic epilepsy of infancy. *Advan neurol* 1998;75:193–206.
14. Dravet C, Bureau M, Guerrini R, et al. Severe myoclonic epilepsy in infants. In: Roger J, Dravet C, Bureau M, Dreifuss FE, Perret A, Wolf P. eds. *Epileptic syndromes in infancy, childhood and adolescence*. 2nd ed. London: John Libbey, 1992:75–88.
15. Dravet C, Bureau M. L'épilepsy myoclonique bénigne du nourrisson. *Rev Electroencephalogr Neurophysiol Clin* 1981;11:438–444.
16. Dravet C, Bureau M, Genton P. Benign myoclonic epilepsy of infancy: electroclinical symptomatology and

differential diagnosis from the other types of generalized epilepsies of infancy. In: Degen R, Dreifuss FE, eds. *Benign localized and generalized epilepsies of early childhood.* Amsterdam: Elsevier Science, 1992:131–135.

17. Giovanardi Rossi P, Parmeggiani A, Posar A, et al. Benign myoclonic epilepsy: long-term follow-up of 11 new cases. *Brain Develop* 1997;19:473–479.

18. Rossi PG, Parmeggiani A., Posar A, et al. Benign myoclonic epilepsy: long-term follow-up in 11 new cases. *Brain Develop* 1997;19:473–479.

19. Lin Y, Itomi K, Takada H, et al. Benign myoclonic epilepsy in infants: video-EEG features and long-term follow-up. *Neuropediatrics* 1998;29:268–271.

20. Dulac O, Plouin P, Chiron C. "Benign" form of myoclonic epilepsy in children. *Neurophysiol Clin* 1990;20:115–129.

21. Lombroso CT. Early myoclonic encephalopathy, early infantile epileptic encephalopathy, and benign and severe infantile myoclonic epilepsies: A critical review and personal contribution. *J Clin Neurophysiol* 1990;7:380–408.

22. Delgado–Escueta AV, Greenberg D, Weissbecker K, et al. Gene mapping in the idiopathic generalized epilepsies: Juvenile myoclonic epilepsy, childhood absence epilepsy, epilepsy with grand mal seizures, and early childhood myoclonic epilepsy. *Epilepsia* 1990;31:S19–S29.

23. Cossette P, Liu L, Brisebois K, et al. Mutation of GABRA1 in an autosomal dominant form of juvenile myoclonic epilepsy. *Nat Genet* 2002;31:184–189.

24. Claes L, Del-Favero J, Ceulemans B, et al. De novo mutations in the sodium-channel gene SCN1A cause severe myoclonic epilepsy of infancy. *Am J Hum Genet* 2001;68:1327–1332.

25. Mikami M, Yasuda T, Terao A, et al. Localization of a gene for benign adult familial myoclonic epilepsy to chromosome 8q23.3-24.1 *Am J Hum Genet* 1999;65:745–751.

26. De Falco FA, Striano P, De Falco A, et al. Benign adult familial myoclonic epilepsy: Genetic heterogeneity and allelism with ADCME. *Neurology* 2003;60:1381–1385.

27. Liu AW, Delgado–Escueta AV, Serratosa JM, et al. Juvenile myoclonic epilepsy locus in chromosome 6p21.2-p11: linkage to convulsions and electroencephalography trait. *Am J Hum Genet* 1995;57:368–381.

28. Lin Y, Itomi K, Takada H, et al. Benign myoclonic epilepsy in infants: Video-EEG features and long-term follow-up. *Neuropediatrics* 1998;29:268–271.

29. Panayiotopoulos CP, Obeid T. Juvenile myoclonic epilepsy: an autosomal recessive disease. *Ann Neurol* 1989;25:440–443.

30. Neubauer BA, Fiedler B, Himmelein B, et al. Centrotemporal spikes in families with rolandic epilepsy: Linkage to chromosome 15q14. *Neurology* 1998;51:1608–1612.

31. Guerrini R, Bonanni P, Nardocci N, et al. Autosomal recessive rolandic epilepsy with paroxysmal exercise-induced dystonia and writer's cramp: delineation of the syndrome and gene mapping to chromosome 16p12-11.2 *Ann Neurol* 1999;45:344–352.

32. Hall SJ, Wallace ME. Canine epilepsy: a genetic counseling programme for keeshonds. *Vet Rec* 1996;138:358–360.

33. Noda A, Hashizume R, Maihara T, et al. NER rat strain: a new type of genetic model in epilepsy research. *Epilepsia* 1998;39:99–107.

34. Fletcher CF, Lutz CM, O'Sullivan TN, et al. Absence epilepsy in tottering mutant mice is associated with calcium channel defects. *Cell* 1996;87:607–617.

35. Burgess DL, Jones JM, Meisler MH, et al. Mutation of the Ca2+ channel beta subunit gene Cchb4 is associated with ataxia and seizures in the lethargic (lh) mouse. *Cell* 1997;88:385–392.

36. Letts VA, Felix R, Biddlecome GH, et al. The mouse stargazer gene encodes a neuronal Ca^{2+}-channel gamma subunit. *Nat Genet* 1998;19:340–347.

37. Nunoya T, Tajima M, Mizutani M. Ahereditary nervous disorder in Fayoumi chickens. *Lab Anim* 1983;17:298–302.

38. Wang XJ, Reynolds ER, Deak P, et al. The seizure locus encodes the Drosophila homolog of the HERG potassium channel. *J Neurosci* 1997;17:882–890.

11

Myoclonic–Astatic Epilepsy of Early Childhood—Definition, Course, Nosography, and Genetics

B. A. Neubauer,* A. Hahn,* H. Doose†, and I. Tuxhorn‡

*Department of Neuropediatrics, Zentrum Kinderheilkunde und Jugendmedizin, University of Giessen, Giessen Germany; †Norddeutsches Epilepsie-Zentrum, Raisdorf, Germany; ‡Epilepsy Center Bethel, Klinik Mara, Bielefeld, Germany

INTRODUCTION

The first concept of myoclonic-astatic epilepsy (MAE) dates back to the 1960s when myoclonic epilepsies of early childhood were separated from infantile spasms and Lennox–Gastaut Syndrome (LGS). The prominent familial aggregation together with the characteristic seizure symptomatology dominated by myoclonic and myoclonic astatic seizures led Doose and co-workers to delineate MAE as a syndrome in its own right (1). Family studies of history and EEG suggested a genetic etiology. This notion of an idiopathic epilepsy was questioned and not accepted however because of the variable course and frequent deleterious course. Severe MAE was, therefore, categorized into the cryptogenic epilepsies by the ILAE Commission. Nevertheless, the discovery of *SCN1A* and *SCN1B* mutations in four unique or rare families with GEFS+ (generalized epilepsy febrile seizure plus) whose phenotype included MAE provide support for the genetic basis of some cases of MAE. Channel gene defects were identified, thereby proving the conceptual robustness of MAE as a genetic disorder. In its early delineation, MAE was mixed with other myoclonias of infancy including SMEI, BMEI, and other unclassifiable cases of myoclonic epilepsies. Further work by various authors have substantially disentangled the many phenotypes and genotypes of myoclonias in infancy from MAE. A more specific syndrome of primary generalized or genetic myoclonic astatic seizures have become evident. Presently modern therapy has significantly improved prognosis, although, in some cases, outcome can still be unpredictable.

DEFINITION

Myoclonic astatic epilepsy, as a rule, occurs in children with an uneventful history. Like most other myoclonic epilepsies of early childhood, it clearly affects more boys than girls. The sex ratio is about 2.7:1 (2). If inclusion criteria only considers children older than 1 year, this ratio might even reach 3:1 (3). Epilepsy starts in 94% in the first 5 years. In 24%, onset of seizures occurs during the first year of life (2,4,5). The observed seizure symptomatology includes myoclonic, myoclonic-astatic, generalized tonic-clonic, tonic seizures with generalized onset, and a nonconvulsive status epilepticus formerly referred to as "status of minor seizures."

SEIZURE SEMIOLOGY

Table 11–1 summarizes the seizure symptomatology of the first 109 diagnosed cases (1,2,4,5).

TABLE 11–1. *Seizure Symptomatology in 109 MAE Cases*

Myoclonic and/or myoclonic astatic	100%
Absences	62%
Febrile convulsions	28%
Generalized tonic-clonic seizures	75%
At onset	34%
During course	41%
Status of minor seizures (nonconvulsive-status)	30%

From Doose H. Myoclonic astatic epilepsy of early childhood. In: Roger J, Bureau M, Dravet C, Dreifuss FE, Perret A, Wolf P. eds. *Epileptic syndromes in infancy, childhood and adolescence.* 2nd ed. London: John Libbey, 1992:103–114. With permission.

In about 60% of cases, epilepsy starts with febrile or afebrile generalized tonic-clonic convulsions. Alternating grand mal and hemi-grand mal are a possible presentation. Some days or a few weeks later, myoclonic and/or myoclonic-astatic seizures appear in abundance, frequently in combination with short absences. At first, this occurs predominantly after awakening. Infrequently sleep-related, tonic axial seizures may manifest during its long course and are not necessarily associated with an unfavorable prognosis. The same holds true for the rare partial seizures that eventually can be observed in MAE.

Myoclonic seizures consist of symmetric, mostly generalized jerks, accentuated in the arms and the shoulders and frequently associated with a simultaneous flexion of the head. The intensity of these seizures is variable and ranges from violent myoclonic jerks with sudden falls to abortive forms merely presenting as short irregular twitches of the face.

Myoclonic-astatic seizures are characterized by a loss of muscle tone preceded by a (short) myoclonia. In polygraphic recordings, the loss of muscle tone corresponds to a silent period in the electromyography (EMG) that is paralleled by the slow wave in the EEG following the spikes or polyspikes of the myoclonus (Fig. 11–1). Myoclonic seizures with and without a discernable myotonia frequently occur together or in series. The myoclonia and the following myotonia equally contribute to the characteristic myoclonic-astatic seizure (6,7) see Chapter 3 and 15 (8).

Absences are seen in more than one-half of the children with MAE. Myoclonic and astatic seizures, when they come in series, are frequently accompanied by absences that are often combined with myoclonic jerks.

A peculiar type of *nonconvulsive-status epilepticus* (status of minor seizures) can be oberved in 36% (1,2,4) to 95% (3) of MAE patients. The characteristic clinical picture is a somnolent, stuporous child with subtle myoclonic seizures, frequently involving the face and the extremities. The child is unresponsive, drools, has slurred speech, or is even aphasic. This status may continue for days if not interrupted by adequate means.

ELECTROENCEPHALOGRAM

Background activity is of special interest in MAE. In cases beginning with GTCS, the EEG may stay entirely normal for weeks. However, in almost all instances, a rhythmic parietally accentuated 4–7 Hz activity develops early in the course (Fig. 11–2B). This rhythmic slowing of background activity was frequently questioned and falsely attributed to drowsiness. In patients with MAE (and other idiopathic generalized epilepsies of early childhood with myoclonic seizures), it represents a constant trait that is not related to the state of vigilance. This has been documented by EEG recordings of children who were kept attentive by displaying cartoons, etc. (8, p. 24). During the early stages, spikes, irregular spikes, and polyspikes may well be absent and appear only after some delay, starting during sleep.

If myoclonic seizures dominate the course at a given time, the EEG shows short paroxysms of irregular spikes and polyspikes (Fig. 11–3D). In children with astatic and myoclonic astatic seizures, 2- to 3-Hz spikes and waves appear (Figs. 11–1 and 11–3A). As the epilepsy progresses, typical absence patterns may appear. At times, all generalized EEG discharges in MAE may show lateralization and "pseudo-foci" (Fig. 11–3B) that may change from side to side, sometimes even during a single recording.

During a status of myoclonic-astatic seizures, the EEG displays continuous spike waves with interposed slow waves (Fig. 11–3A). Especially in younger children, irregular polymorphous

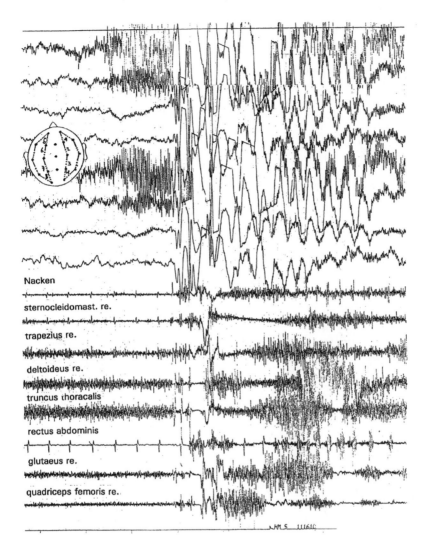

Nacken

sternocleidomast. re.

trapezius re.

deltoideus re.

truncus thoracalis

rectus abdominis

glutaeus re.

quadriceps femoris re.

FIG. 11–1. Polygraphic record of a myoclonic-astatic seizure in MAE. The seizure was induced by startle. Initial spikes are associated with a short myoclonic jerk. The following slow wave is accompanied by a silent period in the deltoid, truncus thoracalis, gluteal and quadriceps femoris muscles. (Recorded in: Schweizerische Epilepsieklinik Zürich, 1992; from Doose H. EEG in childhood epilepsy—Initial presentation and long-term follow-up. Ist ed. Montrouge: John Libbey, 2003. With permission).

hypersynchronic activity, sometimes resembling hypsarrhythmia, is characteristic (Fig. 11–2A).

During nocturnal tonic seizures typical a 10- to 15-Hz spike series can be observed. In distinction to the tonic seizures observed in LGS, the EEG onset is generalized in MAE (Fig. 11–4).

In sleep recordings, grouped paroxysms of irregular spikes and waves are activated. However, ESES (electrical status epilepticus during slow sleep) is never observed.

GENETICS

Doose (1,2,4,5) investigated the families of 107 patients with MAE and demonstrated the role of genetic factors in the pathogenesis of MAE (compare Fig. 11–3A–E). In probands' siblings, probands' parents, and siblings of probands' parents, a seizure incidence of 32% was documented (febrile seizures included). The seizure incidence was higher in siblings than in parents

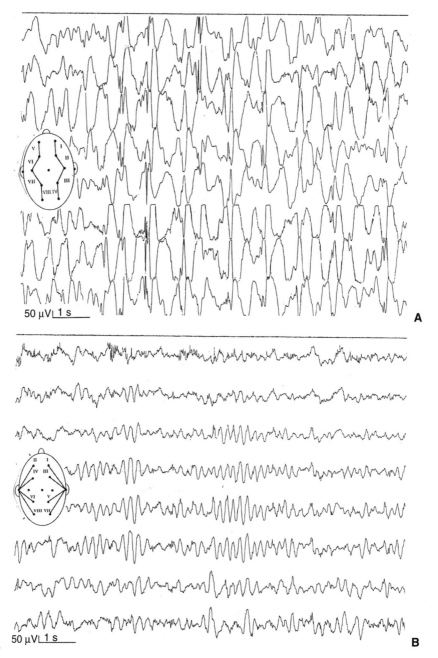

50 µV⎣1 s

A

50 µV⎣1 s

B

FIG. 11–2. Long-term follow up of a patient with MAE. **A:** 5 years. Status of myoclonic astatic seizures. Hypsarrythmia-like EEG pattern with rare spikes. **B:** 5 years. Complete remission 4 weeks later after ACTH treatment. Parietally accentuated theta rhythms. **C:** 11 years. Seizure-free, prominent theta rhythms over the parietal leads. **D:** 22 years. Still free of seizures. Eye closure sensitivity with polyspikes (From Doose H. EEG in childhood epilepsy—Initial presentation and long-term follow-up. Ist ed. Montrouge: John Libbey, 2003. With permission).

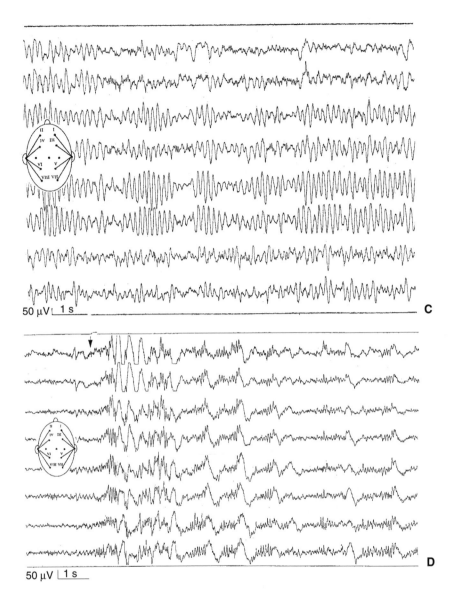

FIG. 11–2. (*Continued*)

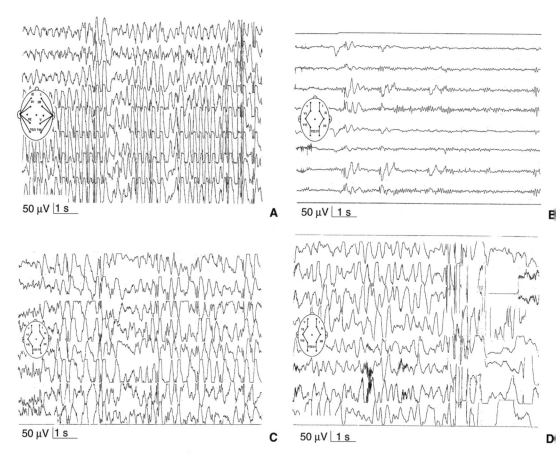

FIG. 11–3. A: 3-year-old girl with MAE. Discontinuous status with 4-Hz rhythms and generalized spike waves. **B:** 17 years. Complete seizure remission since years. Bilateral parietal spikes and waves (pseudo-foci). **C:** 3-year-old daughter of the index patient with MAE. **D:** 4-year-old son of the index patient with short myoclonic seizures during hyperventilation (From Doose H. EEG in childhood epilepsy—Initial presentation and long-term follow-up. Ist ed. Montrouge: John Libbey, 2003. With permission).

(see Table 11–2 for details). Affected siblings showed absences in 25% of cases. The majority of seizures (febrile convulsions and absences) documented in relatives occurred before the 5th year of age. In siblings and parents, epilepsy-associated EEG traits (photosensitivity, 4-7 Hz rhythms, and spike waves) were also found at a significantly increased rate (4). MAE is one of the characteristic seizure syndromes of the GEFS$^+$ phenotype as described by Scheffer and Berkovic (9). In fact, the first families of GEFS$^+$ were ascertained from probands with MAE. In GEFS$^+$ families, four probands with MAE have been found to harbor mutations in *SCN1B, SCN1A,* and *GABRG2* (10–12). Sugawara et al. (13)

reported a case with febrile seizures and drop attacks and found a mutation in the *SCN2A* gene. In the epilepsy syndrome, what the index patient suffers from is not entirely clear, but MAE is a possibility.

DELINEATION (DIFFERENTIAL DIAGNOSIS)

Before the delineation of MAE by Doose and coworkers and its final recognition by the ILAE, it is evident that basically all MAE cases were classified as LGS, which still represents the most important differential diagnosis. Critical features

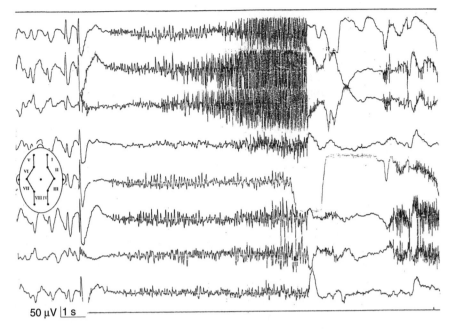

FIG. 11–4. Nocturnal tonic seizure in a 21-year-old patient with MAE. Simultaneous generalized spikes, followed by a short depression and a 5 sec generalized discharge of polyspikes with sudden end. (From Doose H, *EEG in childhood epilepsy—Initial presentation and long-term follow-up.* Ist ed. Montrouge: John Libbey, 2003. With permission).

to discriminate both syndromes will have to focus on the following criteria of MAE:

- History (normal development before seizure onset vs. symptomatic origin)
- Characteristic EEG pattern in MAE as outlined above
- No atypical absences
- No tonic seizures or tonic drop attacks during daytime in MAE (rare exceptions) and a non-focal, generalized EEG pattern during tonic seizures (8,20)

TABLE 11–2. *Familial Incidence of Seizures in 107 Families of Patients with MAE*

	n	%
Brothers } av. 15%	78	18
Sisters	82	12
Fathers	100	7
Fathers' siblings	246	3
Mothers	102	4
Mothers' siblings	221	4

From Doose H, Baier WK. Genetic factors in epilepsies with primarily generalized minor seizures. *Neuropediatrics* 1987;18 [suppl 1]:1–64. With permission.

- High incidence of epilepsy-associated genetic EEG traits (in MAE patients)
- A positive family history in about 30% of cases
- Altogether a generalized EEG pattern in MAE with no constant focal discharges, as a rule, with, however, "pseudo-foci" of variable localization during course

Other syndromes that show overlaps with MAE and vice versa are benign and severe myoclonic epilepsy of childhood. This cannot be resolved to completeness because the concept of MAE does not so much rest on prognosis as it does in benign and severe myoclonic epilepsy of infancy. In our point of view, this is no issue of conflict, for it is evident that all three entities are syndromes in their own right. The electroclinical picture, together with the course, will allow an unambiguous allocation at an early stage in most instances.

Atypical benign partial epilepsy of childhood or Pseudo-Lennox syndrome (14–16) is another possible differential diagnosis of MAE. However, even in cases with parallels in clinical presentation, EEG recordings with characteristic rolandic spikes activated to prolonged generalized discharges during slow wave sleep are never seen in MAE and thereby provide a tool for differentiation. Family (EEG) studies reveal greatly divergent findings in both syndromes (17).

TREATMENT

Revised treatment standards over the last several years have significantly improved outcome and prognosis (18). Valproic acid is still the first choice drug. If it fails to achieve complete remission, the decision which drug to use next depends on the predominant seizure type. If absences prevail, ethosuximide (ESM) should be commenced as the next step. If GTCS represent the leading semiology, bromide is frequently the most effective drug, which is even superior to phenobarbital or primidone (19). Lamotrigine may both be effective and provoke myoclonic seizures in generalized myoclonic epilepsies. Therefore, it may represent a valuable option, but has to be used with caution (20). Based on its broad mechanism of action, topiramate is another possibility. However, no data on its effectiveness in MAE are yet available. Carbamazepine, phenytoin, and vigabatrin should be avoided, for they frequently provoke seizure exacerbation (2,3,21). In cases with refractory nonconvulsive status epilepticus, corticotropin (ACTH) or high-dose steroid–puls therapy may be an alternative (2). Zonisamide, a new antiepileptic drug (AED), which shows some effect in progressive myoclonus epilepsies, awaits conclusive trials for idiopathic myoclonic epilepsies (22).

PROGNOSIS

From the early descriptions of the MAE disorder, it becomes clear that outcome is highly variable. The spectrum ranges from complete remission and totally normal intellectual development to therapy-resistant epilepsy with severe cognitive disabilities (1,2,7,23). Over the years, however, therapeutic possibilities have constantly improved and the danger of seizure and epilepsy aggravation by carbamazepine and phenytoin has been more and more recognized. In a recently published series of 81 patients with MAE, 68% became eventually seizure-free. In this retrospective Japanese series, ACTH, ESM, and ketogenic diet proved especially effective (18). Repetitive nonconvulsive status epilepticus (status of minor seizures) and nocturnal tonic seizures were frequently associated with an unfavorable prognosis (2,18).

REFERENCES

1. Doose H, Gerken H, Leonhardt R, et al. Centrencephalic myoclonic-astatic petit mal. Clinical and genetic investigations. *Neuropediatrie* 1970;2:59–78.
2. Doose H. Myoclonic astatic epilepsy of early childhood. In: Roger J, Bureau M, Dravet C, Dreifuss FE, Perret A, Wolf P. eds. *Epileptic syndromes in infancy, childhood and adolescence.* 2nd ed. London: John Libbey, 1992:103–114.
3. Kaminska A, Ickowicz A, Plouin P, et al. Delineation of cryptogenic Lennox-Gastaut syndrome and myoclonic astatic epilepsy using multiple correspondence analysis. *Epilepsy Res* 1999;36(1):15–29.
4. Doose H, Baier WK. Epilepsy with primarily generalized myoclonic-astatic seizures: a genetically determined disease. *Eur J Pediatr* 1987;146:550–554.
5. Doose H, Baier WK. Genetic factors in epilepsies with primarily generalized minor seizures. *Neuropediatrics* 1987;18 [Suppl 1]:1–64.
6. Oguni H, Fukuyama Y, Imaizumi Y, et al. Video-EEG analysis of drop seizures in myoclonic astatic epilepsy of early childhood (Doose syndrome). *Epilepsia* 1992;33(5):805–813.
7. Oguni H, Uehara T, Imai K. Atonic epileptic drop attacks associated with generalized spike-and-slow wave complexes: Video-polygraphic study in two patients. *Epilepsia* 1997;38(7):813–818.
8. Doose H. *EEG in childhood epilepsy*—Initial presentation and long-term follow up. 1st ed. Montrouge: John Libbey, 2003.
9. Scheffer IE, Berkovic SF. Generalized epilepsy with febrile seizures plus. A genetic disorder with heterogeneous clinical phenotypes. *Brain* 1997;120:479–490.
10. Wallace RH, Wang DW, Singh R, et al. Febrile seizures and generalized epilepsy associated with a mutation in the Na^+-channel beta1 subunit gene SCN1B. *Nat Genet* 1998;19(4):366–370.
11. Wallace RH, Scheffer IE, Barnett S, et al. Neuronal sodium-channel alpha1-subunit mutations in generalized epilepsy with febrile seizures plus. *Am J Hum Genet* 2001;68(4):859–865.
12. Wallace RH, Marini C, Petrou S, et al. Mutant GABA(A) receptor gamma2-subunit in childhood absence epilepsy and febrile seizures. *Nat Genet* 2001;28(1):49–52.
13. Sugawara T, Tsurubuchi Y, Agarwala KL, et al. A missense mutation of the Na^+ channel alpha II subunit gene Na(v)1.2 in a patient with febrile and afebrile seizures causes channel dysfunction. *Proc Natl Acad Sci USA* 2001;98(11):6384–6389.
14. Aicardi J, Chevrie JJ. Atypical benign partial epilepsy of

childhood. *Develop Med Child Neurol* 1982;24(3):281–292.

15. Doose H. Symptomatology in children with focal sharp waves of genetic origin. *Eur J Pediatr* 1989;149(3):210–215.

16. Hahn A, Pistohl J, Neubauer BA, et al. Atypical "benign" partial epilepsy or pseudo-Lennox syndrome. Part I: symptomatology and long-term prognosis. *Neuropediatrics* 2001;32(1):1–8.

17. Doose H, Hahn A, Neubauer BA, et al. Atypical "benign" partial epilepsy of childhood or pseudolennox syndrome. Part II: family study. *Neuropediatrics* 2001;32(1):9–13.

18. Oguni H, Tanaka T, Hayashi K, et al. Treatment and long-term prognosis of myoclonic-astatic epilepsy of early childhood. *Neuropediatrics* 2002;33(3):122–132.

19. Ernst JP, Doose H, Baier WK. Bromides were effective in intractable epilepsy with generalized tonic-clonic seizures and onset in early childhood. *Brain Develop* 1988;10(6):385–388.

20. Guerrini R, Dravet C, Genton P, et al. Lamotrigine and seizure aggravation in severe myoclonic epilepsy. *Epilepsia* 1998;39(5):508–512.

21. Lortie A, Chiron C, Mumford J. The potential for increasing seizure frequency, relapse, and appearance of new seizure types with vigabatrin. *Neurology* 1993;43(11) [Suppl 5]:S24–S27.

22. Uthman BM, Reichl A. Progressive myoclonic epilepsies. *Curr Treat Options Neurol* 2002;4(1):3–17.

23. Dulac O, Plouin P, Chiron C. "Benign" form of myoclonic epilepsy in children *Neurophysiol Clin* 1990;20(2):115–129.

12

Idiopathic Myoclonic-Astatic Epilepsy of Early Childhood—Nosology Based on Electrophysiologic and Long-Term Follow-Up Study of Patients

Hirokazu Oguni,* Kitami Hayashi,* Kaoru Imai,* Makoto Funatsuka,* Masako Sakauchi,* Seigo Shirakawa,* and Makiko Osawa*

*Department of Pediatrics, Tokyo Women's Medical University, Tokyo, Japan

INTRODUCTION

The Commission on Classification and Terminology of the International League Against Epilepsy has most recently proposed benign myoclonic epilepsy in infants (BME) and myoclonic-astatic epilepsy of early childhood (MAE) as distinct subgroups of idiopathic generalized epilepsy and severe myoclonic epilepsy in infants (SME) and cryptogenic LGS (CLGS) as subgroups of generalized epileptic encephalopathy (1). Controversies, nonetheless, continue and are unresolved as to the clinical distinction between these four syndromes. The clinical phenotypes overlap and it is difficult to separate and differentiate between each disorder, especially between MAE and the other three syndromes (2–9). Historically, a number of studies have focused on groups of patients whose epilepsy starts in infancy and whose phenotype seizures consist of myoclonic or astatic attacks of idiopathic etiology. These groups of patients were distinguished from other patients with LGS or West syndromes. (10–16). Most authors support giving the idiopathic epilepsy subtypes in this age range a more favorable prognosis than the latter two malignant syndromes. However, these groups of patients unfortunately suffered from a relatively wide variety of seizure types whose prognosis also varied. Seizure phenotypes ranged from myoclonic seizures alone or astatic seizures alone or myoclonic seizures or astatic seizures in combination with atypical absence and generalized tonic-clonic or clonic seizures (GTCS). Prognosis ranged from very benign to relatively resistant or poor prognosis. Some authors tried to subclassify them into many subdivisions. Others tried to consider them as one syndrome with a wide range of clinical manifestations, based on the conceptual framework of genetically determined corticoreticular epilepsy (3,4,15). Although syndromic classification and the diagnostic limits that border each syndrome are important, more precise information regarding the neurophysiologic characteristics, treatment response, and long-term outcomes in the idiopathic patient group are needed for practical purposes and for further discussions on classification. Here we present the results of our clinical and EEG studies in patients with MAE extensively investigated at Tokyo Women's Medical University. We discuss the nosology of this unique epileptic syndrome based on our own experiences (17–23).

ELECTROPHYSIOLOGIC CHARACTERISTICS OF THE MAIN SEIZURE TYPES

The most important and distinct feature of seizures in MAE appear to be an astatic seizure or epileptic drop attack, repeatedly illustrated in references. The drop attack itself is not a necessary prerequisite for MAE in the original criteria (4). The advent of simultaneous video-EEG technology has disclosed that most epileptic drop attacks seen in clinical practice were caused by brief tonic seizures. Atonic drop attacks, which were originally thought of as a cause of epileptic drop attacks, are extremely rare (24,25). We have been studying the ictal polygraphs of myoclonic or astatic seizures to investigate the neurophysiologic background of these brief motor seizures, and identified true atonic drop attacks

to be a cause of astatic seizures in children with MAE, most of whom were initially treatment resistant, but finally entered into remission (19–23). The number of ictal polygraphs of patients with MAE, which were available for detailed neurophysiologic examinations, amounted to 30, including video-EEG ($n = 5$), polygraph ($n = 2$) and video-polygraph ($n = 23$). Patients with SME, BME, and CLGS were excluded based on the criteria previously defined by ILAE. All attacks occurred intermittently and did not form clusters in the periodic fashion seen in infantile spasms. Analysis of ictal EEGs showed that all attacks corresponded to generalized spike or polyspike-and-wave complexes in contrast to those of tonic drop attacks observed in LGS (26–29).

The main seizure types of MAE were largely divided into atonic and myoclonic types;

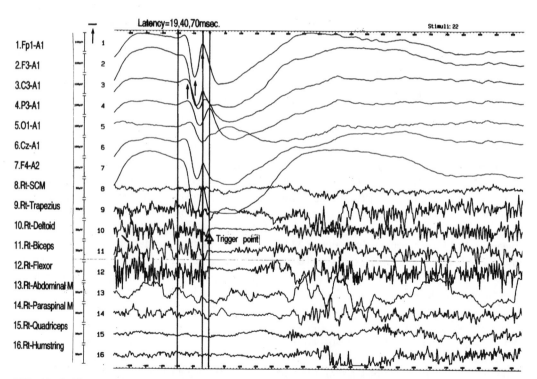

FIG. 12–1. The morphology of generalized spike-and-wave complexes causing atonic drop attacks. The polygrahic data were sampled at 1024 Hz through Rhythm Program (Stellate Inc. Montreal). Twenty-two ictal polygraphs were averaged at the onset of surface EMG interruptions of the right deltoid muscles. The latencies measured between the onset of atonia (right deltoid muscle) and each peak of the negative and positive spike component at F3 consisted of 19, 40, and 70 msec.

myoclonic in 16 cases, atonic with or without preceding minor myoclonia in 11 cases, and myoclonic-atonic in 3 cases. Although atonic seizures were, at times, preceded by minor myoclonic movement of the extremities, the major symptomatology was global atonia causing the patients to fall to the ground, when they were intense enough. In the ictal EEG of atonic seizures, the spike-and-wave morphology was similar, characterized by a positive–negative–deep–positive wave followed by a large negative slow wave (Fig. 12–1). Interestingly, when we compared the morphology of spike-and-wave complexes among atonic seizures of different intensity in two patients, the depth of the second positive component of spike-and-wave complexes corresponded well to the intensity of the attacks; the second component was deeper and the atonic seizures were stronger (22). The difference of the component was very clear when we compared the averaged spike-and-wave com-

plexes between those causing atonia and those without atonia (Fig. 12–2).

The clinical manifestations of atonic seizures were characterized by a sudden collapse of the body forward, with immediate recovery, when the patients were sitting on the floor. When they were standing, their bodies and legs suddenly sagged. In more intense attacks, they collapsed straight downward onto the buttocks with an immediate recovery (Fig. 12–3A and B). Close and repeated analysis of the atonic attacks on video and surface electromyography (EMG) showed minor myoclonic jerks on the extremities preceding the atonic attacks. They were subtle enough to miss if not carefully analyzed. When patients were in the lying position, we only recognized sudden facial changes without any movement of the body or minor movement due to sudden muscle tonus reduction. Surface EMG showed sudden interruption of the ongoing EMG activity extending up to 400 msec (Fig. 12–1). Latency

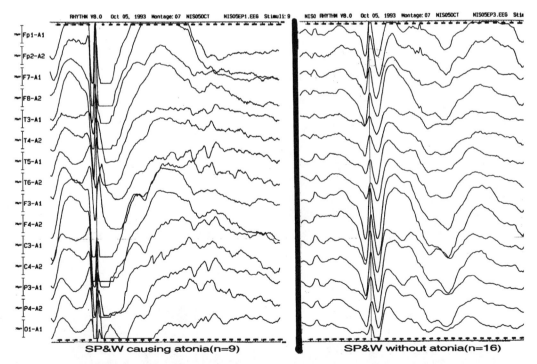

FIG. 12–2. The differences in morphology of spike-and-wave complexes with and without atonia. The morphology of the spike-and wave component was compared between that causing atonia and that without atonia in the averaged spike-and-wave complexes. Note the deep second positive component followed by large and long slow wave in the averaged spike-and-wave complexes causing atonic attack.

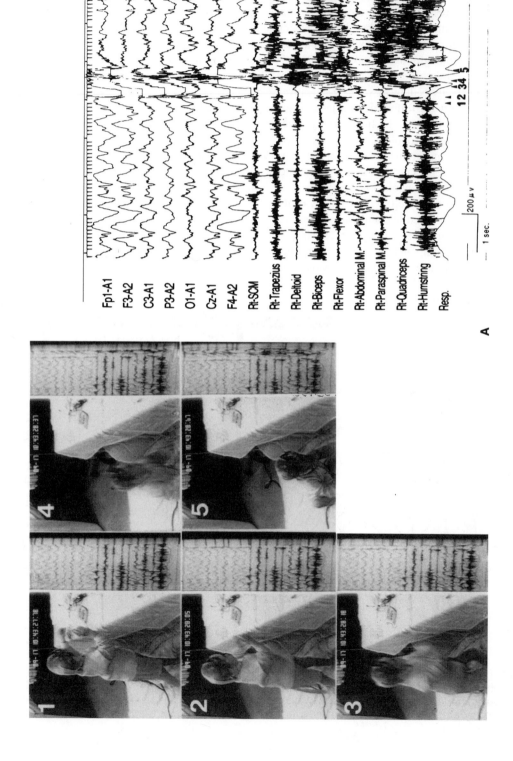

Fp1-A1
F3-A2
C3-A1
P3-A2
O1-A1
Cz-A1
F4-A2
Rt-SCM
Rt-Trapezius
Rt-Deltoid
Rt-Biceps
Rt-Flexor
Rt-Abdominal M.
Rt-Paraspinal M.
Rt-Quadriceps
Rt-Humstring
Resp.

200 µv

1 sec.

1 2 34 5

A

B

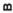

studies measuring onset of these EMG interruptions at various muscles in three cases with MAE demonstrated variable onsets without descending order from proximal to distal muscles (30) (Fig. 12–4). Results suggested that atonia of muscles was a secondary phenomenon, presumably due to inhibition of postural control, rather than an epileptic inhibitory impulse descending through efferent pathways, causing atonia of each of the muscles.

In the predominant myoclonic seizure type, six cases, had a history of falling down during attacks, while the remaining ten cases never had drop attacks. Among six cases with a history of drop attacks, the precise mechanism for falling was a massive propulsion or retropulsion caused by myoclonia of axial muscles in three patients. Myoclonic seizures occurred during wakefulness in ten cases, during sleep in six cases, and in the remaining one case during both sleep and wakefulness. All the attacks occurred intermittently and singly except for one child, who had the myoclonic jerk occurring twice successively. The morphology of spike-and-wave complexes during myoclonia was also similar to the morphology of spike-wave complexes during atonia. However, spike-waves of myoclonias appeared to be more brief during the duration of one complex. In one patient, drop attacks were difficult to distinguish as originating from either myoclonias or atonias when captured in the standing position, due to contamination of movement artifacts on the polygraph (Fig. 12–5). It was much easier to distinguish when they were captured in the lying position because of absence of gravity. We recorded every seizure in standing, sitting, and lying position, in order to distinguish

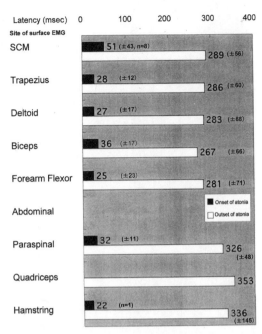

FIG. 12–4. Spreading of the atonic events among the involved muscles during atonic seizures. Latencies were measured between the peaks of the negative spike component at F3 and the onset as well as termination of the EMG interruptions in nine muscles from SCM to hamstring during the atonic drop attacks in the case shown in Fig. 12–3. Eight ictal events were individually studied to identify the efferent system responsible for the atonic seizures. The polygrahic data were sampled at 1024 Hz through Rhythm Program (Stellate Inc. Montreal). The result demonstrated atonia of muscles starting with hamstring, followed by forearm flexor, deltoid, trapezius, and finally SCM, and lasting longer in the distal than the proximal muscles. (From Tanaka T, Tsurumi E, Shirakawa S, et al. Neurophysiological analysis of the epileptic atonic drop attack. *Jpn J EEG EMG* (Jpn) 1998:175. With permission.)

FIG. 12–3. Simultaneous video (A) and polygraphic findings (B) of an atonic drop attack, **A:** Before the seizure, the patient was standing in front of a desk and manipulating a toy (1). He suddenly collapsed straight downward, landing on his buttocks (2–5). Note the semiflexion at the knees (3). The arms also dropped downward (3 and 4). He had already regained consciousness by the time he landed on the floor (5). **B:** The EMG potentials preceding the interrupted EMG potentials were seen polygraphically on the forearm flexor and quadriceps muscles. The EMG discharges of the quadriceps and biceps femoris muscles were restored during the late phase of falling, suggesting that the bodily collapse was probably due not only to global atonia, but also to gravity, such that he immediately recovered once on the floor. Numbers in the photograph corresponded to those of the EEG. (From Oguni H, Uehara T, Imai K. Osawa M. Atonic epileptic drop attacks associated with generalized spike-and-wave complexes—video-polygraphic study in two patients. *Epilepsia* 1997;38:813–818. With permission.)

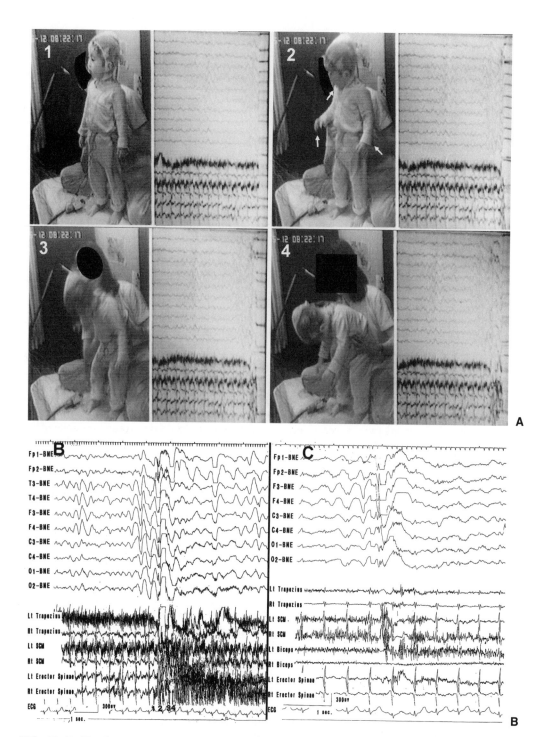

FIG. 12–5. Simultaneous video (**A**) and polygraphic findings (**B**) of the myoclonic astatic seizure **A**: Before the seizure, the patient was standing (1). Suddenly, slight flexion of his head as well as forearms, associated with opening of the mouth, was observed (2). Flexion of the upper trunk at the hip with abduction of both arms, as well as some flexion of both knees, ensued (3). His body was further bent forward, but he did not fall because his mother held him at the waist (4). **B:** Interpretation of the ictal polygraph was difficult because of contamination of many fall-associated artifacts (Numbers indicate seizure sequence). **C:** Another ictal polygraph was captured during semiflexed lying position. On the video, he showed slight flexion of the head and upper trunk against gravity, corresponding

mechanisms underlying falls. As a result, we can determine the exact seizure types underlying drop attacks or astatic attacks even by history-taking from caregivers.

The remaining three patients had myoclonic or myoclonic-atonic seizures, which were characterized by the initial sound "u." The sound was presumably caused by the momentary contracture of the chest with or without subsequent atonia. Myoclonia and atonia appeared to be equal in these three patients as compared to the previous two forms. We have concluded that astatic seizures in MAE are distinguishable from those of LGS.

OTHER SEIZURE TYPES

In our previous long-term follow-up study of 81 patients with MAE (which included these 30 cases), the most frequent accompanying seizures except for myoclonic/atonic seizure (MS/AS) were GTCS seen in 75 patients (23). In 52 of 75 patients, GTCS occurred during both wakefulness and sleep. In contrast to GTCS seen in older children, GTCS with a brief tonic phase or generalized clonic seizures, at times resembling the repetition of massive myoclonic attacks, were frequently recorded. They were characterized by rhythmic opening of the mouth and movement of the arms and legs, which started after a sudden collapse backward on the floor, when the patient was sitting. These attacks were considered generalized clonic seizures rather than repetitive myoclonic attacks because of the presence of a postictal suppression of background activity, even if they were short in duration (22,23). Nocturnal convulsive seizures are generally resistant to treatment and tend to continue for a long time, even after cessation of MS/AS. Generalized tonic-vibrating seizures with a few clonic components during sleep were also confirmed in the late clinical course of the unfavorable outcome group, and were most resistant (8,23).

In some patients, only eye opening with irregular respiration for 10 s or more was recorded, corresponding to generalized multiple spike burst, during sleep and, at times, wakefulness.

Atypical absence seizures corresponding to runs of generalized irregular spike-and-slow waves at 2-3 Hz were seen in 44 patients. Eighteen of these patients also had recurrences of prolonged clouding of consciousness with random segmental myoclonus. Their ictal EEGs showed disorganized marked slow background activity with random spike-and-wave discharges, identical with the status of minor seizures or minor epileptic status (Fig. 12–6). This peculiar seizure tended to start after awakening and lasted for hours.

LONG-TERM OUTCOMES OF PATIENTS WITH MAE

We previously conducted a long-term follow-up study of 7 patients, the age at last MS/AS ranged from 12 to 151 months with a mean of 51 ± 22 months and a median age of 46 months in 77 patients (23). Cumulative percentage remission of MS/AS after onset of attacks reached 40% within 6 months, 63% within 1 year, and 89% within 3 years. Thus, myoclonic-astatic seizures in 89% of 81 patients disappeared within 1 to 3 years despite initial resistance. However, other combined convulsive or nonconvulsive seizures (they were mainly GTCS or GCS) tended to persist after cessation of the myoclonic-astatic seizures. Based on the seizure prognosis, we can tentatively separate patients into three subgroups, favorable, intermediate, and unfavorable outcomes (Table 12–1). However, we have to keep in mind that, even in 55 children with a favorable clinical course (favorable MAE), the attacks were initially resistant to antiepileptic drugs (AEDs), sometimes requiring additional corticotropin (ACTH) or ketogenic treatment. Interestingly, at least 21 patients among the favorable and

FIG. 12–5. (*Continued*) to the EMG discharges at SCM. The ictal EEG was morphologically similar to that of **B**, although this EEG was recorded at 6 cm/sec. [From Oguni H, Fukuyama Y, Imaizumi Y, et al. A video-EEG analysis of drop seizures in myoclonic astatic epilepsy of early childhood (Doose syndrome). *Epilepsia* 1992;33(5):805–813. With permission.]

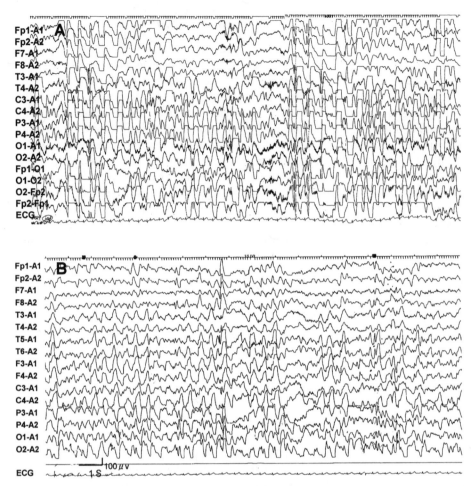

FIG. 12–6. Ictal EEG of minor epileptic status. **A:** The patient was a 2-year 2-month-old girl with favorable MAE. The EEG showed abundant generalized and CP localized spike-and-wave complexes or high-voltage slow wave of varying frequency, corresponding to mild cloudiness of consciousness. **B:** The patient was a 4-year 2-month-old girl with unfavorable MAE. The EEG showed almost continuous high-amplitude irregular slow wave discharges at times mixed with spike discharges. She showed mild cloudiness of consciousness with occasional random myoclonus of the extremities.

TABLE 12–1. *A comparison of various clinical factors among three different outcome groups (N = 81)*

Outcomes[a]	Favorable	Intermediate	Unfavorable	P
N	55	11	15	
Boy/girl	41/14	10/1	10/5	0.3571
Age onset of epilepsy (m)	33 ± 8	32 ± 9	30 ± 11	0.4502
Age onset of MS/AS (m)	36 ± 9	37 ± 14	35 ± 14	0.9878
FH of Epilepsy + FC	4 + 11	1 + 2	6 + 2	*Epi 0.0108*
Seizure type				
Absence	27 (49%)	6 (55%)	10 (67%)	0.4789
Absence status or MES	9 (16%)	1 (9%)	7 (47%)	**0.0222**
Nocturnal seizures	34 (62%)	8 (73%)	10 (67%)	0.7697
Drop attacks	35 (64%)	7 (64%)	10 (67%)	0.9759

(From Oguni H, Tanaka T, Hayashi K, et al. Treatment and long-term prognosis of myoclonic-astatic epilepsy of early childhood. *Neuropediatrics* 2002;33:122–132.)

[a]Abbreviations: MS/AS, myoclonic or atonic seizures; FH = family history; FC = febrile convulsions; MES = minor epileptic status, epi, Epilepsy.

intermediate groups appeared to enter into spontaneous remission, either suddenly or gradually, despite initial resistance to treatment for months or a few years. The attacks, either myoclonic-astatic seizures or nocturnal seizures, disappeared suddenly or progressively without any change in medication.

Approximately one-half of 15 patients with an unfavorable outcome (unfavorable MAE) appeared to be identical to those reported by Kaminska et al. (8) They were characterized by a combination of MA/AS, atypical absence seizures, minor epileptic status, and recurrent GTCS at the early clinical course. Later, these seizures were accompanied by nocturnal GTS or generalized tonic vibrating seizures. Five patients continued to have weekly GTCS only. Eleven patients with an intermediate outcome (intermediate MAE) resembled the clinical course of those with BME, to some extent, experiencing recurrence of GTCS after a long remission period with a mean of 9 years and 2 months. GTCS were controlled easily by reinstitution or increasing the dosage of AEDs. In these patients, the initial clinical course was identical to that of the favorable MAE group.

As to the intellectual outcomes of the 81 patients with MAE, 48 patients or 59% of all the patients showed a normal IQ level at the final follow-up. Sixteen patients or 20% were borderline or had mild retardation, and 17 patients or 21% had less than moderate retardation. The earlier the remission of epilepsy was, the better IQ levels were. Seventeen patients with less than moderate retardation continued to have seizures at the final follow-up.

Among clinical factors, positive family history of epilepsy and incidences of absence status or minor epileptic status appeared to be risk factors for unfavorable outcome (23). Thus, we would like to stress that the prognosis of patients depends on the type of combined seizures rather than the main seizure type being either atonic or myoclonic.

DISTINCTION BETWEEN MAE AND BME

There has been some controversy as to the inclusion criteria of MAE and whether we should limit it to the cases with astatic drop attacks, excluding those without drop attacks, and strictly adhering to the terminology of "myoclonic-astatic" epilepsy (4,7,8,23). In this study, we included the patients who had myoclonic seizures without drop attacks. Some of these patients also had myoclonic seizures during sleep, and ultimate benign outcomes, thus mimicking benign myoclonic epilepsy in infancy except for the presence of recurrent afebrile GTCS or GCS (5) (Fig. 12–7). The discussion of whether we should categorize these patients into the borderland of BME or the spectrum of MAE appeared to be meaningless, because we could not demonstrate a clear difference as to clinical and EEG characteristics as well as to prognosis between the atonic and myoclonic groups (Table 12–2).

We have to stress that astatic or drop attacks are merely the ultimate consequence of disruption

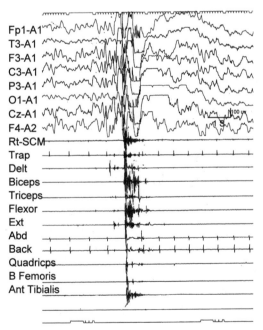

FIG. 12–7. A myoclonic seizure recorded by the video-polygraph. The patient was a 2-year 2-month-old girl with favorable MAE. She had recurrent afebrile GTCS before experiencing nocturnal and daytime myoclonic seizures. This polygraph recorded during sleep showed brief myoclonic EMG discharges involving the whole body. In the video, she had sudden abduction and flexion of both arms and, less intensely, both legs.

TABLE 12–2. *Comparisons of clinical manifestations among the three predominant seizure groups determined by ictal video-polygraphs (N = 30)*

Seizure group	Atonic	Myoclonic-atonic	Myoclonic
N	11	3	16
Male/female	7/4	1/2	9/7
Age of onset of epilepsy (m)	32 ± 10	33 ± 11	27 ± 10
Age of onset of MS/AS (m)	37 ± 13	38 ± 15	32 ± 13
Circadian rhythm (awake/sleep/diffuse)	11/0/0	3/0/0	10/2/4
Drop attack	11	3	6
GTCS	10	3	13
Atypical absence seizures	5	3	6
Minor epileptic status (MES)	2	0	3
Unfavorable prognosis	2	0	8

(From Oguni H, Fukuyama Y, Tanaka T, et al. Myoclonic-astatic epilepsy of early childhood—clinical and EEG analysis of myoclonic-astatic seizures, and discussions on the nosology of the syndrome. *Brain Develop.* 2001;23(7):757–764. With permission.)

of posture control under gravity, and may present as head nodding, sagging or subtle movement if they are mild, forming a spectrum of astasia regardless of myoclonic or atonic seizures. Thus, the most important aspect of nosologic discussion should focus on what type of seizures, atonic, myoclonic or myoclonic–atonic or even brief tonic seizures, produce astatic or drop attacks, and not on presence or absence of astatic or drop phenomenon. Thus, we have included those with myoclonic seizures, which did not make the patients fall or drop to the ground, but only produced subtle astasia.

TREATMENT

In our previous retrospective analysis, ketogenic diet treatment with either classic or MCT types, followed by ACTH, ethosuximide (ESM), clonazepam (CZP), valproate (VPA), and nitrazepam (NTZ), in this order, was most effective for myoclonic-astatic seizures, exhibiting an excellent effect in 58% of the patients (23). Among the AEDs, ESM was most effective in inducing a good or better response in 64% of the patients, achieving results almost comparable with those of ACTH. Supporting the suggestion of Doose, as well as other investigators, that ESM appeared to be the most favorable AED for myoclonic-astatic seizures and that high-dose ESM, in combination with VPA, appears better at controlling myoclonic-astatic seizures (3,4,31). The combination of ESM with VPA

has also been reported to be effective for refractory absence seizures (32). ESM and VPA are considered to have a synergistic effect on absence seizures or bursts of spike-and-wave complexes, which also produce myoclonic and atonic seizures. Better responses to ACTH and ketogenic diet than to ESM should be for the same reason, because both treatments have been shown to be most effective for atypical absence seizures and myoclonic seizures, but not so effective for generalized tonic seizures, which are rare in MAE (33,34). Recently, lamotrigine (LTG) has been successfully tried for some MAE patients (35). Thus, we recommend starting with VPA, and adding high-dose ESM in combination with VPA, if VPA monotherapy fails to control myoclonic-astatic seizures. If they fail to control attacks, we try LTG, CZP or NTZ. When the latter fail, we consider ACTH or ketogenic diet treatment. Although the response to treatments for other seizure types was difficult to evaluate, ketogenic diet treatment also appeared to be effective for convulsive and nonconvulsive seizures. We tried phenyltoin (PHT) for nocturnal convulsive seizures and obtained good results in some patients (*personal experience*).

NOSOLOGIC DISCUSSION OF MAE

In 78% of 81 patients with MAE in our series, the first seizure type was always generalized tonic-clonic or clonic seizures. They started within

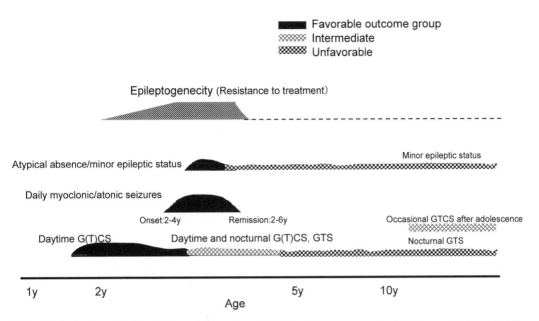

FIG. 12–8. Schematic illustration of age-dependent clinical course and clinical spectrum of MAE. Regardless of predominant seizure types and prognosis, the whole picture of MAE appears to form a clinical and EEG spectrum as shown in this figure. The GTCS starts within 1 to 5 years as a first manifestation and increases in frequency. Atonic or myoclonic seizures then develop and increase in frequency. Atypical absence seizures or minor epileptic status may appear simultaneously. Some nocturnal attacks may also follow, which are commonly resistant to conventional treatment. Then within months or a few years, the seizures suddenly or gradually disappear (black) with a few exceptional cases who continue nocturnal GTS and minor epileptic status (white). Some of the patients experience recurrence of GTCS after a long remission period (gray).

1 to 5 years of age and gradually increased in frequency (23). The interval between the first GTCS and myoclonic-astatic seizures ranged from 0 (days) to 35 months with a median period of 1 month. Treatment-resistant myoclonic-astatic seizures than progressively increased in frequency and finally occurred several to 100 times daily. Atypical absence seizures or minor epileptic status sometimes appeared simultaneously. Occasionally nocturnal attacks also followed. EEG showed slowing of background activity and was full of generalized spike-wave or polyspike-wave discharges, presenting a picture of epileptic encephalopathy. There were some differences in severity between cases. Then, within months or a few years, seizures suddenly or gradually disappeared, with few exceptional cases who continued nocturnal GTS and minor epileptic status. Some patients experienced recurrence of GTCS after a long-remission period.

Neurophysiologic and clinical analysis allows us to illustrate the nosologic framework of MAE (Fig. 12–8). Regardless of predominant seizure types and prognosis, the whole picture of MAE appears to form a clinical and EEG spectrum. If we exclude SME, MAE is considered a unique age-dependent epileptic encephalopathy. Epileptogenesis progresses to a peak within 1 year after onset. Recurrent GTCS, daily myoclonic/atonic seizures, or minor epileptic status are resistant to treatment. They gradually decrease within 2–3 years, when seizures become more easily controlled or they may spontaneously remit.

Myoclonic seizures are subclassified into myoclonic seizures involving proximal muscles not sufficient to cause the patients to fall and more massive seizures causing astatic falling due to strong flexion at the waist or extension of the trunk. There were no differences as to the clinical and EEG characteristics, as well as to the eventual prognosis between atonic and myoclonic groups. The clinical and EEG features of the myoclonic group with favorable prognosis appeared to resemble those with BME, except for the absence of GTCS or absence seizures, suggesting that both conditions share a common underlying pathophysiology. Thus differentiation of the exact seizure type itself, whether it is myoclonic or atonic, may not influence outcome or overall picture of this unique epileptic syndrome. At present, MAE should be recognized as an epileptic syndrome with a relatively wide clinical spectrum, ranging in their main seizure types from myoclonic to atonic seizures. Intellectual outcomes range from favorable to unfavorable. Final prognosis in most patients with MAE, despite initial resistance to antiepileptic drugs, appears to be better when we follow ILAE definitions excluding SME from the original MAE series (36). Although we did not do a systematic analysis, the depth of a positive spike following a negative spike appears to parallel the intensity of atonia. In addition, the atonia itself does not seem to be a direct consequence of spike-wave discharges. In the experimental model of absence seizures, the positive spike component of the spike-and-wave complex was found to correspond to the depth of negative wave or deep excitatory postsynaptic potentials (EPSPs) (37). Epileptic discharges restricted to the deeper laminae of the cortex, reflected as surface positive spike potentials, are shown to be more important in driving spinal motoneurons than the epileptic discharges restricted to the superficial layer of the cortex, reflected as surface negative spike potentials (38). This can reasonably explain the importance of the deep positive component responsible for the neurophysiological cause of atonia. Thus, electrophysiological events underlying MS/AS may be merely a consequence of genetically determined thalamocortical excitability that generates the generalized spike-and-wave complexes. Spike-and-wave, in turn, directly or indirectly produces myoclonic, myoclonic-atonic or atonic seizures, depending on the predominance of inhibition and excitation of neuronal activity (39,40). This can reasonably explain why ESM was best in controlling MS/AS (41,42).

However, we have to wait for advances in molecular biology that could give us a clue to the ultimate understanding of the pathogenesis of MAE. MAE may be a paradigm of a multifactorial disease (4,43,44).

CONCLUSION

Controversy continues regarding the distinction between BME, MAE, SME, and CLGS. These syndromes' clinical characters overlap, making it difficult to separate these disorders from each other, especially between MAE and the other three syndromes. Neurophysiologic as well as long-term follow-up studies of patients with MAE (we excluded the other three ILAE defined syndromes), have provided some evidence subdividing the main seizure types into atonic and myoclonic groups. All attacks corresponded to generalized spike- or polyspike-and-wave complexes. Interictal EEGs showed slowing of background activity and were full of generalized spike-wave or polyspike-wave discharges, presenting a picture of epileptic encephalopathy. There were some differences in severity between cases. With respect to seizure outcome, myoclonic-astatic seizures in 89% of patients disappeared within 1 to 3 years despite initial resistance. GTCS tended to continue. The most effective treatment for myoclonic-astatic seizures was ketogenic diet, followed by ACTH and ESM. The MAE patients were subclassified into favorable, intermediate, and unfavorable forms, according to the ultimate seizure outcomes. We could not demonstrate a clear difference as to the clinical and EEG characteristics as well as the prognosis between the atonic group and myoclonic groups. Although the determination of exact seizure type in MAE is scientifically important, distinguishing between myoclonic or atonic seizures, may not influence the outcome of this unique epileptic syndrome. MAE is considered a unique age-dependent epileptic encephalopathy, whose epileptogenesis progresses to a peak within 1 year after the onset. Recurrent GTCS, daily myoclonic/atonic seizures, or minor epileptic status are initially resistant to treatment. They gradually decrease within 2 to 3 years, when seizures become more easily controlled or spontaneously remit. At present, MAE should be recognized as an epileptic syndrome with a relatively wide clinical spectrum whose main seizure types range from myoclonic to atonic. Intellectual outcomes range from favorable to unfavorable. The final prognosis in most patients with MAE, despite initial resistance, appears to be better when we follow ILAE definitions, excluding SME from the original MAE series.

CASE PRESENTATIONS

Case 1

A 12-year-old boy with favorable MAE. He developed febrile GTCS twice in one day at 2 years and 11 months of age (Fig. 12–9). One and a half months later, he had afebrile GTCS, recurring once every week or two weeks. Subsequently, he developed recurrent daily drop attacks at the age of 38 months. PB, VPA, and CZP did not affect seizures. He was

referred to the hospital and admitted for examination. Although there was no gross neurologic abnormality, he was rather hyperactive and had difficulty concentrating. TK-Binet IQ was 84. Interictal EEG showed slow background activity consisting of centroparietal dominant 6-7 Hz theta activity during wakefulness and frequent intermittent generalized spike-and-wave complexes at 1.5 to 3 Hz during sleep (Fig. 12–10). A video-polygraphic study was performed to investigate his seizures. When he was sitting on the floor, he experienced a sudden collapse of his body forward, with immediate recovery. Surface EMG showed sudden interruption of ongoing electromyographic activity. When he was standing, his body and leg suddenly sagged; in more intense attacks we only recognized sudden facial change without any movement of the body (Fig. 12–3). There were also atypical absence seizures, corresponding to generalized rapid spike bursts. Brain magnetic resonance imaging (MRI), computerized tomography (CT) scan, as well as cerebrospinal fluid (CSF) and metabolic

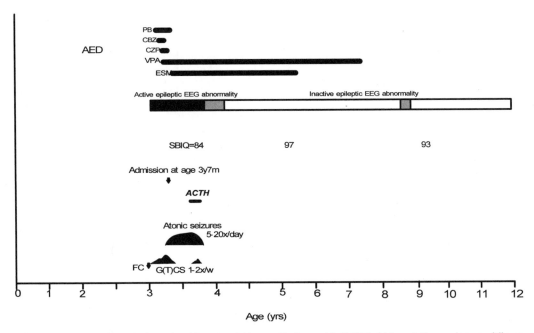

FIG. 12–9. Clinical evolution of a 12-year-old boy with favorable MAE. Abbreviations: dense oblique line, active epileptic EEG abnormality; oblique line, inactive epileptic abnormality; FC, febrile convulsion; GTCS, generalized tonic-clonic seizures or generalized clonic seizures.

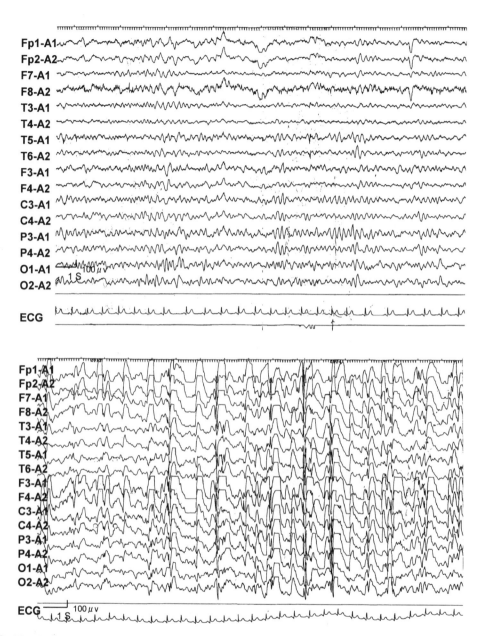

FIG. 12–10. Interictal EEG findings of the patient shown in Fig. 12–9. The upper EEG was recorded during wakefulness and the lower EEG during sleep.

investigation, including organic and amino acid analysis failed to reveal any abnormality. A combination of high-dose ESM (up to 127 μm/ml) and VPA (66 μm/ml) therapy was administered with significant reduction of seizure frequency, but failed to control his atonic attacks

completely. ACTH therapy transiently produced eye-opening seizures during sleep, corresponding to generalized multiple spike-bursts, and GTCS twice. ACTH controlled atonic seizures completely. He has been seizure-free since the age of 46 months. He has enjoyed junior high school. WISC-R performed at 10 years of age showed FSIQ was 97.

Case 2

A 10-year-old girl with favorable MAE. She started to have recurrent afebrile GTCS (once every 2 weeks) at the age of 32 months. A few weeks later, she developed myoclonic seizures, which became daily. She was referred to the hospital at 34 months of age. Myoclonic seizures were characterized by a momentary jerking of both arms and legs and trunk (Fig. 12–7). They occurred mostly during sleep. When attacks were strong, they sometimes produced short breath sounds and the patient was awakened from sleep. Interictal EEG showed slow background activity consisting of diffuse theta and delta activity, and frequent intermittent generalized single and multiple spike-and-wave complexes at 2–3 Hz during wakefulness and sleep. Myoclonic seizures were finally controlled by combination of VPA and ESM at 36 months of age (Fig. 12–11). She has been seizure-free since then. Her IQ was 92 (WISC-R FSIQ) at 9 years of age.

Case 3

A 19-year 3-month-old girl with intermediate outcome. She started to have atonic seizures at 13 months of age. She had daily head-nodding or brief drop attacks despite AED treatment in the local hospital (Fig. 12–12). She also experienced brief generalized clonic attacks. Her development had been stagnant and her Developmental Quotient was 62, equivalent to that of a 2-year-old, when she was first referred to our hospital at 3 years 1 month of age. Her drop attacks were making her susceptible to injuries. When she was standing and playing the organ, she collapsed straight downward onto her buttocks, and hit her head on the organ. When she was sitting, she showed only head-nodding. A videopolygraphic study demonstrated attacks that corresponded to generalized spike-and-wave complexes with a sudden interruption of ongoing EMG discharges. When she was lying on her back, we could observe some myoclonic components preceding the atonic attacks. The atonic seizures were controlled by a combination of VPA and ESM at the age of 38 months. After

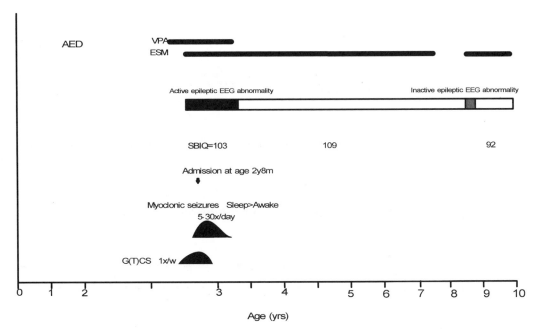

FIG. 12–11. Clinical evolution of a 10-year 5-month-old girl with favorable MAE. Abbreviations are the same as those in Fig. 12–3.

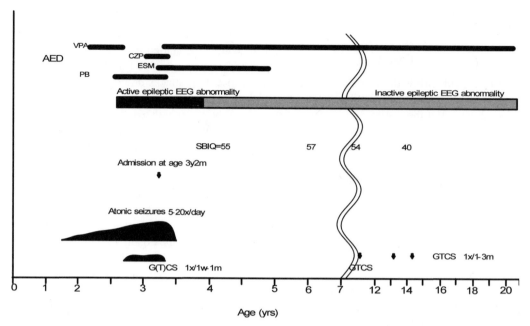

FIG. 12–12. Clinical evolution of a 19-year 3-month-old girl with intermediate MAE.

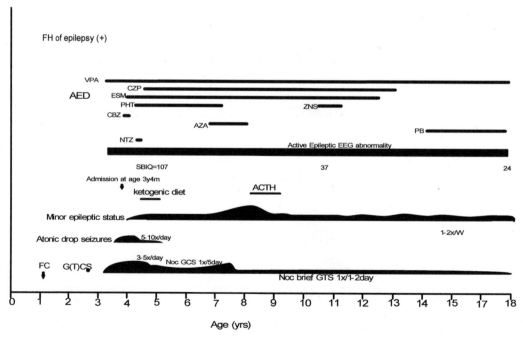

FIG. 12–13. Clinical evolution of an 18-year 5-month-old girl with unfavorable MAE. Abbreviation: Noc GCS, nocturnal generalized clonic seizures.

a long remission period, GTCS developed at 10 years 5 months of age, and continued once every 3 to 6 months, in part, due to drug omissions. Photosensitivity on the EEG also appeared after adolescence.

Case 4

An 18-year-5-month-old girl with unfavorable MAE. Her aunt had epilepsy and received medication. Her mother had a history of FC. The patient had FC at the age of 1 year 7 months. She started to have recurrent GCS at 39 months of age (Fig. 12–13). Myoclonic-astatic seizures developed at the age of 40 months; she was referred to the hospital. A video-polygraphic study captured sudden massive myoclonic attack causing retropulsion of the body, when she was lying on her side. The myoclonic-astatic seizures occurred only a few times a day. She had nocturnal short-lasting generalized tonic-clonic seizures with a prominent clonic component. She also experienced minor epileptic status (MES), characterized by cloudiness of consciousness with ataxia and some myoclonic component. It started upon awakening and persisted for a couple of hours, corresponding to diffuse irregular mixed slow activity and diffuse spike-and-wave complexes. Various AEDs, in addition to ketogenic diet and ACTH treatment, failed to control nocturnal convulsive attacks and MES. Myoclonic-astatic seizures were controlled at 44 months of age. At the age of 7 years, the tonic element was more pronounced in her nocturnal seizures. She has continued to have MES and nocturnal generalized tonic vibrating seizures. Her IQ level decreased from 107 at 3 years of age to 24 at 18 years of age.

REFERENCES

1. Engel J Jr. International League Against Epilepsy (ILAE). A proposed diagnostic scheme for people with epileptic seizures and with epilepsy: report of the ILAE Task Force on Classification and Terminology. *Epilepsia* 2001;42(6):796–803.
2. Dalla Bernardina, B, Capovilla G, Chiamenti C, et al. Cryptogenic myoclonic epilepsies of infancy and childhood; Nosological and prognostic approach. In: Wolf P, Dam M, Janz D, Dreifuss FE, eds. *Advances in Epileptology:* 16th Epilepsy International Symposium. New York: Raven Press, 1986:175–179.
3. Aicardi J. Myoclonic epilepsies of infancy and early childhood. In: Aicardi J, ed. *Epilepsy in children.* New York: Raven Press, 1992:67–79.
4. Doose H. Myoclonic astatic epilepsy of early childhood. In: Roger J, Dravet C, Bureau M, Dreifuss FE, Wolf P, eds. *Epileptic syndromes in infancy, childhood and adolescence.* 2nd ed. London: John Libbey, 1992:103–114.
5. Dravet C, Bureau M, Roger J. Benign myoclonic epilepsy in infants. In: Roger J, Bureau M, Dravet C, Dreifuss FE, Perret A, Wolf P, eds. *Epileptic syndromes in infancy, childhood and adolescence.* 2nd ed. London: John Libbey, 1992:67–74.
6. Dravet C, Bureau M, Roger J. Severe myoclonic epilepsy in infants. In: Roger J, Bureau M, Dravet C, Dreifuss FE, Perret A, Wolf P, eds. *Epileptic syndromes in infancy, childhood and adolescence.* 2nd ed. London: John Libbey, 1992:75–88.
7. Guerrini R, Dravet C, Gobbi G, et al. Idiopathic generalized epilepsies with myoclonus in infancy and childhood. In: Malafosse A, Genton P, Hirsch E, Marescaux C, Broglin D, Bernasconi R, eds. Idiopathic generalized epilepsies: clinical, experimental and genetic aspects. London: John Libbey, 1994:267–280.
8. Kaminska A, Ickowicz A, Plouin P, et al. Delineation of cryptogenic Lennox-Gastaut syndrome and myoclonic astatic epilepsy using multiple correspondence analysis. *Epilepsy Res* 1999;36(1):15–29.
9. Guerrini R, Parmeggiani L, Kaminska A, et al. Myoclonic astatic epilepsy. In: Roger J, Bureau M, Dravet C, Genton P, Tassinary CA, Wolf P, eds. *Epileptic syndromes in infancy, childhood and adolescence.* 3rd ed. London: John Libbey, 2002:105–112.
10. Harper JR. True myoclonic epilepsy in childhood. *Arch Dis Childhood* 1968;43:28–35.
11. Doose H, Gerken H, Leonhardt R, et al. Centrencephalic myoclonic-astatic petit mal. *Neuropediatrie* 1970;2:59–78.
12. Aicardi J, Chevrie JJ. Myoclonic epilepsies of childhood. *Neuropediatrie* 1971;3:177–190.
13. Jeavons PM. Nosological problems of myoclonic epilepsies in childhood and adolescence. *Develop Med Child Neurol* 1977;19:3–8.
14. Aicardi J. Course and prognosis of certain childhood epilepsies with predominantly myoclonic seizures. In: Wada JA, Penry JK, eds. *Advances in Epileptology:* 10th Epilepsy International Symposium. New York: Raven Press, 1980:159–163.
15. Dravet C, Roger J, Bureau M, et al. Myoclonic epilepsies in childhood. In: Akimoto H, Kazamatsuri H, Seino M, Ward A, eds. *Advances in Epileptology:* 13th Epilepsy International Symposium. New York: Raven Press, 1982:135–140.
16. Rossi GP, Gobbi G, Melideo G, et al. Myoclonic manifestations in the Lennox-Gastaut syndrome and other childhood epilepsies. In: Niedermeyer E, Degen R, eds. The Lennox-Gastaut syndrome. New York: Liss, 1988:137–158.
17. Oguni H, Fukuyama Y. A clinical and electroencephalographic study of myoclonic epilepsies in infancy and early childhood: Part 1. On the classification. *J Jpn Epil Soc* (Jpn) 1989;7:67–76.
18. Oguni H, Fukuyama Y. A clinical and electroencephalographic study of myoclonic epilepsies in infancy and early childhood: Part 2. Idiopathic myoclonic epilepsy

with benign prognosis. *J Jpn Epil Soc* (Jpn) 1989;7:77–88.

19. Oguni H, Fukuyama Y, Imaizumi Y, et al. A video-EEG analysis of drop seizures in myoclonic astatic epilepsy of early childhood (Doose syndrome). *Epilepsia* 1992;33(5):805–813.

20. Oguni H, Imaizumi Y, Uehara T, et al. Electroencephalographic features of epileptic drop attacks and absence seizures: a case study. *Brain Develop* 1993;15:226–230.

21. Oguni H, Uehara T, Imai K, et al. Atonic epileptic drop attacks associated with generalized spike-and-wave complexes—video-polygraphic study in two patients. *Epilepsia* 1997;38:813–818.

22. Oguni H, Fukuyama Y, Tanaka T, et al. Myoclonic-astatic epilepsy of early childhood—clinical and EEG analysis of myoclonic-astatic seizures, and discussions on the nosology of the syndrome. *Brain Develop* 2001;23(7):757–764.

23. Oguni H, Tanaka T, Hayashi K, et al. Treatment and long-term prognosis of myoclonic-astatic epilepsy of early childhood. *Neuropediatrics* 2002;33(3):122–132.

24. Egli M, Mothersill I, O'Kane M, et al. The axial spasm—the predominant type of drop seizure in patients with secondary generalized epilepsy. *Epilepsia* 1985;26:401–415.

25. Ikeno T, Shigematsu H, Miyakoshi M, et. al. An analytic study of epileptic falls. *Epilepsia* 1985;26:612–621.

26. Aicardi J. Lennox-Gastaut syndrome. In: Aicardi J, ed. *Epilepsy in children.* New York: Raven Press, 1992:44–66.

27. Dulac O, N'Guyen T. The Lennox-Gastaut syndrome. *Epilepsia* 1993;34[Suppl 7]:7–17.

28. Oguni H, Kitami H, Osawa M. Long-term prognosis of Lennox-Gastaut syndrome. *Epilepsia.* 1996;37[Suppl 3]:44–47.

29. Beaumanoir A, Blume W. Lennox-Gastaut syndrome. In: Roger J, Bureau M, Dravet C, Genton P, Tassinary CA, Wolf P, eds. *Epileptic syndromes in infancy, childhood and adolescence,* 3rd ed. London: John Libbey, 2002:113–135.

30. Tanaka T, Tsurumi E, Shirakawa S, et al. Neurophysiological analysis of the epileptic atonic drop attack. *Jpn J EEG EMG* (Jpn) 1998:175.

31. Wallace SJ. Myoclonus and epilepsy in childhood: A review of treatment with valproate, ethosuximide, lamotrigine and zonisamide. *Epilepsy Res* 1998;29(2):147–154.

32. Rowan AJ, Meijer JWA, de Beer-Pawlikowski N, et al. Valproate-ethosuximide combination therapy for refractory absence seizures. *Arch Neurol* 1983;40:797–802.

33. Vining EP. Clinical efficacy of the ketogenic diet. *Epilepsy Res* 1999;37(3):181–190.

34. Yamatogi Y, Ohtsuka Y, Ishida T, et al. Treatment of the Lennox-Gastaut syndrome with ACTH: Clinical and electroencephalographic study. *Brain Develop* 1979;1:267–276.

35. Dulac O, Kaminska A. Use of lamotrigine in Lennox-Gastaut and related epilepsy syndromes. *J Child Neurol* 1997;12[Suppl 1]:23–28.

36. Proposal for revised classification of epilepsies and epileptic syndromes; Commission on classification and terminology of the international league against epilepsy. *Epilepsia* 1989;30:389–399.

37. Weir B, Sie PG. Extracellular unit activity in cat cortex during the spike-wave complex. *Epilepsia* 1966;7:30–43.

38. Elger CE, Speckmann E-J, Prohaska O, et al. Pattern of intracortical potential distribution during focal interictal epileptiform discharges (FIED) and its relation to spinal field potentials in the rat. *Electroencephalogr Clin Neurolophysiol* 1981;51:393–402.

39. Gloor P. Electrophysiology of generalized epilepsy. In: Schwartzkroin PA, Wheel H, eds. *Electrophysiology of epilepsy.* New York: Academic Press, 1984:107–136.

40. Dulac O, Plouin P, Shewmon A. Myoclonus and epilepsy in childhood: 1996 Royaumont meeting. *Epilepsy Res* 1998;30(2):91–106.

41. Coulter DA, Huguenard JR, Prince DA. Characterization of ethosuximide reduction of low-threshold calcium current in thalamic neurons. *Ann Neurol* 1989;25(6):582–593.

42. Snead OC, 3rd, Depaulis A, Vergnes M, et al. Absence epilepsy: advances in experimental animal models. *Adv Neurol* 1999;79:253–78.

43. Doose H, Baier WK. Genetic factors in epilepsies with primarily generalized minor seizures. *Neuropediatrics* 1987;18:1–64.

44. Scheffer IE, Wallace R, Mulley JC, et al. Clinical and molecular genetics of myoclonic-astatic epilepsy and severe myoclonic epilepsy in infancy (Dravet syndrome). *Brain Develop* 2001;23:732–735.

13

Myoclonic Absences: The Seizure and The Syndrome

Michelle Bureau* and Carlo Alberto Tassinari[†]

*Centre Saint-Paul, Hôpital Henri Gastaut, Marseille, France; [†]Ospedale Bellaria, Bologna, Italy

INTRODUCTION

Myoclonic absences (MA) represent a specific seizure type, whose diagnosis rests on clinical observation and ictal polygraphic and EEG-video recording. Clinically MA are characterized by rhythmic and bilateral jerks of the limbs. The ictal electroencephalogram shows a rhythmic, bilateral, synchronous, and symmetric spike-and-wave discharge at 3 Hz associated with myoclonias rhythmically repeated at 3 Hz and an increasing tonic contraction.

Since the first description by Tassinari et al. in 1969, 1971 (1,2), and later in 1985 (3), the authors stressed the fact that MA represent an individual seizure type and proposed the existence of a specific epileptic syndrome in which MA were the only or the predominant seizure type. It should thus be separated from other forms of generalized epilepsy, such as childhood absence epilepsy (CAE). Indeed, MA were shown to be most often associated with mental retardation and a resistance to medical treatment so that the prognosis was more severe than in idiopathic generalized epilepsy (IGE).

The 1989 International classification of epilepsies and epileptic syndromes eventually recognized that epilepsy with MA was a separate entity and included it in the group of cryptogenic or symptomatic generalized epilepsies (4). This can be found in the new proposed diagnostic scheme for people with epileptic seizures and with epilepsy (5). Epilepsy with MA is maintained in epilepsy syndromes and related conditions.

THE MYOCLONIC ABSENCE: A SPECIFIC SEIZURE TYPE

Clinical Symptomatology

Motor Manifestations

The myoclonias constitute the constant characteristic feature, often associated with more or less tonic contraction. The myoclonias mainly involve the muscles of the shoulders, arms, and legs. The muscles of the face are less frequently involved. When this occurs, they are more evident around the chin and the mouth, whereas twitching eyelids is typically absent or rare.

Due to concomitant tonic contraction, the jerking of the arms is accompanied by a progressive elevation of the upper extremities, giving rise to a quite constant and recognizable pattern. When the patient is standing, falling is uncommon but a backward or forward oscillation is frequently seen. Head and body deviation (without concomitant ocular or oculoclonic deviation) can be observed in some cases. In some cases slight automatic movements were observed.

Impairment of consciousness is of variable intensity, ranging from a complete loss of consciousness to a mild disruption of contact. Sometimes the myoclonias are felt as a very disturbing experience; the subject frequently holds himself, giving the impression of attempting to control the intensity of the jerking. He may recall the words pronounced by the examiner during the seizure.

Autonomic Manifestations

In some cases a change or an arrest of respiration and sometimes a loss of urine can be noted.

- The MA have an abrupt onset and termination
- The duration ranges from 10 to 60 s (longer than usually observed in CAE)
- The frequency is high and MA occur at least several times per day—often tens of times per day. They are often provoked by hyperventilation or awakening. In 14% of cases, they can be elicited by intermittent photic stimulation (ILS). MA can occur during light sleep, sometimes awakening the patient. Episodes of MA status are distinctly rare [1 case among 36 cases reported by Tassinari et al. (6)].

EEG and Polygraphic Symptomatology

The ictal EEG consists of rhythmic spike-and-wave discharge at 3 Hz, bilateral, synchronous, and symmetric, as observed in the absences of CAE. The onset and the end of the spike-waves are abrupt, except in rare cases in which the EEG discharge ends progressively, sometimes with asymmetric delta waves over the frontal areas. In some seizures, typical spike-waves can be intermixed with polyspikes

The polygraphic recording discloses the appearance of bilateral and rhythmic myoclonias, at the same frequency as the spike-waves, beginning about 1 s after the onset of the EEG discharge. Later into the seizure, the myoclonias are associated with a tonic contraction that is maximal on the shoulder and deltoid muscles and that is responsible for the elevation of the arms (Fig. 13–1). The tonic contraction can mask or render the myoclonias clinically less evident; the motor manifestations are thus less

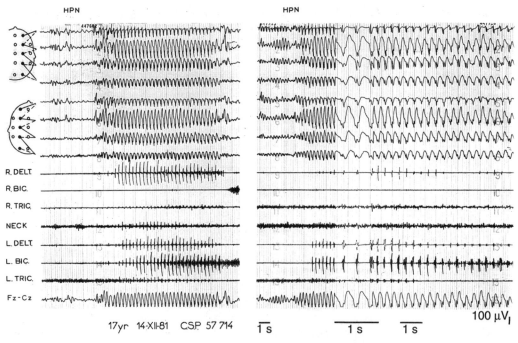

FIG. 13–1. Myoclonic absences (MA) elicited by hyperventilation. **Left:** MA characterized by a 3-Hz spike-and-waves discharge. Note that the rhythmic jerks (recorded on the right and left deltoids, biceps and triceps muscles, and on the neck) appear 1 to 2 s after the onset of the spike-wave discharge and that the tonic contraction appears 3 to 4 s later, mainly on the left deltoid. **Right:** another MA, recorded at 30 mm/s.

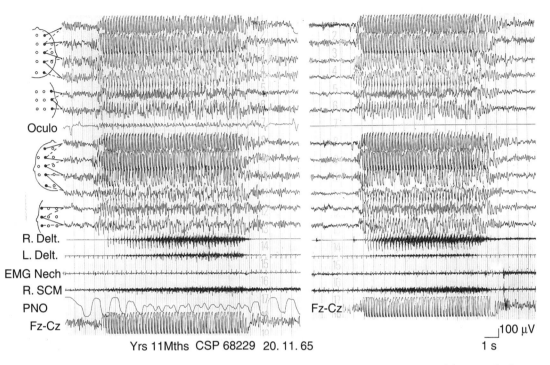

Oculo

R. Delt.
L. Delt.
EMG Nech
R. SCM
PNO
Fz-Cz

Fz-Cz

100 µV

1 s

Yrs 11Mths CSP 68229 20. 11. 65

FIG. 13–2. Myoclonic absences in a 6 year 11 month old boy. Note the asymmetry of the myoclonias and the tonic contraction that is more intense on the right deltoid than on the left.

evident. Sometimes the myoclonias and the tonic contraction are unilateral or clearly asymmetric (Fig. 13–2) (with a jerky rotation of head and trunk) despite the generalized EEG pattern (Fig. 13–3).

Tassinari et al. (1,2) proved, by means of high-speed oscilloscopic recording, that there is a strict and constant relation between the spike-wave discharge and the myoclonias. The detailed morphology of spikes shows a positive transient (7) of high amplitude in strict relationship with the appearance, latency, and amplitude of the myoclonias. Each spike on the EEG is followed on the electromyography (EMG) by a myoclonia with a latency of 15 to 40 msec for the more proximal muscles and of 50 to 70 msec for the more distal muscles. This myoclonia is again followed by a brief silent period (60 to 120 msec) that interrupts the tonic contraction.

At times, the spike-wave in the first second are of smaller amplitude (because the early positive component of the spike is of small amplitude) and are not accompanied by myoclonias (Fig. 13–4).

The awake interictal EEG shows a normal background activity for age in all cases. We have never recorded the sinusoidal slow rhythm in the posterior areas, as has been observed in CAE. Generalized spike-waves are noted in one-third of cases and, more rarely, focal or multifocal anomalies. ILS is without effect except when it elicits MA.

Myoclonic Absences and Sleep

Sleep organization is constantly normal and physiologic patterns (vertex spikes, K complexes, spindles) are present bilaterally and symmetrically. The evolution of interictal spike-wave discharges during sleep is similar to that observed in CAE (8). The MA can occur during stage I of sleep, sometimes awakening the patient (Fig. 13–5). Generalized spike-wave discharges of variable duration (25–10 s), that are sometimes associated with bursts of myoclonias, can be observed during sleep stages II and III. Isolated spikes or irregular spike-waves predominating on one or the other anterior regions are

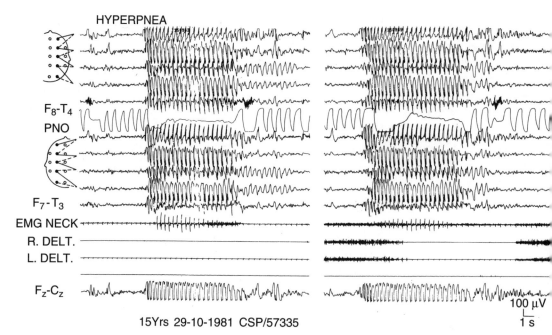

FIG. 13–3. MA elicited by hyperventilation. The myoclonic jerks involve only the neck muscles causing a jerky rotation of head.

frequent during slow sleep. On the other hand, no other interictal discharges are recorded and, particularly, no bursts of fast rhythms at 10 Hz as observed in the Lennox-Gastaut syndrome (LGS).

SEIZURES OTHER THAN MYOCLONIC ABSENCES

In one-third of cases, MA are the only seizure type observed throughout the evolution. In two-third of cases there are other seizures either before the onset or the diagnosis of MA or in association with MA.

Seizures before the onset or the diagnosis of MA were found in 38% of cases. These were, above all, simple absences (in some cases, in fact, these may have been MA that were not recognized), and rare generalized tonic-clonic seizures (GTCS) or convulsive seizures, generally of a clonic type. A lasting febrile convulsion was noted in only one case.

Seizures Associated with MA

GTCS are noted in 45% of cases. They are rare in one-half of the cases (<1 per year), and in the other cases they were very frequent (1 per

month) and occurred without circadian distribution. Simple absences were mentioned in 4% of cases, sometimes accompanied by some eyelid myoclonias. In 33% of cases were mentioned sudden and serious falls, which have, however, never been recorded. Absence status without myoclonias accompanied by spike-wave discharges on the EEG were recorded in 17% of cases. Only one patient in our series has presented a status with rhythmical myoclonias and diffuse spike-wave discharges, which was interrupted by an intravenous injection of diazepam. Only 10% of patients had more than two types of seizures.

DIFFERENTIAL DIAGNOSIS

Polygraphic recording (EEG + EMG) is mandatory when the clinical suspicion of MA is raised. Indeed, the diagnosis of MA rests mainly on the polygraphy that shows spike-wave discharges at 3 Hz in strict relation with severe, diffuse, and rhythmic myoclonias at 3 Hz.

After the first descriptions, several studies contributed to confirm or to exclude the diagnosis of MA and emphasized the importance of the polygraphic recordings (6,9–14). The following

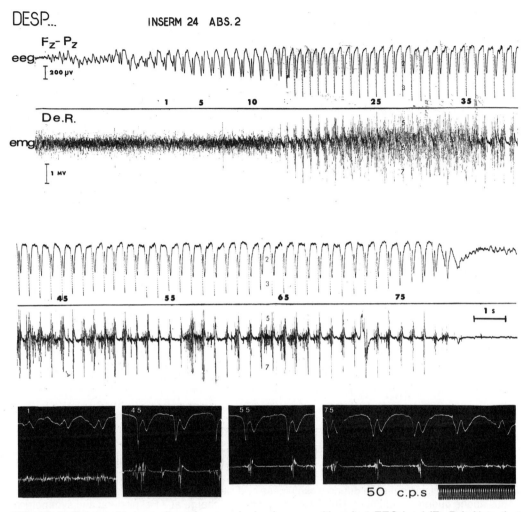

FIG. 13–4. Polygraphic recording of a myoclonic absence with only 1 EEG lead (Fz-Pz). Note that low-amplitude spike-wave precedes the onset of myoclonic jerks and of tonic contraction, which are correlated with an increase of amplitude of the spike-wave. The myoclonias last as long as the spike-wave discharge, while the tonic contraction resolves during the absence.

list illustrates how MA can be differentiated from some other very similar myoclonic seizures based on clinical description alone:

- Generalized clonic seizures accompanied by discharges of polyspike waves and not by 3-Hz spike-waves do not occur in rhythmic bursts and are not associated with an impairment of consciousness.
- Absences with a mild clonic component (classification of the ILAE; 15) in which myoclonias involve only eyelids and facial muscles. In 2001, Cappovilla et al. (14) investigated

12 patients with absence seizures associated with myoclonic manifestations and a spike-wave discharge at 3 Hz, similar to that observed in MA or in typical absences. The myoclonias in their cases were typically restricted to the facial areas (eyebrows, nostrils, perioral regions, chin) or neck muscles, contrary to the MA in which there is a constant and prominent involvement of the proximal limb muscles. Indeed, clinically, all patients reported by Capovilla et al. showed a benign evolution: during follow-up, seven patients withdrew from treatment without relapse. This study

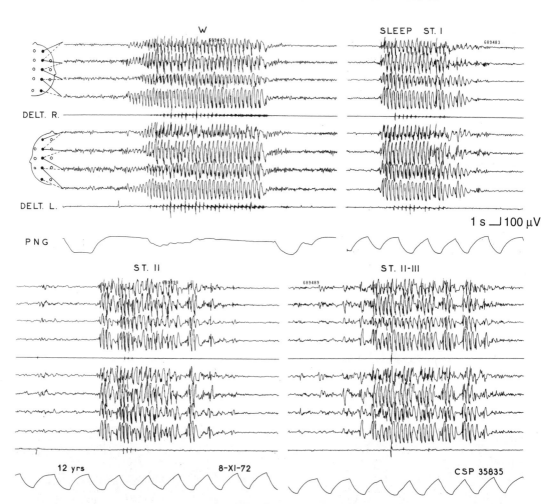

FIG. 13–5. Myoclonic absence during wakefulness and sleep in a 12-year-old girl. **Top left:** Spontaneous abene during wakefulness. Rhythmic spike-wave discharge at 3 Hz, bilateral and symmetrical accompanied by rhythmic myoclonias at the same frequency of the spike-wave. Note the associated contraction and arrest of respiration. **Top right:** MA during stage 1 of shorter duration. **Bottom left and right:** Generalized spike-wave discharge during sleep stages II and III. The spike-wave discharges are irregular, fragmented, and associated with mild and variable myoclonias.

points out the importance of polygraphic recordings to differentiate between absences with myoclonias and MA.

- Partial motor seizures when the motor manifestations of MA are asymmetrical [with head and body turning (Fig. 13–5)] or predominant on one side.

In 1988, Giovanardi Rossi et al. (16) described, under the name of atypical MA, four cases in which the clinical diagnosis could be invoked because of the association, during a seizure, of loss of contact, eyelid myoclonias, and myoclonias of the arms. However, there were atypical clinical phenomena described as slow falls in two cases. The seizures were elicited by the opening or the closure of the eyes in three cases. The EEG was different, above all because of the existence of fast rhythms occurring between the spike-wave discharges or preceding the generalized 3-Hz spike-wave discharges.

Elia et al. (17) studied 14 patients with MA. Among these, seven had chromosomal abnormalities (Angelman syndrome, four, 12p trisomy, two, and inv dup (15), one). In these cases, the MA were atypical because of their early onset, their brief duration, and the mild intensity of the myoclonias and the tonic contraction.

Finally, seizures mimicking MA have been observed in diffuse nonspecific epileptic encephalopathies. In such cases, the polygraphic recording shows atypical features consisting of irregular spike-waves, onset, and offset that are less abrupt or the combination of myoclonic motor phenomena and atonia (12).

In fact, the diagnosis of MA based on the anamnestic description only can be extremely difficult: motor manifestations, i. e., the rhythmic myoclonic movements, can be overlooked, particularly when there is a tonic contraction associated with them. During the evolution and possibly under the effect of treatment, the myoclonias can be of reduced intensity. In such cases, the polygraphic demonstration of MA can be a surprise.

MYOCLONIC ABSENCE EPILEPSY: THE SYNDROME

Myoclonic absences are a characteristic type of seizures, but other factors may justify the recognition of a specific syndrome distinct from other types of generalized epilepsy. From the review of 53 cases (40 cases observed at the Centre Saint-Paul in Marseille and 13 at the Bellaria Hospital at Bologna) some features may be considered distinctive of MA epilepsy. A detailed analysis of these cases was published in the third edition of the book *Epileptic Syndromes in Infancy, Childhood, and Adolescence* (10).

Incidence: Epilepsy with MA is an uncommon type of epilepsy accounting for 0.5 to 1% of all epilepsies observed in a selected population of epilepsies at the Centre Saint-Paul.

Sex ratio: There is a male preponderance (70%) at variance with the female preponderance (60 to 70%) in CAE (18).

Etiologic factors: Present in 35% of the cases (14/40 cases of the Centre Saint-Paul) [prematurity (four cases), perinatal damage (six cases), consanguinity, (two cases), congenital hemiparesis (one case), and partial trisomy of

the long arm of chromosome 14 (one case)]. Chromosomal anomalies have been also reported by other authors (17,19).

Genetic factors: A family history of epilepsy, most often generalized epilepsies, is found in about 20% of cases.

Age at onset: The mean age of onset is 7 years with a range from 11 months to 12 years 6 months. Some cases, beginning during the first year of life, have been reported (20,21).

Neurological state: Neurological state is normal, except in the case of congenital hemiparesis.

Neuroimaging: Neuroimaging is abnormal in 17% of the cases, mostly showing a slight degree of diffuse and aspecific atrophy, without focal lesions.

Seizures: In about one-third of the cases, MA are the only seizure type. In the remaining patients, other seizures occur either before the onset of MA or in association with them. They consist of GTCS, absences, seizures with fall or absence status.

Mental retardation: Mental retardation is noted in 45% of the cases before the onset of MA.

Evolution: A longitudinal study of long-term prognosis performed on the 40 cases of the Centre Saint-Paul (10) shows that MA disappear in 37.5% of the cases (15/40) (Group 1) and that they persist or that epilepsy changes in the other 25 cases (Group 2). Patient follow-up after the onset of epilepsy varied from 3 years 4 months to 29 years with a median of 13 years 2 months.

In Group 1, the mean follow-up after the end of MA is of 11 years 6 months (range 4–15 years) and the follow-up in Group 2 is of 12 years 5 months (7–23 years) after the onset of MA. The different parameters studied show that there are more personal antecedents in Group 1 than in Group 2 (47 vs. 20%). On the other hand, a family history of epilepsy is less frequent in the Group 1 than in the Group 2 (13 vs. 33%). The age of onset of MA is approximately the same in the two groups (mean: 7 years). The main difference concerns the associated seizures that were present in 80% of Group 2 and only in 40% of Group 1. In Group 2, the seizures were mainly represented by GTCS or seizures with falls, while, in Group 1, simple absences were the only associated seizure type.

In Group 2, five patients have shown a disappearance of MA and the appearance of other seizure types, such as atypical absences, without myoclonias and slow spike-waves on the EEG, as well as clinical or subclinical tonic seizures which are accompanied on the EEG by fast rhythms. This resulted in an electroclinical picture similar to that of the LGS. This state was transitory in two cases. MA reappeared afterward and remained the only seizure type with a comparatively benign outcome.

The appearance or worsening of psychomotor retardation was observed in the two groups, but it was more severe and concerned more children in Group 2.

On the other hand, one of the factors predictive of good or bad outcome, i.e., adequate treatment as mentioned by Tassinari et al. (6,12,22), is not confirmed in our long-term study of 40 patients. Indeed, the association in 17 cases of sodium valproate (VPA) and ethosuximide (ESM) at appropriate doses led to a remission in only eight cases (47%). There was no notable difference between the time when the VPA + ESM cotherapy was given and the onset of MA (4 years 2 months, Group 1, and 3 years 6 months, Group 2). The plasma levels in the two groups were quite similar (VPA: 105.5 μg/ml in Group 1 vs. 90 μg/ml in Group 2 and ESM 60 μg/ml vs. 70 μg/ml). Patients with unfavorable outcome had numerous GTCS associated with MA. They had never received phenytoin or carbamazepine, which, in 5 other cases, have been considered factors of worsening.

Thus, the evolution of epilepsy seems to depend primarily on the existence of associated GTCS and is not in relation to the existence of signs of encephalopathy (27% in Group 1 and 9% in Group 2).

TREATMENT

The classical cotherapy VPA + ESM with appropriate plasma levels is more efficient if myoclonic absences are not associated with other seizures types, particularly with GTCS. In some cases, the combination of phenobarbital, VPA, and benzodiazepines leads to a good control of seizures. Manonmani and Wallace (11) and Wallace (23) showed that the combination of VPA or ESM with lamotrigine (LTG) could have a favorable effect in cases that are resistant to classic treatment. Other drugs such as levetiracetam (LEV), topiramate (TPM), or zonisamide (ZNS) may also prove to be of interest.

CONCLUSION

The syndrome of MA represents a particular form of epilepsy of childhood, because of a type of seizure that is observed exclusively in this form. The recognition of the specific seizure type rests on direct clinical observation and polygraphic EEG-video recording. The EEG–EMG pattern of MA is specific and allows differential diagnosis with other generalized seizure types. The diagnosis of MA is sufficient per se for the identification of a syndrome, namely myoclonic absence epilepsy that stands in the international classification of epilepsies and epileptic syndromes (Commission on Classification and terminology of the ILAE, 1989) among cryptogenic or symptomatic generalized epilepsies. There are two forms: a pure form in which MA are the single or the predominant type of seizures and another form in which MA are associated with other seizure types, particularly with numerous GTCS. The latter form has a very poor prognosis, which does not depend on treatment or on the timing of its prescription after the onset of MA, but seems to be related to the existence of associated GTCS.

REFERENCES

1. Tassinari CA, Lyagoubi S, Santos V, et al. Etude des décharges de pointes ondes chez l'homme. II: Les aspects cliniques et électroencéphalographiques des absences myocloniques. *Rev Neurol* 1969;121:379–383.
2. Tassinari CA, Lyagoubi S, Gambarelli F, et al. Relationships between EEG discharge and neuromuscular phenomena. *Electroencephalogr Clin Neurophysiol* 1971;31:176.
3. Tassinari CA, Bureau M. Epilepsy with myoclonic absences. In: Roger J, Dravet C, Bureau M, Dreifuss F, Wolf P, eds. *Epileptic syndromes in infancy, childhood and adolescence.* London: John Libbey, 1985:121–129.

4. Commission on Classification and Terminology of the International League Against Epilepsy: Proposal for revised classification of epilepsies and epileptic syndromes. *Epilepsia* 1989;30:389–399.

5. Engel J, Jr. A proposed diagnostic scheme for people with epileptic seizures and with epilepsy. Report of the ILAE Task Force on Classification and Terminology. *Epilepsia* 2001;42:796–803.

6. Tassinari CA, Bureau M, Thomas P. Epilepsy with myoclonic absences. In: Roger J, Bureau M, Dravet Ch, Dreifuss F, Perret A, Wolf P. eds. *Epileptic syndromes in infancy, childhood and adolescence.* 2nd ed. London: John Libbey, 1992:151–160.

7. Weir B. The morphology of the spike-wave complex. *Electroencephalogy Clin Neurophysiol* 1965;19:284–290.

8. Tassinari CA, Bureau-Paillas M, Dalla Bernardina B, et al. Generalized epilepsies and seizures during sleep. A polygraphic study. In: Van Praag HM, Meinardi H, eds. *Brain and sleep.* Amsterdam: De Erven Bhon, 1974:154–166.

9. Lugaresi E, Pazzaglia P, Franck L, et al. Evolution and prognosis of primary generalized epilepsies of the petit mal absence type. In: Lugaresi E, Pazzaglia P, Tassinari CA, eds. *Evolution and prognosis of epilepsy.* Bologna: Aulo Gaggi, 1973:2–22.

10. Bureau M, Tassinari CA. The syndrome of myoclonic absences. In: Roger J, Bureau M, Dravet Ch, Genton P, Tassinari CA, Wolf P, eds. *Epileptic syndromes in infancy, childhood and adolescence.* 3rd ed. London: John Libbey, 2002:305–312.

11. Manonmani V, Wallace SJ. Epilepsy with myoclonic absences. *Arch Dis Childhood* 1994;70:288–290.

12. Tassinari CA, Michelucci R, Rubboli G, et al. Myoclonic absences epilepsy. In: Duncan JS, Panayiotopoulos CP, eds. *Typical absences and related epileptic syndromes.* London: Churchill Livingstone, 1995:185–195.

13. Salas Puig J, Acebes A, Gonzalez C, et al. Epilepsy with myoclonic absences. *Neurologia* 1990;5:242–245.

14. Cappovilla G, Rubboli G, Beccaria F, et al. A clinical spectrum of the myoclonic manifestations associated with typical absences in childhood absence epilepsy. A video-polygraphic study. *Epileptic Disord* 2001;3:57–61.

15. Commission on Classification and Terminology of the International League Against Epilepsy. Proposal for revised classification of epileptic seizures. *Epilepsia* 1981;22:489–501.

16. Giovanardi Rossi P, Ricciotti A, Melideo G, et al. Atypical myoclonic absences: clinical, electroencephalographic and neuropsychological aspects. *Clin Electroencephalogr* 1988;19:87–94.

17. Elia M, Guerrini R, Musumeci S.A, et al. Myoclonus absence-like seizures and chromosome abnormality syndromes. *Epilepsia* 1998;39:660–663.

18. Loiseau P, Panayiotopoulos CP, Hirsch E. Childhood absence epilepsy and related syndromes. In: Roger J, Bureau M, Dravet C, Genton P, Tassinari CA, Wolf P. eds. Epileptic syndromes in infancy, childhood and adolescence. 3rd ed. London: John Libbey, 2002:285–303.

19. Guerrini R, Bureau M, Mattei MG, et al. Trisomy 12p syndrome: A chromosomal disorder associated with generalized 3-Hz spike and wave discharges. *Epilepsia* 1990;31:557–566.

20. Aicardi J. Typical absences. in the first two years of life. In: Duncan JS, Panayiotopoulos CP, eds. *Typical absences and related syndromes.* London: Churchill Livingstone, 1994:284–288.

21. Verrotti A, Greco R, Chiarelle F, et al. Epilepsy with myoclonic absences with early onset: a follow-up study. *J Child Neurol* 1999;14:746–749.

22. Tassinari CA, Michelucci R. Epilepsy with myoclonic absences: A reappraisal. In: Wolf P, ed. *Epileptic seizures and syndromes.* London: John Libbey, 1994:137–141.

23. Wallace SJ. Myoclonus and epilepsy in childhood: A review of treatment with valproate, ethosuximide, lamotrigine and zonisamide. *Epilepsy Res* 1998;29:147–154.

14

Eyelid Myoclonia and Absence

Athanasios Covanis

Neurology Department, The Childrens Hospital "Agia Sophia," Goudi, Athens, Greece

INTRODUCTION

Jeavons syndrome or the syndrome of eyelid my-oclonia and absence is a type of photosensitive epilepsy. In the literature it is usually included under myoclonic epilepsies, absences or even reflex epilepsies. Although "eyelid myoclonia and absences" (ELMA) has a number of characteristic clinical features that have been stressed by many authors the last decade, it is still underdiagnosed.

Jeavons in 1977 first described ELMA as a separate type of photosensitive epilepsy with this quotation: Eyelid myoclonia and absences show a marked jerking of the eyelids immediately after eye closure and there is an associated brief spike-and-wave activity. The eyelid movement is like rapid blinking and the eyes deviate upwards, in contrast to the very slight flicker of eyelids that may be seen in a typical absence in which the eyes look straight ahead. Brief absences may occur spontaneously and are accompanied by 3 cycles per second spike-and-wave discharges. The spike-and-wave discharges seen immediately after eye closure do not occur in the dark. Their presence in the routine EEG is a very reliable warning that abnormality will be evoked by photic stimulation (1). In 1982 Jeavons changed the term from eyelid myoclonia and absences to eyelid myoclonia with absences (2), which was a mistake as he later admitted (3). The term "eyelid myoclonia with absences" implies that an absence is induced by eye closure, whereas, in fact, absences also occur independently of eye closure, often being induced by hy-

perventilation (3) and intermittent photic stimulation (IPS).

In typical cases, there is marked jerking of the eyelids, which is more pronounced in bright sunlight and some children regarded as having self-induced epilepsy (4–6) appear to have eyelid myoclonia. Binnie et al (1980) commented on the need for prolonged EEG recording for the diagnosis and that eye closure on command failed to induce eyelid myoclonia. In our experience, in all patients, the diagnosis is easily made during routine sleep–wake electroencephalograms (EEG) and, in all children, eye closure on command induces eyelid myoclonia. Following the description of Jeavons, more authors have identified ELMA as a separate entity (7–14). Therapy is less effective than in other photosensitive epilepsies (7).

The classification of epilepsies and epileptic syndromes in 1989 (15) did not include ELMA and the recent diagnostic scheme for people with epileptic seizures and with epilepsies has accepted eyelid myoclonia with or without absences as a new seizure type (16).

DEFINITION

Eyelid myoclonia and absences is a form of idiopathic generalized epilepsy (IGE) with characteristic clinical and EEG features, which comply with the definition of an epileptic syndrome called "Jeavons Syndrome." The combination of clinical and EEG phenomena, which follow eye closure, are unique and pathognomonic of

ELMA: In a previous normal school age child, eye closure in the light induces eyelid flicker, flutter, or jerking in association with generalized EEG discharges. The eyes may open and stare or the eyelids open retract and jerk with an upward deviation of gaze (but never to the side). The discharges are invariably evoked during IPS. This type of discharge does not occur in the dark. The concomitant impairment of consciousness, conspicuous or inconspicuous, is relevant to the duration of the generalized discharge. Myoclonic jerks other than eyelid and generalized tonic–clonic seizures do occur. Females predominate in this condition.

EPIDEMIOLOGY

Prevalence

In 1982, we reported a prevalence of 7.3% among IGE (7). According to our unpublished data, ELMA represents 2.5% of all epilepsies and 11% of IGE. Similar prevalence of 2.7% and 12.9% correspondingly, is reported in adults (13). ELMA is as common as juvenile myoclonic epilepsy (JME), but is underdiagnosed and the mild forms underreported.

Sex Distribution and Age of Onset

As with most of the photosensitive epilepsies, eyelid myoclonia is more common in females. Two studies (7,11) reported a female to male ratio of 3.7:1 and 4:1, respectively. In another study (13) of 11 patients, all were female.

The age of onset is similar to that of childhood absence epilepsy (CAE) and earlier than most photosensitive epilepsies. An onset ranging from 2 to 14 years (mean 5.8 ± 2.3 y) has been reported (7,11,13). In our experience, based on 50 patients with ELMA, the female to male ratio is 3.2:1 and the age of onset from 2.5 to 14 years (mean 7.2 ± 2.7 y).

ETIOLOGY

Eyelid myoclonia and absences is an idiopathic generalized photosensitive epilepsy syndrome with characteristic clinical and EEG features. In contrast to the other syndromes, which have myoclonic jerks, absences, and generalized tonic–clonic seizures in different proportion in their phenotype, eyelid jerking is a unique feature of this syndrome. There is a familial preponderance and the concordance rate is high (17). In our population of 50 ELMA patients, the family history was positive for epilepsy in 28%. Among them there were nine families of probands with Jeavons syndrome and first-degree relatives with ELMA or IGE. The concordance rate was 78%. From these families, it is difficult to be specific about the mode of inheritance, although they suggest some dominant alleles.

PATHOPHYSIOLOGY

Jeavons syndrome is genetically determined and expressed in childhood. In order for the genetic predisposition to be manifest clinically, it needs the simultaneous operation of two additional factors: the spontaneous or on-command slow eye closure and the visual light input. Eye closure is a brief, less than a 3-msec phase during which the upper and lower eyelids touch. The hyperexcitable cortical area alone can generate spontaneous generalized discharges without apparent clinical phenomena, e.g., during sleep. A strong intermittent light input in a predisposed person without eye closure, can induce discharges, which may be associated with absences, e.g., during IPS with the eyes open. Eye closure in a predisposed person *cannot* generate discharges without light input, e.g., in total darkness. The eyelid movements are under voluntary, automatic, reflex, autonomic, and emotional control. The cortical area representing eye closure lies in the precentral gyrus adjacent to the hand area (18), which is involved in self-induced epilepsy. The "cortical factor" involved in spontaneous or on-command eye closure seems to be important as passive slow eye closure in the presence of light does not induce discharges or eyelid myoclonia in a predisposed person, except in some cases of early onset. Blinking, which is a brainstem reflex, does not trigger clinical and EEG phenomena. Similar observations are observed in self-induced epilepsy where the cortical hand area is involved. EEG and clinical phenomena are induced by hand waving, voluntary oɪ on-command in the presence of light. Passive hand waving or waving the examiners hand in front of the eye(s) in the presence of light does not induce discharges and clinical phenomena in a predisposed person.

Some authors believe that in ELMA there is a malfunction of alpha-rhythm generator (19) or a malfunction of the magnocellular and parvocellular system (20). However, alpha rhythm is produced on passive eye closure.

We have studied video-EEGs in a population of 50 children with ELMA and have observed two patterns of eye closure:

1. The normal quick blink pattern: The normal quick blink pattern, a positive wave is recorded in the frontal areas. The downward portion (eye closing) and the upward portion (eye opening) deflection of the positive wave lasts about 100 msec each. The eye closure phase is very brief—there is no plateau and no clinical and EEG phenomena.

2. The abnormal eye closure pattern: In the abnormal eye closure pattern, the eyes close slowly either spontaneously or on-command. Three main patterns are observed (a) Eyes close freely with no initial contraction and a slight flicker or flutter of the eyelids is observed at closure, which is associated with generalized alpha-theta rhythm with or without spikes in the EEG. The palpebral fissure is slightly opened. Occasionally, the upper lid will fling open and jerk, associated with slight upward deviation of gaze and brief generalized irregular spike-wave discharge. (b) The command to close the eyes is associated with an initial mild eyelid contraction of 30- to 70-msec duration before the eyelids begin to close. The closing phase—downward deflection of the positive wave—lasts 100 to 200 msec. At the end of the eye closure phase, an eyelid contraction is observed, which lasts 100 to 350 msec (plateau) before the eyes attempt to open. At the end of eye closure and during the upward deflection of the positive wave, which lasts from 150 to 500 msec, the eyelids flicker, flutter, or jerk in association either with a generalized alpha-beta rhythm of 10 to 30 mv or higher-amplitude irregu-

lar spike-wave discharges, respectively. The central posterior spread of the discharge occurs with a delay of less than 100 msec. The stronger the contraction at eye closure, the stronger the jerking during the process of eye opening and the more precise the generalized and irregular spike-and-wave discharges (GSWDs), The longer the GSWDs, the more likely the process to be repeated, as the child tries to follow the command "close your eyes" and more clear brief absences are observed. After a few repeats of the clinical and EEG phenomena, the eyes remain open. The child no longer attempts to follow the command to close the eyes. (c) The command to close the eyes is characterized by repeated eyelid contractions, associated with GSWDs, which prevent the eyes from closing. Eyes close 500 to 700 msec after the command or the initiation of the discharge and then open quickly and stare. The closing of the eyelids is associated with the slow wave and the opening with the spike of the spike-wave complex.

CLINICAL AND ELECTROENCEPHALOGRAM MANIFESTATIONS

"... There is marked jerking of the eyelids associated with 3c/s SWDs o PSWDs often irregular, immediately after eye closure and invariably positive response on IPS. The mean age of onset is 6 years and female predominate...."
Jeavons PM. DMCN 1977

Eyelid myoclonia and absences or Jeavons syndrome with or without GTCS or other myoclonic jerks is associated with characteristic EEG features during eye closure, sleep, drowsiness, hyperventilation, and IPS and constitutes a separate syndrome.

Seizures Types

Three types of seizures characterize Jeavons syndrome: myoclonic, absences, and generalized tonic–clonic seizures. Occasionally, a tonic spasm of the eyelids is observed as a component of the marked jerking.

Myoclonic seizures are of two types: eyelid myoclonia and myoclonic jerks other than eyelid.

Myoclonic Seizures

Eyelid Myoclonia

Eyelid myoclonia of variable intensity is, by definition, always present. The eyelids may tremble, flicker, flutter or fling open and jerk with a concomitant upward deviation of the eyes and a brief absence. In bright sunlight jerking of the eyelids may be very pronounced and some of the children regarded as having self-induced epilepsy appear to have ELMA (5,6). In certain cases of typical forms of ELMA, a brief *tonic spasm* is observed, either in the preseptal palpebral portion of the obicularis oculi muscle, which prevents the closing movement for a few milliseconds, or in the pretarsal portion at eye closure, just before the eyelids open and jerk. Eyelid myoclonia occur, as a rule, immediately after eye closure, simultaneously with the EEG discharges. The movements are rhythmic, repetitive, slight or marked, single or multiple, even in the same patient. The tremor-like or flutter-like movements are associated in the EEG with beta-alpha rhythm occasionally intermixed with brief spike-wave discharge, when a stronger jerk interferes with the mild movements. These phenomena can be easily interrupted by eye opening. The marked jerking of the eyelids may be a single event lasting from 0.5 to 3 s or may be repeated a few times before the child succeeds to keep the eyes open and relax, sometimes with a sigh of relief. Each clinical event is associated in the EEG with generalized 3- to 5-Hz spike-wave or polyspike-wave discharge of the same duration. The repetition gives the discharges a discontinuous or fragmented pattern. Each jerk is related to the spike and the eye closing with the slow wave of the spike-and-wave complex.

The eyelid myoclonias are very frequent and easily diagnosed, but often misinterpreted for tics.

Myoclonic Jerks Other Than Eyelid

Myoclonic jerks other than eyelid myoclonia are rarely reported by the children or observed by the parents. In adults with ELMA, infrequent myoclonic jerks of the upper limbs occurred in 54.5% of the patients either independently or together with the eyelid myoclonia (13). In our population of 50 children with ELMA (mean age 7 $\pm$ 2.7 y), myoclonic jerks occurred in 34% of the cases and were mainly observed on eye closure. Myoclonic jerks and absences, if present, are usually evoked during IPS, simultaneously with eyelid myoclonia and the irregular generalized spike-wave discharge induced by eye closure. The head may jerk to one side or be drawn to one side like a magnet. Other head movements like nodding, shaking or backward jerks are also observed. The myoclonic jerk may be preceded or followed by eye opening and staring. It may be followed by a massive jerk associated with a second GSWD, if the IPS is not switched off. The intensity of head jerk varies from a subjective feeling to very strong movement. The jerks may also occur in either the arm or shoulder, but rarely occur in the lower extremities.

Absences

Absences in ELMA are probably present in all cases but very difficult to discover as they are usually very brief, lasting less than a second. In order to see the transient eye glare, it is necessary to evaluate video-EEGs very meticulously. It may only be obvious as a hesitation or a gap in counting.

Absences without eyelid myoclonia are usually observed during hyperventilation or IPS with the eyes open in association with generalized spike-wave discharge. The absences very rarely last more than a few seconds and typical absences are not seen or are very infrequent (14).

Generalized Tonic–Clonic Seizures

Generalized tonic–clonic seizures (GTCS) occurred in 50% of our population of children and were the usual referral symptom. In the mild forms of ELMA, which go untreated for many years, GTCS are infrequent, occurring once or twice in a lifetime. In the rest, the diagnosis of ELMA is made after the first GTCS and treatment is initiated. The usual precipitating factors are sleep deprivation and drowsiness, fatigue, drug-resistant forms or inappropriate medication, and flashing lights. In older children, alcohol abuse, associated with sleep deprivation, is an additional precipitating factor.

Other Clinical and EEG Characteristics

Sleep EEG

In ELMA, during sleep, the EEG is either minimally abnormal with focal polyspikes and polyspike-and-wave complexes, usually over the frontal regions. EEG is characterized by generalized spike or polyspike-and-wave discharges, brief or of longer duration, and fragmented with additional focal polyspike complexes. During these discharges eyelid jerking and absences or other myoclonic jerks are not usually observed. However, a slight trembling of the eyelids may be observed in close-up video recording. Rarely, the eyes may open during the discharge and close again toward the end or immediately after the discharge.

The spontaneous EEG discharges, condensed during drowsiness and hyperventilation are seen in at least 60% of cases with ELMA. The discharges seen after eye closure are of longer duration.

Intermittent Photic Stimulation

EEG discharges after eye closure during IPS are seen in all patients as in the resting record. However, on IPS, these discharges are more precise and are also evoked with eyes open. Discharges on IPS with eyes open may induce absences without eyelid myoclonia and on eye closure with eyelid myoclonia. In some cases, eye closure during IPS provokes myoclonic jerks of the upper body. In our population of 50 children, photosensitivity was seen in 92% and in 76% was marked. Those children, which did not evoke discharges during IPS (8%), were of the younger age group (range 0.5 to 3.5 years) and unable to cooperate. The avoidance of the stimulus by not looking or by moving the head away from the stimulus and closing the eyes induces discharges, which cannot be accurately attributed to IPS. The positive response during IPS is relevant to the technique and the type of photostimulator (21,22). The EEG ideally should be sleep–wake after sleep deprivation.

CLINICAL VARIETIES OF JEAVONS SYNDROME

Mild Form

On eye closure, the eyelids tremble, flicker or flutter with slight opening of the palpebral fissure, associated with theta/alpha/beta rhythm in the EEG. Occasionally, during prolonged video-EEG recordings, eyelids may fling open and jerk as the patient stares. The majority of patients never seek medical advice and when they are discovered by accident are reluctant to follow treatment. A few may recall one or two generalized seizures in their lifetime. Few rarely report myoclonic jerks, which are usually recorded during IPS. All patients are of normal intelligence.

ELMA of Early Onset

Early-onset eyelid myoclonia has the characteristic clinical and EEG features of the syndrome. It can, thus, be easily differentiated from the other forms of absence or myoclonic epilepsy syndromes of early onset. In this young age group, eyelid tonic contraction at eye closure is common and photosensitivity is expressed early. The repeated eye closure phenomena, in some children, are very disturbing, as is the bright light. The child often rubs his eyelids or puts his arms in front of his eyes. Blinking by confrontation and passive eye closure may occasionally induce discharges in this young age group. The response to therapy, which is, in all cases, polytherapy and prognosis are worse compared with the other forms of ELMA. More than 75% have moderate to severe educational problems.

Classical ELMA

In typical Jeavons syndrome cases, there is marked jerking of the eyelids, often with upward deviation of the eyes. The jerking follows eye closure and there is a simultaneous generalized and irregular spike-and-wave discharge in the EEG. In all cases, eyelid myoclonia is associated with absences and all show usually marked photosensitivity. In few cases, during IPS, the head instead of jerking is sometimes drawn to one side, as if by a magnet. Some of the children admit that the feeling on eye closure is pleasant. This form of ELMA, if not treated early, may lead to a habitual urge for eye closure during periods of inactivity or boredom.

ELMA—Juvenile Myoclonic Epilepsy Form

The presenting symptom is myoclonic jerks of the arms, which occur particularly on eye closure and become more pronounced during hyperventilation and IPS. Simultaneous eyelid clonic movements with absences may occur. Generalized tonic–clonic seizures do occur as in ELMA and JME.

CASE HISTORIES

Since Jeavons Syndrome is not well documented in the literature, several case histories are illustrated. Emphasis is given to families with at least two members concordant with ELMA.

Family 1

Proband was 10.5 years, when first seen, because of frequent shivering myoclonic jerks. He has had recurrent eyelid jerking with upward deviation of his eyes and infrequent myoclonic jerks of the upper limbs or head since the age of 9. The sleep–wake video-EEG showed generalized, often irregular spike-wave/polyspike-wave discharges on eye closure, which were associated with eyelid jerking and absences with or without concomitant myoclonic jerks of the upper limbs. Eye opening almost completely attenuated the discharges. The clinical and EEG phenomena condensed during hyperventilation. The photosensitivity range was from 5 to 60 f/s. The discharges were always evoked on eye closure, but also with the eyes open or closed. Clinically the discharges were associated with eyelid myoclonia, absences, and myoclonic jerks. The past history and developmental milestones were normal. His subsequent school performance was poor.

Therapy with VPA alone was clinically and 80% electroencephalographically successful for 6 years. When VPA was not taken regularly eyelid jerking reappeared.

The routine examination of his sister at the age of 15 years demonstrated eyelid flutter on eye closure. The video-EEG showed GSWDs a few seconds after eye closure and a photosensitivity range from 5 to 45 f/s, with concomitant eyelid myoclonias, absences, and jerks of the right shoulder. She refused therapy. She had minor educational problems.

Family 2

A boy with severe mental retardation and partial seizures presented at the age of 9. His 36-year-old mother was noticed to have eyelid fluttering or jerking on eye closure. On direct questioning she admitted that she used to "play her eyelids" since childhood, but never had GTCS or jerks. The boy's 22-year-old brother had frequent eyelid jerking, which started at the age of 3. At the ages of 2.5 and 4 years old, he had two afebrile episodes with loss of consciousness. At the age of 11.5 years, he had five GTCS within 8 months. The EEG at that time showed GSWDs on eye closure, particularly during hyperventilation and IPS with concomitant eyelid and other jerking. He was given carbamazepine (CBZ) and later phenobarbitone with poor compliance. When we saw him at the age of 22, he was taking VPA, but infrequently. He continued to have eyelid jerking on eye closure and his video-EEG on awake, showed brief fast/spiky discharges on eye closure with eyelid jerking and a photosensitivity from 14 to 30 f/s with eyelid myoclonias. He never complied with treatment. As his mother and, unlike his brother, he is of borderline intelligence. He continues to have eyelid jerking. He says: " my eyes are hurting me, when I stop blinking."

Family 3

This patient was discovered to have eyelid myoclonia during a routine EEG, which was requested by the pediatrician for immaturity at the age of 4.5 years. She was noticed to have tonic eyelid contraction at eye closure each time she closed her eyes. At times, her eyelid will fling open and jerk with a very transient absence. Her mother commented that she knew about this condition for the past 18 months, particularly while she was watching television. The sleep–wake video-EEG showed irregular 3- to 3.5-Hz spike-waves/polyspike-wave discharges of 0.5- to 2-s duration on eye closure with eyelid myoclonia and occasional jerks involving the head or massive. The photosensitivity range was 5 to 45 f/s with concomitant clinical phenomena. During IPS her mother complained of dizziness. She was taken to the next room where she had a GTCS for the first time in her life. She was 28-years-old. Her video-EEG showed eyelid myoclonias on eye closure with irregular spike-wave discharges. She was photosensitive. VPA was prescribed both for her and her daughter. She was noncompliant and her daughter's therapy was not regular. She is now 38 years old, of borderline intelligence, and her 15-year-old daughter has severe educational problems.

Family 4

This patient presented at the age of 12.5 years, after a GTCS provoked by drowsiness. She recalls rare myoclonic jerks since the age of 12, particularly during the summer, when she was looking at the sun's reflection on seawater. She also remembers some unilateral jerks involving the upper limbs. Her sleep–wake video-EEG showed polyspike-wave complexes in the frontal regions and single or up to 3-s duration and generalized polyspike-wave discharges, which were maximal over the frontal regions during sleep. Hyperventilation increased the generalized 3- to 5-Hz polyspike-wave discharges of 1- to 3-s duration, which were almost always after eye closure and associated with eyelid flutter and some jerks of the head or arms. The photosensitivity range on eye closure was 1 to 60 f/s and with the eyes open 7 to 30 f/s. Most of the discharges were typical, with concomitant eyelid flutter and spontaneous eye opening and stare. Some frequencies evoked myoclonic jerks. She was put on levetiracetam (LEV).

Her 33-year-old mother was noticed to have eyelid flutter on eye closure. On direct questioning, she remembers that her father and his sister also had eyelid fluttering or jerking on eye closure. Her waking EEG showed, during hyperventilation, brief discharges of fast activity or irregular spike-wave discharges on eye closure with eyelid flutter. She never asked for medical advice and never had any GTCS or myoclonic jerks.

Family 5

The patient was seen at the age of 14, following a GTCS while she was in a discotheque. The right arm suddenly started jerking and she dropped a spoon that she was holding. She stood up but fell on the floor and had a GTCS lasting 3 minutes with postictal confusion. On examination, we noticed eyelid jerking on eye closure and this was also observed during the conversation by the parents and others.

From past history, she had two febrile GTCS at the ages of 3 and 4. The EEGs showed on eye closure 14- to 16-Hz activity intermixed with generalized 3-Hz spike-wave discharges of up to 5-s duration. The discharges occurred immediately after eye closure or about 1.5 s after eye closure. During hyperventilation, the discharges became more frequent and increased in duration. The IPS was uncomfortable for her. Discharges were evoked from 5 to 35 f/s with eyes open and on eye closure. All discharges on eye closure were associated with eyelid flutter or eyelid jerking with or without absences (staring). During counting, concomitant with some brief discharges, the intensity of her voice was reduced. Discharges on eye closure with clinical phenomena also occurred while she played video games. She did not comply with the suggested therapy.

The mother reported that her husband, who was now deceased, had eyelid movements on eye closure and that her other 15-year-old daughter also showed the same condition. The sister's EEG revealed generalized discharges of mixed frequencies on eye closure; the photosensitivity range was 10 to 35 f/s. She is not being treated.

Case 6

She was referred to us at the age of 8.5 years by a child psychiatrist who assessed her for educational problems. Past and developmental history were normal. At the age of 6, she started having eyelid jerking with absences, but the parents believed that she was having tics. The sleep–wake video-EEG confirmed discharges and clinical phenomena on eye closure, which became worse during hyperventilation and IPS. The photosensitivity range was 5 to 40 f/s. This girl's attempts to control the clinical phenomena were very obvious during the recording.

The response to VPA monotherapy was complete and has remained so for the past 7 years. However, her performance at school remains at low level. The EEGs of her brothers at the ages of 4 and 7 years old, were normal.

Case 7

He presented at the age of 10 years old because of myoclonic jerks of the arms on eye closure, like an electric current; he also reported dropping things. Eyelid jerking with upward deviation of the eyes was noticed by his family members a few months prior to the onset of the myoclonic jerks. He had many eyelid jerking and 2 to 3 myoclonic jerks per day. The sleep–wake video-polygraphic EEG showed irregular discharges of 2.5- to 4-Hz spike-wave of 1- to 1.5-s duration and eyelid myoclonia with or without absences. Focal frontal polyspike-and-wave complexes were seen during drowsiness. Hyperventilation condensed discharges. Myoclonus of the arms was induced by eye closure. During IPS between the frequencies 5 to 20 f/s on eye closure evoked typical discharges; he felt very uncomfortable. The test was stopped. While playing a video game, he exhibited many discharges with the eyes open and on eye closure together with myoclonic jerks of the arms. The jerks progressively became more frequent and he appeared confused and unable to concentrate.

This boy's past and developmental history were uneventful. The mother had febrile seizures in childhood. The bright sunlight was very uncomfortable for her. An EEG at the age of 29 was normal. His father had also a negative EEG at the age of 38. His sister had two febrile GTCSs within 24 hours at the age of 21 months. Her sleep–wake EEGs at ages of 2 years 3 months and 6 years showed some irregular spike-wave discharges on eye closure and a photosensitivity range from 22 to 25 f/s.

The following are of some interest from the father's history. A male first cousin of his father died at the age of 9 during a seizure. One aunt sleep walks and has epilepsy; another aunt sleep talks. One male first cousin has acquired hemiplegia and epilepsy. His grandfather and grandmother sleep walked and sleep talked, respectively. Two sisters of his grandmother had epilepsy. One died at the age of 14 during a seizure and the other continues to take antiepileptic therapy at the age of 63.

Case 8

She started having typical eyelid myoclonias and absences at the age of 5 years old. The main provocative factors were fatigue, television viewing, and bright sunlight in the presence of different patterns. She had tried a number of AEDs unsuccessfully and when we saw her at the age of 8 years and 5 months she was taking primidone (PRM), valproate (VPA), and clonazepam (CZP). The EEG showed generalized polyspikes-and-wave discharges, particularly on eye closure and a photosensitivity range of 10 to 50 f/s associated with eyelid myoclonias and absences. VPA monotherapy of up to 40 mg/kg/day improved clinical symptoms and spontaneous discharges vanished. However, eyelid myoclonia in the presence of bright sunlight and during IPS has persisted, although with less intensity. The combination of VPA with ethosuximide (ESM), lamotrigine (LTG), and levetiracetam (LEV) did not help and were withdrawn. Her photosensitivity range varies between 10 and 30 f/s. Alternative measures for photosensitivity have helped, particularly during the summer.

ATYPICAL FORMS

Case 9

He presented at the age of 4.5 years because of jerking eyelids, myclonic jerks, and GTCS. He was on carbamazepine (CBZ). He started having GTCS at the age of 6 months, which were a very frequent and the predominant type of seizure. Phenobarbitone was less successful than CBZ, which initially controlled the GTCS. Eyelid jerking and other myoclonic jerks became apparent at the age of 2.5, when the GTCS were somehow better controlled. The EEG at the age of 4.5 showed very frequent brief and irregular generalized 2- to 3-Hz spike-wave and polyspike-wave discharges, particularly on eye closure with concomitant eyelid jerking and occasional jerk of the upper limbs. Focal spikes or polyspikes or polyspike-wave complexes were also seen. Discharges were seen during IPS, but were very difficult to correlate with IPS. He probably had a photosensitivity range from 2 to 60 f/s. He was developmentally retarded for his age. CBZ was withdrawn and VPA was introduced, with under a 50% result. The subsequent combination with LTG and ethosuximide (ESM) temporally improved the clinical picture. The combination of VPA, LTZ, and LEV has not improved the seizures more than 40%. The EEG remains very abnormal with clinical eyelid phenomena during EEG, particularly during eye closure. However, GTCS have improved more than 80% and the EEG improved from 50% to 80%. He has a moderate to severe mental retardation.

Case 10

This 8-year-old girl came to see us from Bulgaria because of frequent eyelid jerking. At the age of 6.5 years, she had her first generalized seizure. Seven months later, she started having jerks, up to 20 per day. Following an EEG she was put on low doses of VPA and, subsequently, CZP was added with no improvement. The generalized seizures started occurring after awaking. CBZ stopped the generalized seizures but the eyelid myoclonias were made more obvious. From the age of 8 to 9 we performed four awake EEGs after sleep deprivation and one sleep–awake record. All video-EEGs showed very frequent generalized 2.5- to 3-Hz spike and polyspike-and-wave discharges, regular or irregular, usually up to 5 s duration but occasionally to 10- and 20-s duration with or without clinical phenomena. Sodium valproate 30 mg/kg/day reduced seizure activity by 80%. Adding ESM or nitrazepam (NTZ) did not help. We followed-up for 1 year. Subsequently, 14 months after her last EEG, she stopped having seizures and 2 months later, on

mother's wishes, the treatment was discontinued with no relapses for 8 years. The last visit was 2 years ago at the age of 16. The awake EEG after sleep deprivation was normal.

DIAGNOSIS AND DIFFERENTIAL DIAGNOSIS OF EYELID MYOCLONIA AND ABSENCES

The diagnosis of ELMA is easy for those who have seen the unique clinical and EEG phenomena induced simultaneously with eye closure. The sleep–wake video-polygraphic EEG is necessary in order to confirm the diagnosis and elucidate the combined symptoms. Photosensitivity is essentially a laboratory finding and can be established only by using the correct photostimulator, methodology, and interpretation (21,22).

In children and some adults, eyelid trembling or fluttering is often seen on eye closure and should be differentiated from the mild forms of ELMA by the findings in the EEG. Some overlap does exist.

Self-Induced Epilepsy

Self-induced epilepsy is rarely reported in the literature. In 1932, Radovici et al (23) reported a mentally retarded patient, waving one hand, with fingers outstretched in front of the eyes. The phenomenon of self-induction is regarded as rarity: it occurs in 1:10000 EEGs (24) or 1:1000 patients with epilepsy (25) or 1:100 photosensitive patients (21). When photosensitive patients are placed in a well-lit room, self-induction occurs in 24% to 30% of the cases (26,27). Typically, the patient looks at the sun or bright light source and waves one hand, with the fingers apart, rapidly across the eyes. The examiner, waving a hand in front of the patient's eyes in the same fashion does not produce clinical and EEG phenomena. Myoclonic jerks in self-induced epilepsy invariably involve the waving hand. Eye closure, particularly during IPS, may be followed by eye opening, stare, and head jerking. The head jerks in similar fashion as in ELMA. The involvement of the lower extremities is more frequent than in ELMA. Other photosensitive patients may voluntarily close their eyes (28) or are attracted by the television triggering factors (21). It is, therefore, obvious that photosensitivity is the common path for self-induction. Eyelid myoclonia and absences and self-induced epilepsy have similarities and dissimilarities.

Similarities

- Both are a photosensitive form of epilepsy.
- Both occur on a hereditary basis. There is clinical heterogeneity and variability in intelligence.
- In order for both disorders to manifest, the co-existence of three factors are necessary: The genetic predisposition, the voluntary or on-command act of eye closure or hand waving, and the presence of light input.
- In both, the clinical phenomena become more pronounced in bright sunlight and do not occur in total darkness.
- Passive eye closure or hand waving does not induce discharges in the majority of cases.
- In self-induced epilepsy, some discharges and clinical phenomena on IPS are induced by eye closure but typical eyelid myoclonias are not seen.

Dissimilarities

- In ELMA, clinical and EEG phenomena are induced by eye closure while in self-induced epilepsy it is induced by hand waving.
- Eye closure and hand cortical areas are adjacent.
- In ELMA, females predominate, while in self-induced epilepsy males predominate.
- All self-induced patients invariably provoke their seizures. Only in a few cases with ELMA with marked photosensitivity and borderline IQ or the treatment failures, may seizures be self-induced. These patients close their eyes in order to avoid the disturbance of the bright light, falling into the trap of inducing discharges and clinical phenomena. If the feeling is pleasant, they may try to feel it again, particularly during conditions of boredom and anxiety. All patients who self-induce their seizures feel upset and guilty when they are discovered. The majority of ELMA patients, who only have educational difficulties or discrete

cognitive impairment, refer to their eyelid jerking as a nuisance, disturbing, and embarrassing phenomenon, which, under certain circumstances, they are unable to control. They are relieved when therapy is successful and show a good compliance. Binnie and Jeavons (29) consider ELMA to be a type of photosensitive epilepsy, but make the point that ELMA must be differentiated from self-induced epilepsy. A few years later, Binnie (30) and Panayiotopoulos (31) produced arguments in favor of or against self-induction in ELMA, respectively.

COMMENTS

Eyelid myoclonia and self-induced epilepsy are separate entities with some overlap. In both conditions, electrical activity is generated in the eye closure area (pretcentral gyrus) and hand areas, respectively. In turn, those areas send impulses to eyelids and hand to jerk. The stronger the genetic defect, the easier the accessory reflex to develop/elicit. Patients with lower IQ exploit the pleasure by self-induction more than those with normal intelligence. The normal patient finds eyelid jerking a nuisance and embarrassing condition, which prevents them from enjoying life. The latter patients are relieved and happy when therapy controls photosensitivity and show excellent compliance. Patients with marked photosensitivity who do not respond completely to therapy are unable to protect themselves.

ABSENCE SEIZURES IN OTHER FORMS OF IDIOPATHIC GENERALIZED EPILEPSIES

The association of eye closure with absences, jerks and generalized spike or polyspike-wave discharges is seen in some other myoclonic epilepsy syndromes, which have absence seizures in their phenotype, particularly evoked by IPS. The eyes may open and stare or even the eyelids may blink, but do not retract and jerk like in ELMA. The predominant type of seizures are myoclonic jerks. In typical absence epilepsies, the seizures are not an eye closure phenomenon, last longer than 3 s, eyes possibly deviating to one side (never in ELMA), and are not abolished by eye opening. The typical absences are not reproducible by eye closure.

Occipital Epilepsies

In occipital epilepsies, idiopathic or symptomatic, some forced eyelid closure or blinking may occur as an ictal event or herald a secondary generalized seizure (32,33). In occipital epilepsy, slow spike-and-wave complexes appear on eye closure in the posterior regions and continue in long runs as far as the eyes remain closed. Eyelid flutter may be observed, but never eyelid contraction and jerking. On eye opening, there is a partial or complete attenuation of the discharges. GSWD do not characterize occipital epilepsies and the spike of the spike-wave component is smoother, as in all forms of benign focal epilepsies.

Tics

Tics transient or chronic are common in childhood and male subjects are more likely to exhibit them (34). There is genetic and clinical heterogeneity. The motor manifestations are stereotype, involuntary, sudden, inappropriate, nonprepositional, absurd, irresistible, and of variable intensity (35).

Patients with eyelid myoclonia and those who make grimaces to avoid eye closure are referred to the psychologists for tics or mannerisms. Some authors believe that eye ball roll, eye closure, and eye blinking are ticlike symptoms, which cause the absences and the discharges of ELMA in those who are photosensitive (36). The authors do not explain the spontaneous discharges and the frequent discharges occurring during sleep in the majority of patients or why generalized SW discharges are not seen in typical Gilles de la Tourette syndrome, also a common disorder. They also stress the beneficial effect of proconvulsive dopamine antagonists. This hypothesis cannot explain the complete clinical response with antiepileptic drugs, once the EEG discharges are controlled.

Those who have seen tics or eyelid myoclonia and absences have no problem in separating the two conditions. Tics are not an eye closure phenomenon. The tic children may blink or even close their eyelids in a spasm, but their eyes never open automatically, jerk in a rhythmic way or stare. In ELMA, slow eye closure, voluntary or on command, induces characteristic clinical and EEG phenomena.

THERAPY AND PROGNOSIS

Eyelid myoclonia and absences respond worse to monotherapy than other forms of photosensitive epilepsies and better than self-induced epilepsy. Many authors have stressed the difficulty in response of ELMA (7,13). In our recent experience with 50 patients, the response to VPA monotherapy is 72% in 1994 (12) as compared with 53% in 1982 (7). This difference is probably due to early diagnosis and treatment with the most appropriate AED, which is sodium valproate. Early success prevents chronicity, which may lead to self-induction, noncompliance and intractability. In resistant forms, eyelid jerking is usually resistant to therapy, particularly during IPS. In mild untreated forms, eyelid jerking may also continue after the disease ceases in the form of an eyelid tic.

Tonic–clonic seizures, absences, or myoclonic jerks respond easier to therapy. In monotherapy failures, VPA is combined with lamotrigine (LTG) levetiracetam (LEV), ethosuximid (ESM), or even benzodiazepines. Eyelid myoclonia and absences is underdiagnosed and comparable studies are lacking. Monotherapy comparative studies of VPA, LEV, and LTG are also nonexistent and should be done in the future. Carbamazepine (CBZ), oxcabazepine (OXC), vigabatrin (VGB), tiagabine (TGB), and phenytoin (PHT) are not indicated in ELMA. Experience with topiramate (TPM) is lacking.

ELMA is a life-long disorder and its prognosis is similar to that of juvenile myoclonic epilepsy with photosensitivity. The majority of ELMA patients have specific educational problems. The earlier the age of onset, the worse the prognosis. Almost all our early-onset children needed remedial teaching. The mild forms have best prognosis as far as cognitive functions.

REFERENCES

1. Jeavons PM. Nosological problems of myoclonic epilepsies in childhood and adolescece. *Develop Med Child Neurol* 1977;19:3–8.

2. Jeavons PM. Myoclonic epilepsies: Therapy and prognosis. In Akimoto H, Kasamatsuri H, Seino M, Ward A. eds. *Advances in Epileptology*. New York: Raven Press 1982:141–144.

3. Jeavons PM. Eyelid myoclonia and absences:The history of the syndrome. In: Duncan JS, Panayiotopoulos CP. eds. *Eyelid myoclonia with absences*. London: John Libbey, 1996:13–15.

4. Ames FR. Self induction in photosensitive epilepsy. *Brain* 1971;94:781–798.

5. Binnie CD, Darby CE, De Korte RA, et al. Self-induction of epilepsy seizures by eye closure: incidence and recognition. *J Neurol Psych* 1980;43:386–389.

6. Darby CE, De korte RA, Bennie CD, et al. The self-induction of epileptic seizures by eye closure. *Epilepsia* 1980;21:31–41.

7. Covanis A, Jeavons PM, Gupta AK. Sodium valproate: Monotherapy and polytherapy. *Epilepsia* 1982;23:693–720.

8. Gobbi G, Tinuper P, Tassinari CA, et al. Eyelid myoclonia absences. *Bollettino-Lega Italiania Contro L' Epielessia* 1985;51/52:225–226.

9. Gobbi G, Bruno L, Mainetti S, et al. Eye closure seizures. In: Beaumanoir A, Gastaut H, Naquet R. eds. *Reflex seizures and reflex epilepsies*. Medicine et Hygiene, Geneva, 1989:181–191.

10. Dalla Bernadina B, Sgro V, Fontana E, et al. Eyelid myoclonia with absences. In: Beaumanoir A, Gastaut H, Naquet R. eds. *Reflex seizures and reflex epilepsies*. Geneva: Medicine et Hygiene, 1989:193–200.

11. Appleton RE, Panayiotopoulos CP, Acomb BA, et al. Eyelid myoclonia with absences: an epilepsy syndrome. *J Neurol Neurosurg Psych* 1993;56:1312–1316.

12. Covanis A, Skiadas K, Loli N, et al. Eyelid myoclonia with absences. *Epilepsia* 1994;35(7):13.

13. Giannakodimos S, Panayiotopoulos CP. Eyelid myoclonia with absences in adults: a clinical and video-EEG study. *Epilepsia* 1996;37:36–44.

14. Ferrie CD, Agathonikou A, Parker A, et al. The spectrum of childhood epilepsies with eyelid myoclonia. In: Duncan JS, Panayiotopoulos CP. eds. *Eyelid myoclonia with absences*. London: John Libbey, 1996:39–48.

15. Commission on Classification and Terminology of the International League Against Epilepsy. Proposal for revised classification of epilepsies and epileptic syndromes. *Epilepsia* 1989;30:389–399.

16. Engel J, Jr. A proposed diagnostic scheme for people with epileptic seizures and with epilepsy: Report of the ILAE Task Force on Classification and Terminology. *Epilepsia* 2001;42:796–803.

17. Bianchi A and the Italian LAE Collaborative Group. Study of concordance of symptoms in families with absence epilepsies. In: Duncan JS, Panayiotopoulos CP. eds. *Typical absences and related epileptic syndromes*. London: Churchill Communication Europe, 1995:328–337.

18. Leyton ASF, Sherrington CS. Observations of the excitable cortex of the Chimpanzee orangutan and gorilla. *Q J Exp Physiol* 1917;11:135–222.

19. Panayiotopoulos CP, Giannakodimos S, Chroni E, et al. Observations on families with eyelid myoclonia with absences. In: Duncan JS, Panayiotopoulos CP, eds. *Eyelid myoclonia with absences*. London: John Libbey, 1996:93–106.

20. Wilkins A. Towards an understanding of reflex epilepsy and absence. In: Duncan JS, Panayiotopoulos CP, eds. *Typical absences and related epileptic syndromes*. Churchill Communications Europe, London, 1995:196–205.

21. Jeavons PM, Harding GFA. *Photosensitive Epilepsy. Clinics in Developmental Medicine*. London: Heinemann, 1975:No. 56.

22. Trenite DG, Binnie CD, Harding GFA, et al. Medical technology assessment photic stimulation standards of screening methods. *Neurophysiol Clin* 1999;29(4):318–324.

23. Radovici A, Misirliou V, Gluckman M. Epilepsie réflexe provoquée par excitations aptiques des rayons solaires. *Rev Neurol* 1932;1:1305–1308.

24. Wadlington WB, Riley HD. Light-induced seizures. *J Pediat* 1965;66:300–312.

25. Andermann K, Oaks G, Berman S, et al. Self-induced epilepsy. *Arch Neurol* 1962;6:49–79.

26. Darby CE, De Korte RA, Binnie CD. The self-induction of epileptic seizures by eyeclosure. *Epilepsia* 1980b;21:31–42.

27. Kasteleijn-Nolst Trenité DGA, Binnie CD, Overweg J, et al. Treatment of self-induction in epileptic patients. In: Beaumanoir A, Gastaut H, Naquet R. eds. *Reflex seizures and reflex epilepsies*. Geneva: Medicine et Hygiene; 1989:439–445.

28. Green JB. Self-induced seizures: Clinical and electroencephalographic studies. *Arch Neurol* 1966;15:579–586.

29. Binnie CD, Jeavons PM. Photosensitive epilepsies. In: Roger J, Bureau M, Dravet Ch, Dreifuss FE, Perret A, Wolf P. eds. *Epileptic syndromes of infancy, childhood and adolescence*. London: John Libbey, 1992:299–305.

30. Binnie CD. Differential diagnosis of eyelid myoclonia with absences and self-induction by eye closure. In: Duncan JS, Panayiotopoulos CP. eds. *Eyelid myoclonia with absences*. London: John Libbey, 1996:89–92.

31. Panayiotopoulos CP, Giannakodimos S, Agathonikou A, et al. Eyelid myoclonia is not a maneuver for self-induced seizures in eyelid myoclonia with absences. In: Duncan JS, Panayiotopoulos CP. eds. *Eyelid myoclonia with absences*. London: John Libbey, 1996:93–106.

32. Panayiotopoulos CP. *Benign childhood partial seizures and related epileptic syndromes*. London: John Libbey, 1999.

33. Williamson PD, Thadoni VM, Darcey TM, et al. Occipital lobe epilepsy: Clinical characteristics, seizure spread patterns and results of surgery [review]. *Ann Neurol* 1992;31:3–13.

34. Tanner CM, Goldman SM. Epidemiology of Tourette syndrome. *Neurol Clin N Amer* 1997;15:395–402.

35. Shapiro E, Shapiro AK. Semiology, nosology and criteria for tic disorders. *Rev Neurol* 1986;142:824–832.

36. Kent L, Blake A, Whitehouse W. Eyelid myoclonia with absences: Phenomenology in children. *Seizure* 1998;7(3):193–199.

15

Childhood Absence Epilepsy Evolving to Juvenile Myoclonic Epilepsy: Electroclinical and Genetic Features

Marco T. Medina,*,† Reyna M. Durón,*,† María E. Alonso,‡ Charlotte Dravet,§
Lourdes León,‖ Minerva Lopez-Ruiz,¶ Ricardo Ramos-Ramirez,¶
Ignacio Pascual Castroviejo,† Karen Weissbecker,‡‡ B. Westling,†
Katerina Tanya Perez-Gosiengfiao,** Sonia Khan,‡‡ Gregorio Pineda,‖
Ryoji Morita,§§ Astrid Rasmussen,‡ Jaime Ramos Peek,‖‖‖ Sergio Cordova,¶
Iris E. Martínez-Juarez,†,¶ Francisco Rubio-Donnadieu,¶ Adriana
Ochoa-Morales,‡ Aurelio Jara-Prado,‡ Julia N. Bailey,† Miyabi Tanaka,†
Dongheng Bai,† Jesús Machado-Salas,† and Antonio V. Delgado-Escueta†

*National Autonomous University of Honduras, Tegucigalpa, Honduras; †California Comprehensive
Epilepsy Program, David Geffen School of Medicine at UCLA, Los Angeles, California;
‡Neurogenetics and Molecular Biology, Instituto Nacional de Neurología y Neurocirugía, Tlalpan,
Mexico; §Centre Saint-Paul-Hôpital Henri Gastaut, Marseille, France; ‖Hospital Angel Leaños,
Guadalajara, Mexico; ¶Neurology and Neurosurgery Unit, Mexico General Hospital, Mexico City,
Mexico; **Department of Pediatrics, Autonoma University, Madrid, Spain; ††Tulane University
Medical Center, New Orleans, Louisiana; ‡‡Neurosciences Department, Riyadh Armed Forces
Hospital, Saudi Arabia; §§Laboratory for Neurogenetics, RIKEN Brain Science Institute, Saitama,
Japan; ‖‖‖Faculty of Medicine, Universidad Nacional Autónoma de México, University City, Mexico;
¶¶National Institute of Neurology and Neurosurgery, Mexico City, Mexico

INTRODUCTION

The common idiopathic generalized epilepsies such as juvenile myoclonic epilepsy (JME), childhood absence (CAE), and grand mal (GM) on awakening are likely to be etiologically and genetically heterogenous (1–7). The same clinical phenotype may be caused by various single-gene defects or two or more genes interacting in epistasis and with environmental factors. JME begins around puberty with bilateral or unilateral, single or repetitive arrhythmic myoclonic jerks, which occur predominantly in shoulders and arms, usually after awakening or sleep deprivation, and with no associated disturbance of consciousness (8–12). Of JME patients 95% to 97% have grand mal, clonic–tonic–clonic or tonic–clonic convulsions. The interictal EEG shows diffuse 3.5- to 6-Hz polyspike-wave complexes and ictal EEG shows diffuse high-amplitude polyspikes during myoclonias (8–15). JME is most often inherited and sex distribution is reported to be equal or female preponderant, depending on the geographic and racial ethnic source (11–13,16–20).

In the original descriptions of JME, absences were considered a minor feature, as they occur in less than 30% of patients (10,12,14). When present, absences occurred rarely or in clusters with long periods of no attacks called *spanioleptic*.

197

In recent studies, however, frequent absences numbered 1 to 200 per day, called *pyknoleptic*, have been recognized in JME (2,10,11,20–22). When the phenotypes of JME probands were analyzed, pyknoleptic absences were described in late childhood in 27%, in adolescence in 23%, and after 18 years in 5% (1,2). Durner et al. (4,5,23) and Greenberg et al. (6,7) claim that such absences and JME are inherited separately, which implies that separate genes are responsible for absences and myoclonia/grand mal.

Such pyknoleptic absence seizures have probably been responsible for our failure to isolate and identify JME genes. Families with subsyndromes of childhood absence epilepsy, such as CAE which evolves to JME or CAE with eyelid myoclonia and grand mal, or photogenic CAE with myoclonia and grand mal, are often mixed with families of classic JME in linkage mapping. Mixing these various subsyndromes together occur due to various reasons, one of which is the overlap of age at which absence epilepsy starts. Pyknoleptic absence in CAE usually begins between 2 and 12 years of age (2,9), while absences in JME have been reported between 8 and 18 years of age (14,24). Absences of the pyknoleptic variety with 3-Hz spike wave complexes have been reported in 4.6% (8,21), 5% (13), 7.5% (25), and up to 15% (9) of JME cases.

In this chapter, we describe the syndrome of childhood absence epilepsy persisting into adolescence with grand mal and myoclonias in 45 probands. We also describe the seizure phenotypes of 91 affected nonproband family members. We provide, in addition, results of a genome wide screen in a 100-member multiplex/multigenerational family ascertained through a proband with CAE evolving to JME. Results did not support linkage to seven known epilepsy loci, indicating this syndrome is a disorder distinct and separate from presently known epilepsy syndromes.

METHODS

Patient and Family Database

Forty-five families (985 members) were ascertained through a proband with pyknoleptic childhood absence epilepsy that persisted with grand-

mal and myoclonic seizures. Of the families, 29% (13/45) were multiplex/multigenerational, 27% (12/45) were multigenerational only, and 16% (7/45) were multiplex (Fig. 15-1). Of the families (13/45), 28% were simplex. Clinical diagnoses of seizure types and electrocephalographic diagnoses were independently verified by at least two epileptologists. Originally recruited for family studies in JME, these families were subsequently separated as a syndrome distinct from typical JME because of the onset of pyknoleptic absences during childhood (1,2,26). These families were evaluated from 1978 to 2004 in epilepsy clinics from Los Angeles (28 families), Mexico (10 families), Honduras (3 families), Saudi Arabia (3 families), and Spain (1 family). Two of the families evaluated in Los Angeles were originally from Iran and Australia, but were residing in the United States.

Inclusion criteria included (a) epilepsy that started in childhood with pyknoleptic absences (1–200 attacks per day) during 3-Hz spike-wave complexes; interictal EEG consisted of 3-Hz spike and wave and/or 3- to 6-Hz polyspike-wave complexes; (b) absences persisting beyond childhood; (c) myoclonic and tonic–clonic or clonic–tonic–clonic grand-mal seizures that started after absences, and (d) normal neurologic examination and brain imaging. Types, age at onset, and evolution of seizures through adolescence and adulthood were evaluated. The diagnosis of seizure types was based on the International League Against Epilepsy classifications of seizures and syndromes (27–29).

An extended pedigree was constructed for each family. All available affected relatives were interviewed and examined to determine their clinical diagnoses; EEGs were reviewed as available. Of the probands, 58 had neuroimaging studies—31% (14/45) had cerebral tomography scan, 18% (8/45) had brain magnetic resonance, 7% (3/45) had both tomography and magnetic resonance studies, and 18% (8/45) had positron emission tomography (PET). The number of relatives affected in nuclear and extended families, their sex, seizure types, and age at onset were registered.

Maternal or paternal transmission was determined by the pedigree findings. Exclusion criteria consisted of (a) progressive neurologic

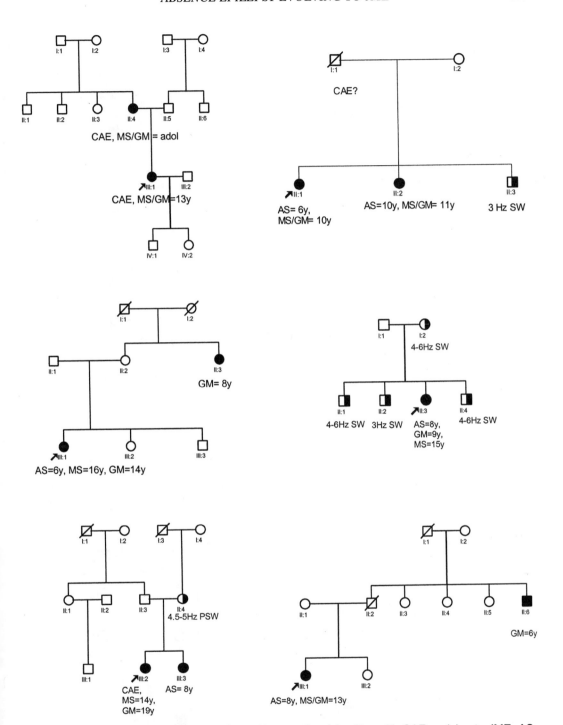

FIG. 15–1. Examples of multiplex and/or multigenerational families with CAE evolving to JME. AS, absences seizures; GM, grand mal; MS, myoclonic seizures; EM, eyelid myoclonia, SW, spike wave, TLE, temporal lobe epilepsy, FS, febrile seizures; PSW, polyspike-wave; EEG, electroencephalogram; JME, juvenile myoclonic epilepsy.

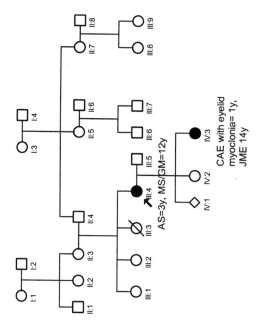

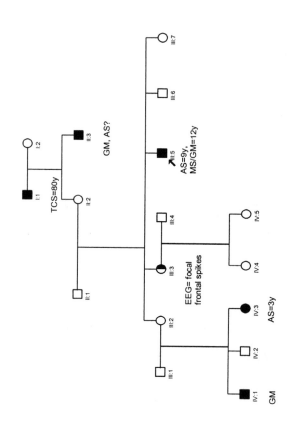

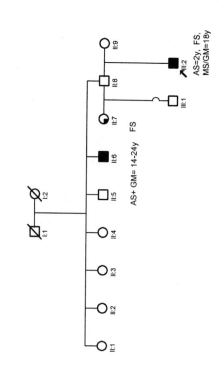

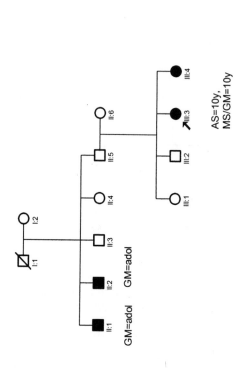

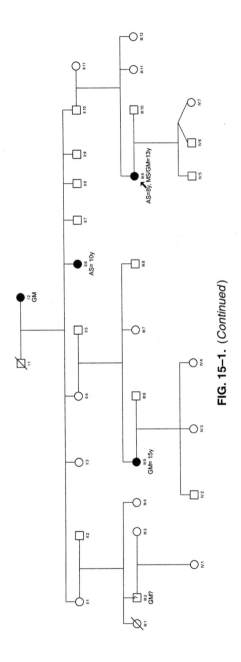

FIG. 15–1. *(Continued)*

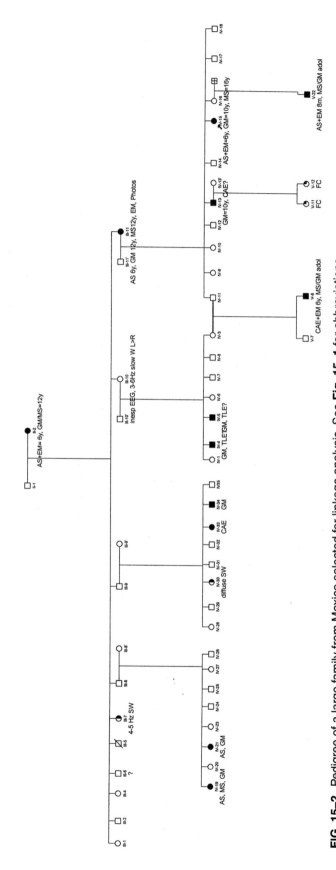

FIG. 15–2. Pedigree of a large family from Mexico selected for linkage analysis. See **Fig. 15–1** for abbreviations.

deterioration; (b) myoclonic absences; (c) typical or classic JME; (d) typical CAE that remits in adolescence, and (e) photogenic epilepsy with female preponderance. Of the patients (84%), 38 had follow-up to adolescence or adulthood.

One Large Family from Mexico Selected for Linkage Study

One large family whose pedigree structure and measures of informativeness (maximum expected LOD score) suggested strong power for linkage were selected to begin genome screening (Fig. 15–2). This large family was from Guadalajara, Mexico and had 100 members, 15 of whom were affected. This family was ascertained through a 15-year-old female proband with CAE evolving to JME. The proband and all nonproband members had 30- to 45-min electroencephalograms using disc electrodes applied according to the 10 to 20 system using colloidion or paste. Power test for this pedigree was simulated using the existing pedigree structure, affection status, and the program SLINK (Ott, 1989) (30). Assuming an autosomal dominant model, we simulated 1000 replicates. Based on quadratic interpolation, average maximum simulated LOD score was 4.5 ± 1.83.

Loci Studied

Because of genetic linkage between classic JME and chromosome 6p12.1 (3,23,31–34), we initially screened the family from Guadalajara (Mexico) with chromosome 6 microsatellites. Subsequently, we performed a 10 to 20 cM genome screen using gel-based radiation microstellites from Research Genetics Inc. (Weber and May, 1989) (35) and fluorescent microstellite markers (ABI Prism genotyping system software, Perkin Elmer, Cyprus, CA). Data for reference families, primer sequences, allele sizes, and frequencies of each marker were obtained from the Genome Database or CEPH Database. Two-point and multipoint analysis used the LINKAGE Software Package (Version 5.21, 1998) (36,37). An autosomal dominant model with 70% penetrance and a disease frequency of 0.001 were used. We assumed no phenocopy, no muta-

tion, and equal recombination between male and female.

Analysis of Familial Aggregation of Seizures and Epilepsy

For segregation analysis, each relative was examined separately for history of epilepsy and degree of relatedness. First-degree relatives were parents and siblings (brothers and sisters), second-degree relatives were uncles, aunts, nieces and nephews, and third-degree relatives included cousins. In addition, offsprings were analyzed separately from the other first-degree relatives. According to hospital and clinic records, CAE with or without grand mal accounts for 2% to 15% of all epilepsies (1,2,40). For risk calculations, we used the cumulative or lifetime prevalence of having epilepsy reported from the Rochester study (3%) (38,39), and considering that at least 2.2% of all epilepsies are CAE and 1.5% are JME (40), we estimated a prevalence of 0.0066% for CAE and a prevalence of 0.045% for JME in general population. Familial aggregation of both absences and myoclonic seizures were compared in the 32 multiplex-multigenerational pedigrees. Seizure types in nonproband members were compared with those of 92 classic JME families. Relative risk for every seizure type in families of CAE evolving to JME was compared with those of JME families.

RESULTS

Probands

Thirty-one families (69%) were of Caucasoid ethnic origin, while fourteen (41%) were mixtures of European and American Indians. Females were preponderant among probands (29 females and 16 males or 1.8F:1M ratio). Figure 15–3 shows the age at onset of seizure types in probands. Childhood absence seizures were documented as the first seizure in all probands, starting at the average age of 6.9 ± 1.8 years (1 to 11 years) in 41 probands. In four other probands, parents could only describe absences as starting *"during or before elementary school."* By the time probands were enrolled in family studies,

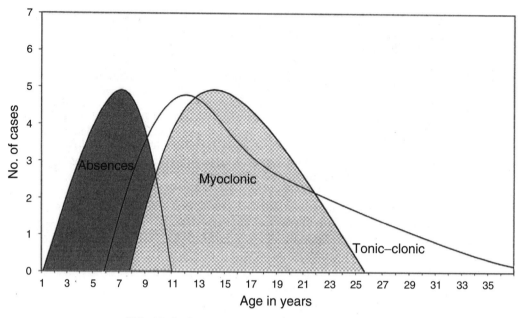

FIG. 15–3. Age at onset of seizures in 45 probands.

they were either adolescents or adults (mean age 26.2 years with range 11 to 60 years), providing opportunity to observe the evolution of absences seizures that started during childhood. In 36 probands older than 20 years (80%), absences had persisted an average 22 ± 11 years (range 5 to 52 years).

Tonic–clonic seizures appeared for the first time at 12 years (range 2 to 37 years). Tonic–clonic convulsions were the chief persisting complaint in 21%. In probands older than 20 years, convulsive tonic–clonic seizures had been chronically recurring for 15 ± 6 years (range 3 to 23 years). All patients, except one, had at least one grand-mal seizure. The most common trigger factors for seizures were sleep deprivation in 33% (15/45), stress in 29% (13/45), light stimuli from TV, computers, and video games in 20% (9/45), and hyperventilation in 18% (8/45). Menses were reported as a trigger factor by 38% of female patients.

Myoclonias started at the mean age of 14 years (range 8 to 47 years) as sudden and involuntary jerks of shoulders and upper extremities, sometimes also affecting trunk, head, neck, and lower extremities. Drops due to severe myoclonic jerks

or astatic seizures were not reported in probands. The most common description involved mild to moderate symmetrical, sudden lightning jerks of hands, forearms, and shoulders inward or upward, often causing the individual to drop items. Myoclonic seizures had persisted for 2 to 26 years (mean 12 years) in probands older than 20 years. Myoclonic seizures as the most prominent seizure type were observed in only six patients (13%). Myoclonic seizures preceded grand-mal convulsion in 18%. More often, they started simultaneously with tonic–clonic seizures in adolescence (40% of patients).

Neurologic Examination and Neuroimaging

Apart from seizures, all probands were otherwise neurologically normal. Neurologic examinations at enrollment and during the follow-up period remained normal. Five cases (11%) had prominent jaw jerk reflexes. Neither brain computed tomography (CT) nor magnetic resonance imaging (MRI) studies showed structural abnormalities among probands, except for one female who had an arteriovenous malformation (angioma venosum) in one frontal lobe, which was considered an incidental finding. Interestingly, two out of eight probands who underwent positron emission tomography (PET) were reported to have hypometabolism in one temporal lobe. One of them was the proband who had a frontal lobe arteriovenous malformation.

Electroencephalographs of Probands

Thirty probands (67%) had routine electroencephalograms (EEG), eight (17%) had EEG telemetry, and seven (16%) had video-EEG studies. Abnormalities were found in 95% of 37 probands (Fig. 15–4). The most common findings were 2- to 5-Hz single spike-and-slow wave complexes (78%) associated with absences. Of the probands, 54% had interictal 4- to 6-Hz polyspike-wave complexes, and 22% had interictal bursts of diffuse fast low amplitude 15- to 25-Hz rhythms in wakeful state. Background activity was normal in all cases. Bursts of 3- to 5-Hz single spike-wave and/or 4- to 6-Hz

polyspike-wave were induced during hyperventilation in 29% of probands and during photostimulation in 22%. Myoclonias were associated with polyspikes or polyspike-wave complexes. Figures 15–5A-D show examples of these EEG traits. We recorded and videotaped myoclonic jerks associated with diffuse high-amplitude polyspikes and 4- to 5-Hz diffuse polyspike-wave complexes during video-EEG telemetry.

Family Members

Thirty-two probands (or 72%) reported seizures in their family members. Epileptic seizures affected 91 nonproband family members and abnormal EEG with spike wave or poly-spike wave complexes affected 8 other asymptomatic members (Figs. 15–6 and 15–7). There was no gender preponderance amongst nonproband affected members (10.6% of females vs. 9.8% males in multiplex/multigenerational families). Absences only or absences with myoclonias or grand mal were seen in 45%, 29% had convulsive grand mal

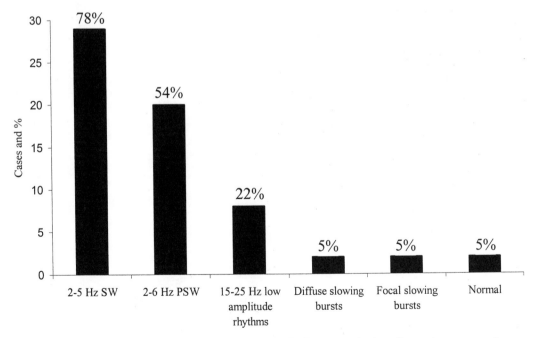

FIG. 15–4. EEGs of 37 probands. The most common finding were single spike-and-wave complexes, 14/37 (47%) had the classic 3-Hz single spike-wave discharges and 14% had both spike-wave (SW) and polyspike-wave (PSW) discharges.

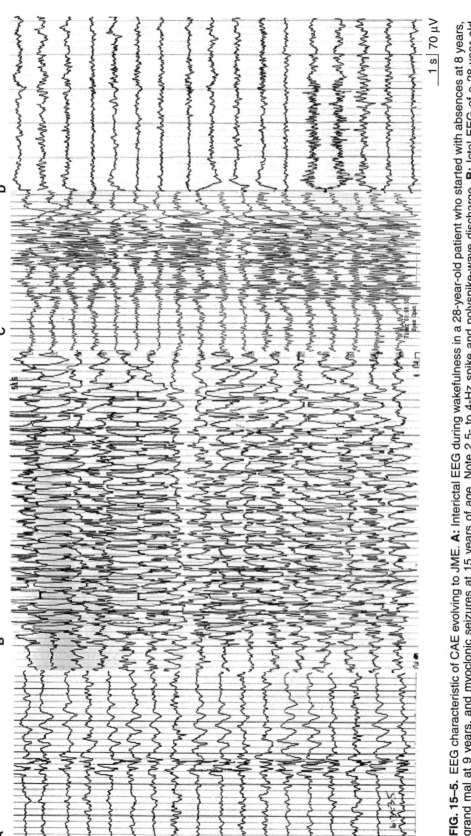

FIG. 15–5. EEG characteristic of CAE evolving to JME. **A:** Interictal EEG during wakefulness in a 28-year-old patient who started with absences at 8 years, grand mal at 9 years, and myoclonic seizures at 15 years of age. Note 2.5- to 4-Hz spike and polyspike-wave discharge. **B:** Ictal EEG of a 28-year old female who had absences with eyelid myoclonia during elementary school and myoclonias/grand mal at 13 years of age. A burst of 2.5- to 4-Hz spike-wave discharges during staring and unresponsiveness. **C:** Ictal EEG during myoclonic jerks in both arms in a 29 year-old who suffered absences since 3 years of age, grand mal since 12 years, and myoclonias since 14 years. Bilateral diffuse polyspike wave discharge of 4- to 5- Hz was preceded by diffuse 15-Hz polyspikes. **D:** An interictal burst of rapid low-voltage polyspikes in a 14-year-old patient whose absences started, when she was 7 years old, myoclonias when 8 years, and grand mal when 12 years.

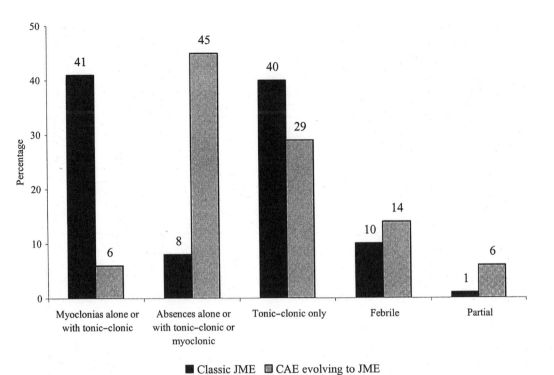

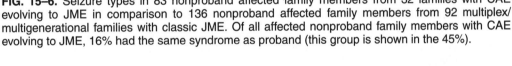

FIG. 15–6. Seizure types in 83 nonproband affected family members from 32 families with CAE evolving to JME in comparison to 136 nonproband affected family members from 92 multiplex/ multigenerational families with classic JME. Of all affected nonproband family members with CAE evolving to JME, 16% had the same syndrome as proband (this group is shown in the 45%).

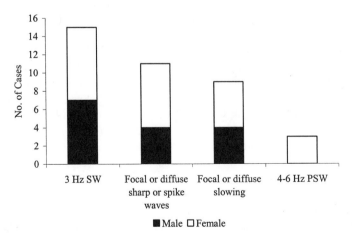

FIG. 15–7. EEG in 38 affected family members from 16 families with CAE evolving to JME. Eight of them (21%) were asymptomatic. SW, spike-waves; PSW, polyspike-waves.

TABLE 15–1. *Frequency of epileptic seizures among first- and second-degree relatives of probands with CAE evolving to JME*

Epilepsy syndrome and seizure types in relatives CAE evolving to JME (32 families)	First-degree affected		Second-degree affected (aunts, uncles, nieces, nephews) n (%)	Total n (%)
	(Parents and sibs) n (%)	Offspring n (%)		
Myoclonias with/without tonic–clonic	1 (2.9)		1 (4.5)	2 (6.3)
Tonic–clonic only	8 (24.0)	1 (100)	8 (36.4)	17 (27.8)
Absences, myoclonias and tonic–clonic	19 (56.0)		6 (27.2)	25 (40.5)
Febrile	5 (14.7)		4 (18.1)	9 (15.2)
Symptomatic localization related	—		—	—
Not validated seizure/epilepsy type	1 (2.9)		3 (13.6)	4 (7.6)
Total affected relatives by degree	34 (100.0)	1 (100)	22 (100.0)	57 (100)
Total relatives and percentage of affectedness by degree	34/161 (21.1)	1/12 (8.3)	22/141 (15.6)	79/415 (19.0)

only, and 6% had myoclonias only or myoclonias plus grand mal. Some members had febrile or partial seizures (Fig. 15–6).

CAE evolving to JME was documented in 12 (13%) of all nonproband clinically affected members (7 females and 5 males). Maternal transmission was observed in 62% of cases vs. 38% of paternal transmission. When checking for parental affectedness, 9/45 (20%) mothers had seizures vs. 2/45 (4%) of fathers. As in probands, the most common abnormal EEG findings were diffuse single or multiple spike waves (Fig. 15–7).

Analyses of familial aggregation of seizures showed that first-degree relatives in families with CAE evolving to JME have a 94- to 188-fold risk of having any seizure type over the risk in the general population (Tables 15–1 and 15–2). The risk of having myoclonic seizures (JME) was also augmented for parents and second-degree relatives (15 to 36 times higher than in general population). This data contrasts with classic JME, in which relatives have increased risk for myoclonias and less risk for absences. The risk of having other seizure types was slightly increased in relatives from both syndromes.

Long-Term Outcome of Seizures in Probands

Absence seizures appeared in childhood heralding the disorder in all 45 probands. In only five cases did grand-mal seizures appear in childhood; yet they did not precede absences. Myoclonic seizures appeared during childhood

in only three cases and, again, did not precede absences. In 38 cases (84%), myoclonias or grand-mal convulsions or both appeared for the first time during adolescence. In five cases, grand-mal convulsions or myoclonias appeared after 21 years of age. During 10–20 years of follow-up, absences continued to be the chief complaint in 48% probands. Absences mixed with tonic-clonic or myoclonic seizures were the chief complaint in 17%, tonic–clonic seizures only in 21%, and myoclonic seizures only in 14%. Absences occurred at least once a day (range 1 to 200 per day).

In 48% of patients, the appearance of the first grand-mal seizure prompted the start of antiepileptic drug treatment. Nineteen probands (42%) had been considered to have refractory partial seizures until the correct diagnosis of an idiopathic generalized epilepsy syndrome prompted valproate (VPA) treatment. Other drugs that had been previously used without success were phenytoin (PHT) (49%), carbamazepine (CBZ) (42%), phenobarbital (PB) (21%), gabapentin (GBP) (8%), and oxcarbacepine (OXC) (2%). Ethosuximide (ESM) had been used in 12%, but seizure control was not achieved.

Data and long-term follow-up were available in 35 cases. Only 8.6% of probands (3/35) taking antiepileptic treatment reported no seizures in adulthood. VPA monotherapy significantly reduced grand-mal tonic–clonic seizures in 80% of patients. However, absences alone or in

TABLE 15–2. *Risk of seizures in relatives of probands with CAE evolving to JME*

Subsyndrome	Relatives with pyknoleptic CAE			Relatives with JME			Relatives with other seizure type		
	No.	%	Relative risk	No.	%	Relative risk	No.	%	Relative risk
CAE evolving to JME									
Parents	4/64	6.2	94	1/64	1.6	36	6/64	9	3.1
Siblings	12/97	12.4	188	0	0	0	11/97	11	3.8
Second-degree relatives	7/141	5.0	76	1/141	0.7	15	14/141	10	3.5
Offspring	1/12	8.3	126	0	0	0	0/12	0	0
Classic JME									
Parents	2/158	1.3	20	5/158	3.1	69	13/158	8.2	3
Siblings	2/296	0.7	11	18/296	6.1	136	12/296	4	1.4
Second-degree relatives	1/705	0.1	1.5	6/705	0.9	20	22/705	3	1
Offspring	0	0	0	2/58	3	77	3/58	5.8	1.7

Reference rates used were cumulative or lifetime prevalence of having epilepsy reported from the Rochester study (3%) (38,39), a prevalence of CAE of at least 2.2% of all epilepsies, and a prevalence of JME of at least 1.5% of all epilepsies (40). According to these data, we can estimate a prevalence of 0.00045 for JME and at least 0.00066 for CAE in general population.

TABLE 15–3. *Exclusionary LOD scores between the large Mexican pedigree and the 6p12-11 locus of JME*

Loci	0.00	0.10	0.20	0.30	0.40	Z_{max}	θ_{max}
D6S1541	−7.67	−0.31	0.39	0.41	0.19	0.41	0.30
D6S272	−3.44	−0.12	0.27	0.27	0.11	0.27	0.20
D6S465	−0.60	0.36	0.52	0.39	0.15	0.52	0.20
D6S1714	−4.83	−0.83	−0.24	0.01	0.06	0.06	0.40
D6S1960	−5.55	−1.54	−0.66	−0.23	−0.04	−0.04	0.40
D6S1573	−9.23	−1.20	−0.23	0.05	0.07	0.07	0.40
D5S295	−1.79	0.00	0.16	0.24	0.19	0.24	0.30
D6S294	−4.01	0.00	0.41	0.42	0.24	0.42	0.30
D6S257	−7.46	−2.14	−0.69	−0.11	0.04	0.04	0.40

combination with myoclonia and rare tonic–clonic seizures persisted as breakthrough seizures, which were closely associated with trigger factors. Because of persisting or refractory seizures, polytherapy was needed in 11.4% of cases. VPA was combined either with clonazepam (CZP), lamotrigine (LTG), levetiracetam (LEV), zonisamide (ZNS), or felbamate.

Linkage Analysis

LOD scores did not support linkage between the Mexican family and chromosome 6p12–11. LOD scores were exclusionary (−9 to −3, with theta = 0) for D6S257, D6S294, D6S1573, D6S1960, D6S1714, and D6S272 (Table 15–3). We did not find significant linkage between this family and seven other known epilepsy loci reported in literature although LOD scores were not exclusionary (Table 15–4), e.g., 2q22 (41), 15q14 (42), 6p21.3 (43), and 5q (44). LOD scores were exclusionary for the benign adult familial myoclonic epilepsy loci in 8q23 (45), and partial epilepsy with variable foci in 22q11 (46). A 10-cM genome scan for the Mexican family identified several "hot-spot" regions that are now being flooded with microstellites separated by 1–2 cM (these results will be reported separately).

DISCUSSION

According to our cohort, the syndrome of CAE evolving to JME is a female-preponderant, autosomal-dominant lifelong syndrome that is more often transmitted by mothers. Absences as the sole phenotype or in combination with other seizure types are the most common persisting seizure type in probands. Absences alone are also the most common seizure phenotype in non-proband family members. One-third of probands have absences with eyelid myoclonia and the EEG most commonly shows 2.5- to 5-Hz single spike-wave complexes; 4- to 6-Hz polyspike-wave complexes and 15- to 25-Hz low-amplitude rhythms may also be present.

Analysis of familial aggregation of seizures in CAE evolving to JME show increased risk for absence epilepsy in other family members. The relative risks for absence in parents, siblings, offspring, and second-degree relatives exhibit a genetic pattern, with risks decreasing with increasing distance of relationship. This suggests the probable effect of a major gene that may also express as JME. To date, there is no locus identified for CAE evolving to JME and our genome scan did not show linkage to any of the known JME loci reported in medical literature (3,33,34,41–46).

We suggest that CAE evolving to JME belongs under the rubric of absence epilepsies for the following reasons: (a) it starts with absences with 3-Hz single spike-and-slow wave in childhood, (b) absences are the most common seizure type in affected members, (c) absences are the most common persisting seizure type in probands, (d) like typical CAE, the affected persons are most often female and transmission is predominantly maternal, and (e) despite treatment with VPA mono- or polytherapy, absences persist lifelong.

Linkage analysis performed by our laboratory have now identified three subvarieties of absence

TABLE 15-4. *Known chromosome loci published for JME, BAFME, and partial epilepsy with variable foci*

Phenotype	Known loci	Gene	No. of families and country	LOD score and recombinantion value (θ)	Reference	LOD scores obtained for the markers in those regions (Z_{max})[a]
1 Classic JME	6p12-11	In study	Los Angeles, CA, 31 México, 1 Belize	4.21 (0.10)	3,34	−9.23
2 Classic JME	2q22-23	CACNB4	1 patient, French–Canadian		41	0.89
3 JME without childhood pyknolepsy	15q14	CHRNA4?	32, Europe	4.42 (α0.65)	42	−2.87
4 JME with absence	6p21.3	BRD2 (RING 3)	20 Probands		43	0.4
5 JME with absence	5q	GABRA1	1, French–Canadian	—	44	0.18
6 Benign adult familial myoclonic epilepsy (BAFME)	8q23.124.1	—	1, Japan	4.3	45	0.91
7 Partial epilepsy with variable foci	22q11-q12	—		6.53	46	−12.45

Results obtained in the genome scan performed in the large Mexican family with CAE evolving to JME showed negative or exclusionary LOD scores for these loci.
[a]All with recombination frequencies (θ) of 0.0.

syndromes namely (a) remitting CAE in chromosome 15q11-12 (47), (b) CAE that persists into adulthood with tonic–clonic convulsions in chromosome 8q24 (1,2,48–50), and (c) CAE evolving to JME (1,2,49). Other subsyndromes of absence epilepsies probably exist, such as absence epilepsy of early childhood starting before 5 years of age (51), myoclonic absence epilepsy in which myoclonias occur simultaneously with absence seizures (52), eyelid myoclonia with absences (53), and juvenile absence epilepsy (54–56). There is some agreement on the nosology of these absence subsyndromes, but identifying their chromosomal loci and epilepsy causing mutations would help substantiate their entities (57–65).

Pyknoleptic absence persisting with grand mal has been reported to occur in 12% to 32% of cases (48,66–71). Some authors have reported CAE to precede JME: 7/65 (11%) by Panayiotopoulos (72) 3/11 (25%) by Asconape and Penry (10) 17% by Wirrel et al. (68–70), and 45/258 (18%) in our studies. However, with the exception of our present results, no family studies have been published that determines the seizure phenotypes of family members, gender preponderance, mode of transmission and long-term outcome. In the past, some authors considered absences starting in childhood as an incidental component of JME (24).

Our long-term follow-up shows one character that differentiates CAE evolving to JME from classic JME: 80% of probands have satisfactory treatment with VPA because grand-mal convulsions significantly decrease, but only 8.6% are completely seizure-free and patients chronically complain of absence seizures. In probands or relatives with classic JME, the main and persisting seizure types are myoclonias with or without tonic–clonic seizures. In classic JME, absences are rarely present in relatives and, when present, they are mostly spanioleptic. In contrast, in the syndrome of CAE evolving to JME, absences are pyknoleptic and often accompanied by eyelid myoclonia (31% of cases). Eyelid myoclonia is not found in classic JME (8,10,12,65). Our data also show that when myoclonic seizures are present in CAE evolving to JME, they are not a predominant feature.

Another differentiating feature in CAE evolving to JME and probably a predictor of chronicity are the combined EEG findings of 3-Hz single spike waves, 3.5- to 6-Hz polyspike wave complexes and low-voltage 15- to 25-Hz frequencies ("runs of rapid spikes"). Other authors have reported similar bursts of 15- to 25-Hz frequencies in patients with idiopathic generalized epilepsy with absences persisting into adulthood, that sometimes show drug resistance (10,73–75). This EEG trait has also been found in other idiopathic syndromes like idiopathic childhood myoclonic-astatic epilepsy (MAE), in which about one-half of cases have persisting seizures or recurrences during adolescence (Medina et al., *unpublished*). The presence of high-voltage polyspikes-and-bursting polyspike-and-slow wave complexes during sleep have also been reported to imply poor prognosis (76). We did not perform overnight sleep studies in our patients. Fast high-amplitude discharges between 8- to 20-Hz during slow-wave sleep are also considered as one of the criteria for Lennox-Gastaut syndrome (LGS) (77–80). In general terms, it has been suggested that 15- to 25-Hz rhythmic discharges are markers for nonremittance (73–75).

There have been several long-term follow-up studies of pyknoleptic CAE that persist into adulthood (66–71,81–83). To date, however, there is no or meager data on the prognosis and treatment response of CAE evolving to JME. Charlton and Yahr (67), Sato et al. (66), Wirrel et al. (68–70) observed the following predictive factors for chronicity: low intelligence quotient, presence of slow background in EEG, positive family history of seizures, history of absence status, early onset of absence seizures, and failure of initial antiepileptic treatment. Details on the evolution of the different seizure types were not available in these earlier reports by these authors.

Our present studies provide a long-term follow-up even to the sixth decade of life, allowing us to ascertain behavior of illness and modification by drug therapy. In our cohort, when seizures of probands older than 20 years were analyzed, it showed that absences could persist for at least 22 years, myoclonias for 12 years, and tonic–clonic seizures for 15 years, indicating a chronic epilepsy.

In conclusion, our clinical and genetic studies support the concept of a female preponderant syndrome that starts as CAE, with eyelid myoclonia persisting and evolving into adolescence with grand-mal and myoclonic seizures. The disorder affects more mothers than fathers and is transmitted more by females than males. Genome scan in a 100-member family did not support linkage to any of the known JME loci in chromosome 6p11-12, 6p21.3, 2q22-23, 15q14, and 5q. Our results thus indicate a subsyndrome distinct from remitting CAE, and classic JME, a syndrome that rightly belongs to the absence epilepsies. Identification of absence-causing mutations in this syndrome should substantiate this clinical entity.

REFERENCES

1. Delgado-Escueta AV, Medina MT, Serratosa JM, et al. Mapping and positional cloning of common idiopathic generalized epilepsies: juvenile myoclonus epilepsy and childhood absence epilepsy. *Adv Neurol* 79:351–374.
2. Delgado-Escueta AV, Alonso M, Medina MT, et al. The search for epilepsy genes in juvenile myoclonic epilepsy: Discoveries along the way. In: Schmitz B, Sander T. eds. *Juvenile myoclonic epilepsy: The Janz syndrome*. Petersfield: Wrightson Biomedical, 2000:145–170.
3. Liu AW, Delgado-Escueta AV, Gee MN, et al. Juvenile myoclonic epilepsy in chromosome 6p12-p11: locus heterogeneity and recombinations. *Am J Med Genet* 1996;63:438–446.
4. Durner M, Zhou G, Fu D, et al. Evidence for linkage of adolescent-onset idiopathic generalized epilepsies to chromosome 8 and genetic heterogeneity. *Am J Hum Genet* 1999;64:1411–1419.
5. Durner M, Keddache MA, Tomasini L, et al. Genome scan of idiopathic generalized epilepsy: Evidence for major susceptibility gene and modifying genes influencing the seizure type. *Ann Neurol* 2001;49:328–335.
6. Greenberg DA, Durner M, Keddache M, et al. Reproducibility and complications in gene searches: Linkage on chromosome 6, heterogeneity, association, and maternal inheritance in juvenile myoclonic epilepsy. *Am J Hum Genet* 2000;66:508–516.
7. Greenberg DA, Durner M, Resor S, et al. The genetics of idiopathic generalized epilepsies of adolescent onset: Differences between juvenile myoclonic epilepsy and epilepsy with random grand mal and with awakening grand mal. *Neurology* 1995;45(5):942–946.
8. Janz D. Epilepsy with impulsive petit mal (juvenile myoclonic epilepsy). *Acta Neurol Scand* 1985;72:449–459.
9. Salas-Puig J, Gonzalez C, Tunon A, et al. Epilepsia Mioclónica juvenil: Aspectos electroclinicos. *Boll Lega It Epil* 1988;62/63:199–201.
10. Asconape J, Penry JK. Some clinical and EEG aspects of benign juvenile myoclonic epilepsy. *Epilepsia* 1984;25:108–114.
11. Oller-Daurella L, Oller LFV. *5000 Epilépticos-Clínica y Evolución*. Barcelona, Spain: ESPAXS, S.A. Publicaciones Médicas, 1994:169–170.
12. Delgado-Escueta AV, Enrile-Bacsal F. Juvenile myoclonic epilepsy of Janz. *Neurology* 1984;34:285–294.
13. Mai R, Canevini MP, Pontrelli V, et al. L'epilessia mioclonica giovanile di Janz: Analisi prospettica di un campione di 57 pazienti. *Boll Lega It Epil* 1990;70/71:307–309.
14. Wolf P. Juvenile myoclonic epilepsy. In Roger J, et al. eds. *Epileptic syndromes in infancy, childhood and adolescence*. London: John Libbey, 1992.
15. Genton P, Gelisse. Juvenile myoclonic epilepsy. *Arch Neurol* 2001;58.
16. Greenberg DA, Delgado-Escueta AV, Maldonado HM, et al. Segregation analysis of juvenile myoclonic epilepsy. *Genet Epidemiol* 1988;5:81–94.
17. Doose H, Neubauer BA. Preponderance of female sex in the transmission of seizure liability in idiopathic generalized epilepsy. *Epilepsy Res* 2001;43:103–114.
18. Mehndiratta MM, Aggarwal P. Clinical expression and EEG features of patients with juvenile myoclonic epilepsy (JME) from North India. *Seizure* 2002;11:431–436.
19. Vijai J, Cherian PJ, Sylaja PN, et al. Clinical characteristics of a South Indian cohort of juvenile myoclonic epilepsy probands. *Seizure* 2003;12:490–496.
20. Jain S, Tripathi M, Srivastava AK, et al. Phenotypic analysis of juvenile myoclonic epilepsy in Indian families. *Acta Neurol Scand* 2003:107:356–362.
21. Janz D, Durner M, Beck-Mannagetta G. Family studies on the genetics of juvenile myoclonic epilepsy (epilepsy with petit mal). In: Beck-Mannagetta G, Anderson VE, Doose H, Janz D. eds. *Genetics of the epilepsies*. Springer-Verlag, Berlin, 1989:43–52.
22. Panayiotopoulos C, Obeid T, Waheed G. Absences in juvenile myoclonic epilepsy: A clinical and video-electroencephalographic study. *Ann Neurol* 1989; 25:391–397.
23. Durner M, Sander T, Greenberg DA, et al. Localization of idiopathic generalized epilepsy on chromosome 6p in families of juvenile myoclonic epilepsy patients. *Neurology* 1991;41:1651–1655.
24. Thomas P, Genton P, Gelisse P, et al. Juvenile myoclonic epilepsy. In: Roger J, Bureau M, Dravet C, Dreifuss FE, Perret A, Wolf, P. eds. *Epileptic syndromes in infancy, childhood and adolescence*. London: John Libbey, 2002:335–355.
25. Tsuboi, T, Christian W. On the genetics of primary generalized epilepsy with sporadic myoclonous of impulsive petit-mal type. *Humangenetik* 1973;19:155–182.
26. Delgado-Escueta AV, Medina MT, Serratosa JM, et al. Mapping and positional cloning of common idiopathic generalized epilepsies: Juvenile myoclonus epilepsy and childhood absence epilepsy. In: Delgado-Escueta AV, Wilson WA, Olsen RW, Porter RJ. eds. *Jasper's basic mechanisms of the epilepsies. Advances in Neurology.* 3rd ed. Vol. 79. Philadelphia: Lippincott Williams & Wilkins, 1999:351–373.

27. Commission on Classification and Terminology of the International League Against Epilepsy. Proposal for revised clinical and electrographic classification of epileptic seizures. *Epilepsia* 1981;22:489–501.

28. Commission on Classification and Terminology of the International League against Epilepsy. Proposal for revised classification of epilepsies and epileptic syndromes. *Epilepsia* 1989;30:389–399.

29. Commission on Epidemiology and Prognosis, International League Against Epilepsy. Guidelines for epidemiological studies on epilepsy. *Epilepsia* 1993;34(4):592–596.

30. Ott J. Computer-simulation methods in human linkage analysis. *Proc Natl Acad Sci USA* 1989;86:4175–4178.

31. Greenberg DA, Delgado-Escueta AV, Widelitz H, et al. Juvenile myoclonic epilepsy (JME) may be linked to the BF and HLA loci on human chromosome 6. *Am J Med Genet* 1988;31:185–192.

32. Weissbecker KA, Durner M, Janz D, et al. Confirmation of linkage between juvenile myoclonic epilepsy locus and the HLA region of chromosome 6. *Am J Med Genet* 1991;38:32–36.

33. Liu AW, Delgado-Escueta AV, Serratosa JM, et al. Juvenile myoclonic epilepsy locus in chromosome 6p21. 2-p11: Linkage to convulsions and electroencephalography trait. *Am J Hum Genet* 1996;57:368–381.

34. Bai D, Alonso ME, Medina MT, et al. Juvenile myoclonic epilepsy: Linkage to chromosome 6p12 in Mexico families. *Am J Med Genet* 2002;113:268–274.

35. Weber LJ, May PE. Abundant classes of human DNA polymorphism, which can be typed using the polymerase chain reaction. *Am J Hum Genet* 1989;44:388–396.

36. Ott J. A computer program for linkage analysis of general human pedigrees. *Am J Hum Genet* 1974;28:528–529.

37. Terwilliger JD, Ott J. *Handbook of human genetic linkage.* Baltimore: Johns Hopkins University Press, 1994:126–216.

38. Hauser W, Hesdorffer D. *Epilepsy: Frequency, causes and consequences.* Maryland: Epilepsy Foundation of America, 1990:93–118.

39. Annegers JF. The Epidemiology of Epilepsy. In: Wyllie E. ed. *The treatment of epilepsy. Principles and practice.* Philadelphia: Lea & Febiger, 1993:157–164.

40. Manford M, Hart YM, Sander JW, et al. The National General Practice Study of Epilepsy. The syndromic classification of the International League Against Epilepsy applied in a general population. *Arch Neurol* 1992;49:801–808.

41. Escayg A, De Waard M, Lee D, et al. Coding and noncoding variation of the human calcium-channel beta(4)-subunit gene CACNB4 in patients with idiopathic generalized epilepsy and episodic ataxia. *Am J Hum Genet* 2000;66:1531–1539.

42. Elmslie FV, Rees M, Williamson MP, et al. Genetic mapping of a major susceptibility locus for juvenile myoclonic epilepsy on chromosome 15q. *Hum Mol Genet* 1997;8:1329–1334.

43. Pal DK, Evgrafov OV, Tabares P, et al. BRD2 (RING3) is a probable major susceptibility gene for common juvenile myoclonic epilepsy. *Am J Hum Genet* 2003;73:261–270.

44. Cossette P, Liu L, Brisebois K, et al. Mutation of GABRA1 in an autosomal dominant form of juvenile myoclonic epilepsy. *Nature Genet* 2002;31:184–189.

45. Mikami M, Yasuda T, Terao A, et al. Localization of a gene for benign adult familial myoclonic epilepsy to chromosome 8q23.3-q24.1. *Am J Hum Genet* 1999;65:745–751.

46. Lan Xiong L, Labuda M, Li D, et al. Localization of a gene determining familial partial epilepsy with variable foci to chromosome 22q11-q12. *Am J Hum Genet* 1999;65:1698–1710.

47. Tanaka M, Castroviejo IP, Olsen R, et al. Linkage analysis between subsyndromes of childhood absence epilepsy and the GABA A receptor beta 3 subunit gene on chromosome 15q11. 2-12. *Epilepsia* 2000;41[Suppl 7]:250.

48. Fong C, Shan P, Huang Y, et al. Childhood absence epilepsy in and Indian (Bombay) family maps to chromosome 8q24. *Neurology* 1998;50:A357.

49. Delgado-Escueta AV, Perez-Gosiengfiao KB, Bai D, et al. Recent developments in the quest for myoclonic epilepsy genes. *Epilepsia* 2003;44[Suppl.11]:13–26.

50. Delgado-Escueta AV, Serratosa JM, Liu A, et al. Progress in mapping human epilepsy genes. *Epilepsia* 1994;35[Suppl 1]:S29–S40.

51. Chaix Y, Daquin G, Monteiro F, et al. Absence epilepsy with onset before age three years: A heterogeneous and often severe condition. *Epilepsia* 2003;44(7):944–949.

52. Tassinari CA, Lyagoubi S, Santos V, et al. Etude des décharges de pointes ondes chez l'home II: Les aspects cliniques et électroencéphalographiques des absences myocloniques. *Rev Neurol* 1969;121:379–383.

53. Appleton RE, Panayiotopoulos CP, Acomb BA, et al. Eyelid myoclonia with typical absences: an epilepsy syndrome. *J Neurol Neurosurg Psych* 1993;56 (12):1312–1316.

54. Bartolomei F, Roger J, Bureau M, et al. Prognostic factors for childhood and juvenile absence epilepsies. *Rev Neurol* 1996;24(132):930–936.

55. Oller L. Prospective study of the differences between the syndromes of infantile absence epilepsy and syndromes of juvenile absence epilepsy. *Epilepsia* 1993;34 [Suppl 3]:S42–S48.

56. Porter RJ. The absence epilepsies. *Epilepsia* 1993; 34[Suppl 3]:S42–S48.

57. Guilhoto LM, Manreza ML, Yacubian EM. Syndromic classification of patients with typical absence seizures. *Arq Neuropsiquiatr* 2003;61(3A):580–587.

58. Baykan B, Gokyigit A, Gurses C, et al. Recurrent absence status epilepticus: clinical and EEG characteristics. *Seizure* 2002;11(5):310–309.

59. Agathonikou A, Panayiotopoulos CP, Giannakodimos S. Typical absence status in adults: Diagnostic and syndromic considerations. *Epilepsia* 1998;39(12):1265–1276.

60. Reutens DC, Berkovic SF. Idiopathic generalized epilepsy of adolescence: are the syndromes clinically distinct? *Neurology* 1995;45(8):1469–1476.

61. Tiacci C, D'Alessandro P, Cantisani TA, et al. So-called petit mal status: Epileptic syndrome or seizure type? *Ital J Neurol Sci* 1995;16(5):279–294.

62. Obeid T. Clinical and genetic aspects of juvenile absence epilepsy. *J Neurol* 1994;241(8):487–491.

63. Gordon N, Aird RB. Idiopathic childhood absences, a system disorder: Its diagnosis and differentiation. *Develop Med Child Neurol* 1991;33(8):744–748.

64. Holmes GL, McKeever M, Adamson M. Absence seizures in children: clinical and electroencephalographic features. *Ann Neurol* 1987;21(3):268–273.

65. Roger J, Bureau M, Dravet C, Dreifuss FE, Perret A, Wolf P, eds. *Epileptic syndromes in infancy, childhood and adolescence.* London: John Libbey, 1992.

66. Sato S, Dreifuss F, Penry J. Prognostic factors in absence seizures. *Neurology* 1976;26:788–796.

67. Charlton M, Yahr M. Long-term follow-up of patients with petit mal. *Arch Neurol* 1967;16:595–598.

68. Wirrel EC, Camfield CS, Camfield PR, et al. Long-term prognosis of typical childhood absence epilepsy: remission of progression to juvenile myoclonic epilepsy. *Neurology* 1996;47:912–918.

69. Wirrel E, Camfield C, Camfield D, et al. Prognostic significance of failure of the initial antiepileptic drugs in children with absence epilepsy. *Epilepsia* 2001;42(6):760–763.

70. Wirrell EC. Natural history of absence epilepsy in children. *Can J Neurol Sci* 2003;30(3):184–188.

71. Bouma PA, Westendorp RG, van Dijk JG, et al. The outcome of absence epilepsy: A meta-analysis. *Neurology* 1996;47(3):802–808.

72. Panayiotopoulus CP, Agathonikou A, Koutroumanidis M, et al. Eyelid myoclonia with absences: the symptoms. In Duncan J, Panayiotopoulos CP. eds. *Eyelid myoclonia with absences.* London: John Libbey, 1996: 17–26.

73. Gastaut H, Zifkin B, Mariani E, et al. The long term course of primary generalized epilepsy with persisting absences. *Neurology* 1986;36:1021–1028.

74. Michelucci R, Ruboli G, Passarelli D, et al. Idiopathic generalized epilepsy with persisting absence seizures in adult life: electroclinical patterns. *J Neurol Neurosurg Psych* 1995;61:441–447.

75. Fakhoury T, About-Khalil B. Generalized absence seizures with 10-15 Hz fast discharges. *Clin Neurophysiol* 1999;110:1029–1035.

76. Guye M, Bartolomei F, Gastaut JL, et al. Absence epilepsy with fast rhythmic discharges during sleep: an intermediary form of generalized epilepsy? *Epilepsia* 2001;42(3):351–356.

77. Gastaut H, Roger J, Soulayrol S, et al. Childhood epileptic encephalopathy with diffuse slow spike-waves. *Epilepsia* 1966;7:139–179.

78. Dulac O, N'Guyen T. The Lennox-Gastaut syndrome. *Epilepsia* 1993;34[Suppl 7]:S7–17.

79. Bonani P, Parmeggiani L, Guerrini R. Different neurophysiologic patterns of myoclonus characterize Lennox-Gastaut syndrome and myoclonic astatic epilepsy. *Epilepsia* 2002;43(6):609–615.

80. Bartolomei F, Roger J, Bureau M, et al. Prognostic factors for childhood and juvenile absence epilepsies. *Eur Neurol* 1997;37(3):169–175.

81. Wolf P, Inoue Y. Therapeutic response of absence seizures in patients of an epilepsy clinic for adolescents and adults. *J Neurol* 1984;231(4):225–259.

82. Fois A, Malandrini F, Mostardini R. Clinical experiences of petit mal. *Brain Develop* 1987;9(1):54–59.

83. Sato S, Dreifuss FE, Penry JK, et al. Long-term follow-up of absence seizures. *Neurology* 1983;33(12):1590–1595.

16

Photosensitivity: Genetics and Clinical Significance

B. A. Neubauer,* St. Waltz,† M. Grothe,† A. Hahn,* I. Tuxhorn,‡
T. Sander,§ G. Kurlemann,‖ and U. Stephani†

*Department of Neuropediatrics, Zentrum Kinderheilkunde und Jugendmedizin, Giessen, Germany;
†Department of Neuropediatrics, Klinik für Neuropädiatrie der Universität, Kiel, Germany;
‡Epilepsy Center Bethel, Klinik Mara, Bielefeld, Germany; §Gene Mapping Center (GMC),
Max-Delbrück-Centrum, Berlin, Germany; ‖Department of Neuropediatrics, University of Münster,
Münster, Germany

INTRODUCTION

In some of the generalized idiopathic epilepsy (IGE) syndromes, especially those with the strongest genetic background, photosensitivity is found at a significantly increased rate compared to the normal population and to cohorts of patients with focal or symptomatic epilepsy. Photic stimulation may elicit a cortical response ranging from occipital spikes only to generalized spike-waves discharges (type 1 to 4) during EEG recording. In the past, most authors have only recognized generalized discharges as "true" photosensitivity, for its close association with epilepsy. However, family studies demonstrate a common genetic basis for all four types of photosensitivity and favor an autosomal dominant mode of inheritance. In patients with photosensitive epilepsy, cortical control of contrast gain has been found severely impaired. A dopaminergic mechanism was demonstrated neuropharmacologically. The high prevalence of photosensitivity in the normal population, its occurrence in neurodegenerative disorders, and its detection in individuals suffering from idiopathic epilepsies with confirmed defects of different ion-channel genes makes genetic heterogeneity most likely. In a sample consisting of 37 nuclear pedigrees, we conducted a linkage candidate study investigating the loci of EPM1, EPM2, and DRD1 to DRD5 and formerly reported loci of idiopathic epilepsies on 1p, 2q36, 3p14, 3q26, 4p, 6p11, 6p21.3, 8p11, and 15q14. Finally, none of the investigated loci surpassed the limit of proved or suggestive evidence for linkage.

DEFINITION OF PHOTOSENSITIVITY

Intermittent photic stimulation (IPS) may elicit different types of cortical responses. Photic driving or photic following, a phase-locked wave form frequently observed at stimulation frequencies ranging from 8 to 10 Hz, has no pathologic implication. Apart from this, several types of cortical responses have been labeled photoparoxysmal response or photosensitivity by different authors. The modalities of stimulation are critical for diagnostic sensitivity. This topic is covered by ample literature (1). An early description of flashlight-induced seizure stimulation dates back to Walther and Walther (2), who found the optimal stimulation frequency to range from 12 to 18 Hz. Bickford et al. (3) finally defined generalized spike-wave activity as the "Photoconvulsive Response," which is the most frequent description cited. This type of photoparoxysmal response has a close association to epilepsy, especially when it is self-sustaining beyond the period of stimulation (4). However it is known, that this is only the most drastic type of response: Doose and colleagues graded photosensitivity into four types [Doose et al. (5,6), Waltz et al. (7), Doose and Waltz (8)]. Type 1 is characterized by purely occipital spikes within the occipital alpha rhythm. In type 2, parietooccipital spikes are followed by a biphasic slow wave. Type 3 consists of parietooccipital spikes followed by a biphasic slow wave spreading to the frontal region. In type 4, which is synonymous to the photoconvulsive response of Bickford, gen-

eralized spike-wave and polyspikes occur (Fig. 16–1). This classification was not based on formal definition, but on different types of photoparoxysmal responses found in a multiplex of families of patients with epilepsy. The trait is age dependent with a maximum penetrance and expression between the ages of 9 to 16 years and is more frequent in girls than in boys (9). It may be mentioned that the so-called photomyoclonic or photomyogenic response is not related to the photoparoxysmal response. It consists of strictly stimulus synchronous cloni of the periorbital muscle groups, while the EEG, besides the muscle artifacts, remains unremarkable (10).

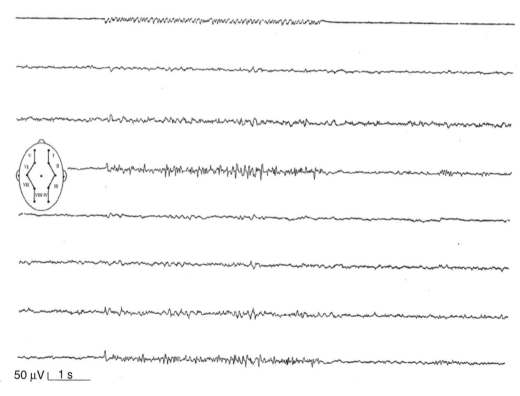

A   50 µV ⌞ 1 s

FIG. 16–1. A: Photoparoxysmal response of 34-year-old mother of an epileptic boy with type 1. Photic stimulation evokes small occipital spikes. B: Photoparoxysmal response of 18-year-old-sister of an epileptic boy with type 2. Photic stimulation evokes biphasic slow waves with interposed spikes over the posterior areas. C: Photoparoxysmal response of 10-year-old girl with type 3. Photic stimulation evokes generalized biphasic and polyphasic sharp transients with interposed spikes. Discharge ends while stimulation continues. D: Photoparoxysmal response type IV. Generalized spike wave and polyspike wave discharge. A sibling showed the identical response to light stimulation. (From Doose H, *EEG in epilepsy*. lst ed. Montouge, France: John Libbey, 2003. With permission).

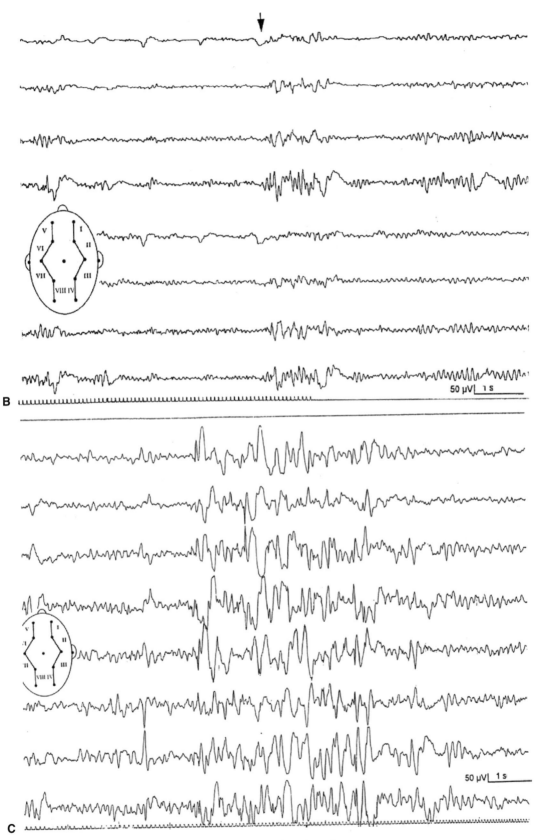

FIG. 16-1. (*Continued*)

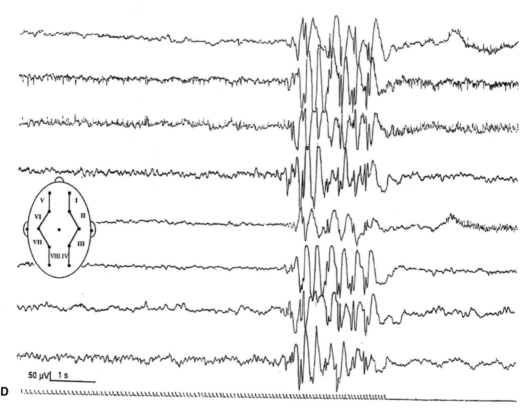

50 µV| 1 s

D

FIG. 16–1. (*Continued*)

PHOTOSENSITIVITY AND EPILEPSY

Starting from the historic definition of photosensitivity, it is now obvious that only the type 4 response is strongly associated with seizures. Binnie (1) argues with Reilly and Peters (4) that in the setting of an EEG laboratory of an epilepsy unit, the *a priori* probability for epilepsy might be 50 times higher than in the normal population. Under these circumstances, a type-4 photosensitivity has a high prognostic value concerning the risk of seizures, possibly reaching up to 80%. Precise numbers given by different authors are difficult to compare for a variety of technical and ascertainment biases. If the setting of an EEG laboratory in an epilepsy unit is left and only healthy individuals are investigated, the epilepsy risk may possibly be much lower, even in type-4 photosensitivity. If all four types of photosensitivity are considered jointly

and nonepileptic children are included (family studies), the relative risk might not be higher than 3% (8).

Categorically, epilepsy in individuals with photosensitivity can be divided into pure photosensitive epilepsy, epilepsy with photosensitivity, and photosensitivity in the EEG only, not accompanied by any documented seizures. It should be noted that only 50% of probands with a type-4 photosensitivity, who experience a video documented, mostly self-limiting seizure, will have a recollection of this (11,12); these reports include generalized tonic–clonic seizures in 84%, absences in 6%, and partial motor seizures in 1.5%. Television or videogame epilepsy is the most prominent example of seizures induced by optic stimulation (13). Photosensitivity is found as a frequent feature in several epilepsy syndromes like JME, eyelid myoclonia with absences, severe myoclonic epilepsy (Dravet syndrome), and myoclonic-astatic epilepsy (Doose syndrome). Some authors argue that, depending on the mode and intensity of photic stimulation in patients with juvenile myoclonic epilepsy (JME), the photoparoxysmal response may be provoked in up to 90% of patients (14), while 30% is the order of magnitude documented under the standard stimulation procedure (15). It is also known that a number of progressive myoclonus epilepsies are almost invariably associated with photosensitivity (1). In Lafora disease and Unverricht–Lundborg syndrome, the photoparoxysmal response closely resembles the one observed in idiopathic epilepsies.

PATHOMECHANISM

The cortical reaction to photic stimuli is most likely controlled by a complex network, which involves several mechanisms and components. The precise pathophysiology of photogenic-induced EEG discharges or seizures is far from clear. However, some basic aspects have been elucidated. It is known that stroboscope flashes with a frequency ranging from about 10 to 20 Hz are most provocative and that a distinct proportion of probands with confirmed photosensitivity also shows pattern sensitivity (16). This may serve as a model that is apparently more suited for neurophysiologic investigation of photosensitivity than pure flash stimulation by itself. It has been shown by Wilkins et al. (17) [concisely reviewed by Binnie (1)] that at least 40% black–white contrast with lined contours at a special frequency of 2 to 4 cycles per degree are most epileptogenic. Binocular fusion, steady neuronal synchronization (pattern may not drift through the visual field), and oscillation support the generation of occipital discharges.

In a series of experiments in 11 patients with photosensitive epilepsy (PSE), Porciatti and coworkers (18) showed that increased contrast of the presented stimulus resulted in an almost constant increase of steady-state VEP amplitude. In normal controls, this response leveled out into a plateau at a much lower contrast of the stimulus and could not be increased to the level observed in the probands. The authors concluded that the cortical mechanism for controlling responses to contrast gain at low temporal frequency and high luminance is severely impaired in patients with PSE. It has also been shown, that apomorphine (a dopaminergic drug) abolishes photosensitivity transiently (19,20). There has been a debate concerning the question whether occipital spikes only (i.e., type 1) and generalized discharges (i.e., type 4), both elicited by visual stimuli, represent different grades of expression of one common mechanism, or are two discrete entities. Several authors have addressed this question and have shown that different modes of stimulation affect the propagation of both responses in a diverging manner (21). However, in our opinion, the conclusion that both responses result from entirely separate mechanisms is too far reaching. Indeed, results obtained by family studies clearly demonstrate common genetic components in both types of responses (7).

GENETICS

The photoparoxysmal response (PPR) is genetically determined. Over the last decades, case studies of more than 10 independent pairs of monozygotic twins concordant for photosensitivity were reported [e.g., Herrlin (22)]. Based on the fact that these twin pairs were not ascertained systematically and because negative concordant twin pairs will most likely fail to be reported, the degree of heritability cannot be deduced from these reports. Different stimulation techniques and diverging trait definitions render data of family studies difficult to compare. Doose and Gerken (23) studied the EEG of 645 siblings of mostly epileptic patients to determine the heritability of different EEG traits. The siblings of photosensitive probands with and without epilepsy showed a high rate of cortical response to photic stimulation. In consecutive studies Waltz et al. (7) and Doose and Waltz (8) graded the photoparoxsymal response into four types on the basis of family studies (Fig. 16–1). It was demonstrated that the incidence of PPR in siblings of probands with PPR type 4 was identical to the incidence found in siblings of probands with types 1–3. Furthermore, the quantitative expression of photosensitivity turned out to be age dependent. Relatives up to the age of 10 years displayed significantly more often type 3 and type 4 discharges than siblings older than 15 years did. Taken together, these data clearly show that the four different types of PPR represent different levels of expression of the identical genetic trait (8).

Waltz and Stephani (24) extended these studies and further investigated the mode of inheritance of the PPR. They analyzed two types of families. In the first group, one of the parents was known to be photosensitive and the rate of photosensitive offspring was determined. It was found that 50% of the siblings were positive. The authors concluded that photosensitivity is transmitted as an autosomal dominant trait. The second group of families was defined by one positive proband with both parents showing no photosensitivity. In this group, only 15% of the siblings of the proband were positive for the trait. Taken into account that both parents were not investigated at the age of maximum expression, which will render some trait carriers false-negative, and considering the fact that 7.6% of the general population shows a PPR (sporadic rate), this finding again is compatible with the drawn conclusion. Much earlier, Watson and Marcus (25), in a similar study, reported different numbers and affected/unaffected ratios, but also concluded an autosomal mode of inheritance. However, their study does not mention the age of the relatives investigated.

MOLECULAR GENETICS

In a significant group of patients with severe myoclonic epilepsy (Dravet Syndrome) *de novo* mutations of the *SCN1A* gene are the causative gene defect (26). Practically all affected children are photosensitive. To our knowledge no systematic study is available that determined the precise proportion of photosensitivity in carriers of *SCN1A* mutations. In two cases of ours with established *SCN1A* gene defects, photosensitivity was present. Recently, in some few families with juvenile myoclonic epilepsy, *GABRG2* and *CLCN2* mutations have been identified. The carriers of the defective gene again were photosensitive (27–29; Heils, *personal commun*).

A stunning case study was recently reported by van Esch et al. (30). In a boy with refractory photosensitive epilepsy, a complex rearrangement of chromosome 2, including 12 distinct breakpoints and one small inversion, were found. The defined breakpoints may serve as target loci for further linkage studies or candidate gene approaches in family collectives.

In our own sample consisting of 37 pedigrees (Fig. 16–2), several candidate loci were investigated by linkage analysis. Parametric and nonparametric two- and multipoint LOD scores and heterogeneity testing was performed by the GENEHUNTER package 1.3 (31). Haplotype relative risk (HRR) and transmission disequilibrium testing (TDT) was performed by the ANALYSE package (32,33). Analysis was performed as an "affected only study" rendering penetrances virtually unimportant. Genotyping was done using standard protocols on an ABI Prism 377 (Applied Biosystems).

Progressive Myoclonus Epilepsies

In summary, the obtained results in EPM1 and EPM2 analyzed under an autosomal mode of inheritance as reported by Waltz and Stephani (24) practically exclude both loci as major contributors to the phenotype in the investigated sample. Assuming autosomal recessive inheritance, EPM1 cannot be excluded formally; however, results close to "0" are far from the limits of suggestive linkage (34) (Tables 16–1, 16–2).

Inclusion of genotype information of two flanking polymorphisms on each locus in order to maximize information content did not reveal different results (data not shown). LOD scores with and without heterogeneity, HRR, and TDT also did not show a significant deviation from the expected mean. DRD 1–5 do not contribute to the phenotype, at least in the majority of families investigated (Table 16–3).

Candidate Loci of the Idiopathic Epilepsies on Chromosomes 1, 2, 3, 4, 8, 19, and 20

Several chromosomal loci have yielded positive linkage results in family collectives of idiopathic epilepsies. Many of these findings have not been

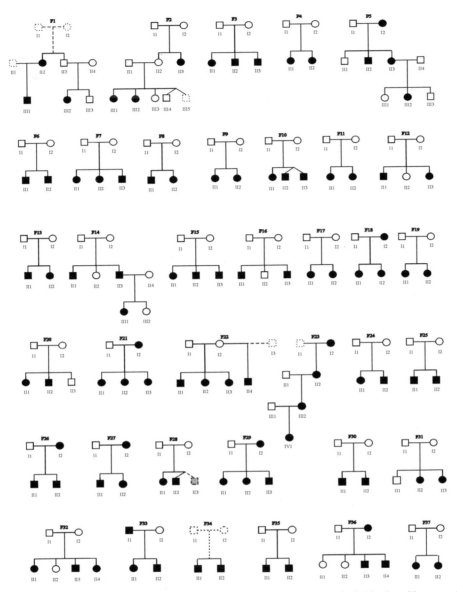

FIG. 16–2. Pedigree structure of 37 families. Solid symbols indicate individuals with proved photoparoxysmal response (type 1–4); unfilled symbols indicate "affection status unknown;" dotted lines, no DNA available.

reproduced in independent samples and have not resulted in conclusive identification of causative alleles or even gene defects. This feature seems to be inherent to many complex traits and probably depends on different ethnic origin of the included families, differing inclusion criteria, and limited sample size. In this study, we investigated loci on chromosome 1p, 2q36, 3p14, 3q26, 4p, 6p11, 6p21, 8p11, 8q24, 14q23, and 15q14 (35–43) (Tables 16–4 and 16–5).

On chromosome 1p positive scores were obtained, however all of the above tested loci did not surpass the proposed limit of suggestive linkage (34). Heterogeneity testing, HRR, and TDT studies did not obtain different results (data not shown).

TABLE 16–1. *Unverricht–Lundborg type (EPM1 on 21q22.3)*

Polymorphism	Autosomal dominant	Autosomal recessive	Z_{all} score/ p value
Two-point LOD scores			
D21S49	− 1.79	0.00/0.53 ($\theta = 0.1$)	1.12/0.13
PFKL	− 2.25	− 0.68	0.85/0.20
D21S171	0.04/1.10 ($\theta = 0.1$)	0.30/0.85 ($\theta = 0.1$)	1.99/0.02
Multipoint LOD scores			
D21S49	− 2.71	− 0.02	1.96/0.03
PFKL	− 2.94	− 0.21	1.90/0.03
D21S49	− 3.02	− 0.57	1.76/0.04

If maximization over theta increased the LOD score higher than 0, it is indicated in brackets. 21q22.3 map: cen D21S49-1cM-PFKL-1cM-D21S171 qter

TABLE 16–2. *Lafora disease (EPM2 on 6q24)*

Polymorphism	Autosomal dominant	Autosomal recessive	Z_{all} score/ p value
Two-point LOD scores			
D6S292	− 3.93	− 2.99	− 0.06/0.52
D6S403	− 3.81	− 3.58	− 0.38/0.64
D6S311	− 3.73	− 2.42	− 0.39/0.35
Multipoint LOD scores			
D6S292	− 4.49	− 3.53	0.12/0.45
D6S403	− 4.43	− 4.27	0.00/0.50
D6S311	− 3.36	− 2.33	0.78/0.21

6q24 map: cen D6S292-6cM-D6S403-4cM-D6S311 qter (Dib et al. 1996).

TABLE 16–3. *Dopamine receptor loci (DRD1–DRD5)*

Locus	Polymorphism	Autosomal dominant	Autosomal recessive
5q34-q35	DRD1	− 3.94	0.75
11q22.2-q22.3	DRD2	− 3.52	− 2.39
3q13.3	DRD3	− 0.56	− 0.89
11p15.5	DRD4	− 1.39	− 1.00
4p15.3-4p15.1	DRD5	− 1.16	1.19

TABLE 16–4. *Two-point LOD scores*

	Polymorphism	Autosomal dominant	Autosomal recessive	Z_{all} score/ p value
1p	D1S430	0.54/1.34 ($\theta = 0.1$)	− 1.91	1.72/0.04
	D1S226	− 1.72	− 2.54	1.12/0.13
	D1S207	0.19/1.71 ($\theta = 0.1$)	− 2.49	2.28/0.01
2q36	D2S371	− 1.07	− 2.87	0.64/0.26
	D2S143	− 2.50	− 3.25	0.81/0.21
	D2S2382	− 0.81	− 1.31	1.29 /0.10
3p14	D3S1261	− 4.25	− 3.59	0.27/0.39
	D3S1598	− 5.13	− 3.36	0.27/0.36
3q26	D3S1574	− 3.80	− 2.82	0.47/0.32
	D3S3725	− 3.63	− 2.80	0.87/0.19
4p	D4S2996	− 6.46	− 3.93	0/0.5
	D4S3000	− 6.08	− 3.25	0/0.5
	D4S409	− 2.71	− 1.25	0.45/0.32
8p11	D8S535	− 3.70	− 0.68	0.50/0.31
	D8S1758	− 5.35	− 3.70	0.40/0.65
	D8S1791	− 1.91	− 0.42	1.74/0.04

TABLE 16–5. *Multipoint LOD scores*

	Polymorphism	Autosomal dominant	Autosomal recessive	Z_{all} score/ p value
1p	D1S430	0.32/1.82[a]	− 3.07	2.33/0.01
	D1S226	− 1.87	− 4.00	1.84/0.034
	D1S207	− 0.082/1.37[a]	− 3.21	2.14/0.017
2q36	D2S371	− 2.94	− 3.57	0.87/0.19
	D2S143	− 3.46	− 3.79	0.97/0.17
	D2S2382	− 1.17	− 2.45	1.65/0.05
3p14	D3S1261	− 4.92	− 4.10	0.32/0.37
	D3S1598	− 6.63	− 4.10	0.00/0.51
3q26	D3S1574	− 5.31	− 3.16	0.70/0.24
	D3S3725	− 4.94	− 3.12	0.82/0.21
4p	D4S2996	− 6.87	− 4.44	0/0.5
	D4S3000	− 8.05	− 4.30	0/0.5
	D4S409	− 4.83	− 2.07	0.11/0.45
8p11	D8S535	− 6.11	− 2.61	0.40/0.34
	D8S1758	− 6.78	− 3.85	0/0.5
	D8S1791	− 4.20	− 2.54	1.00/0.16

[a] Allowing for genetic heterogeneity.

Candidate loci on 6p21.3, 6p11, and 15q14 were evaluated in the same manner. Analysis of haplotypes at D15S1010, D6S1650, and D6S257 gave clearly positive LOD and Z_{all} scores in two- and multipoint testing, initially clearly surpassing the criteria of suggestive linkage. An extension study including seven additional families, however, reduced the scores clearly. Testing in an independent sample will be necessary to evaluate the relevance of this finding.

Currently an international consortium is under way to complete a systematic genome scan in a much larger sample of families. It can be expected that these results will establish the basis for the identification of genes involved in the pathogenesis of photosensitivity.

REFERENCES

1. Binnie CD. Epilepsies with photosensitivity to flicker. In: Engel J, ed. Epilepsy, a comprehensive textbook. Philadelphia: Lippincott Raven, 1998:2491–2505.
2. Walter VJ, Walter, WG. The central effects of rhythmic sensory stimulation. *Electroencephalogr Clin Neurophysiol* 1949;1:57–86.
3. Bickford RG, Sem-Jakobsen CW, White PT, et al. Some observations on the mechanism of photic and photometrazole activation. *Electroencephalogr Clin Neurophysiol* 1952;4:275–282.
4. Reilly EL, Peters JF. Relationship of some varieties of electroencephalographic photosensitivity to clinical convulsive disorders. *Neurology* 1973;23(10):1050–1057.
5. Doose H, Gerken H, Hien-Volpel KF, et al. Genetics of photosensitive epilepsy. *Neuropediatrie* 1969;1(1):56–73.
6. Doose H, Gerken H, Volzke E, et al. Investigations on the genetics of photosensitivity. *Electroencephalogr Clin Neurophysiol* 1969;27(6):625.
7. Waltz S, Christen HJ, Doose H. The different patterns of the photoparoxysmal response—A genetic study. *Electroencephalogr Clin Neurophysiol* 1992;83(2):138–145.
8. Doose H, Waltz S. Photosensitivity—genetics and clinical significance. *Neuropediatrics* 1993;24(5):249–255.
9. Doose H. *EEG in Childhood Epilepsy.* Ist English ed. Montouge, France: John Libbey, 2003:54–71.
10. Rabending G, Klepel H. Photoconvulsive and photomyoclonic reactions: age-dependent, genetically determined variants of enhanced photosensitivity. *Neuropediatrie* 1970;2(2):164–172.
11. Kasteleijn-Nolst Trenite DGA, Binnie CD, Meinardi H. Photosensitive patients: symptoms and signs during intermittent photic stimulation and their relation to seizures in daily life. *J Neurol Neurosurg Psych* 1987;50:1546–1549.
12. Jeavons PM, Harding GFA. *Photosensitive epilepsy.* London: Heinemann, 1975.
13. Ishida S, Yamashita Y, Matsuishi T, et al. Photosensitive seizures provoked while viewing "pocket monsters," a made-for-television animation program in Japan. *Epilepsia* 1998;39(12):1340–1344.
14. Appleton R, Beirne M, Acomb B. Photosensitivity in juvenile myoclonic epilepsy. *Seizure* 2000;9(2):108–111.
15. Gooses R. *Die Beziehung der Photosensitivität zu den verschiedenen Syndromen.* In. Berlin, 1984.
16. Kasteleijn-Nolst Trenite DGA. Photosensitivity in epilepsy: electrophysiology and clinical correlates. *Acta Neurol Scand [Suppl]* 1989;125:3–149.
17. Wilkins AJ, Binnie CD, Darby CE. Visually-induced seizures. *Prog Neurobiol* 1980;15(2):85–117.
18. Porciatti V, Bonanni P, Fiorentini A, et al. Lack of cortical

contrast gain control in human photosensitive epilepsy. *Nat Neurosci* 2000;3(3):259–263.

19. Quesney LF, Andermann F, Gloor P. Dopaminergic mechanism in generalized photosensitive epilepsy. *Neurology* 1981;31(12):1542–1544.

20. Quesney LF, Andermann F, Lal S, et al. Transient abolition of generalized photosensitive epileptic discharge in humans by apomorphine, a dopamine-receptor agonist. *Neurology* 1980;30(11):1169–1174.

21. Harding GF, Fylan F. Two visual mechanisms of photosensitivity. *Epilepsia* 1999;40(10):1446–1451.

22. Herrlin K. Epilepsy, light sensitivity and left-handedness in a family with monozygotic triplets. *Pediatrics* 1960;25:385–399.

23. Doose H, Gerken H. On the genetics of EEG-anomalies in childhood. IV Photoconvulsive reaction. *Neuropediatrie* 1973;4:162–171.

24. Waltz S, Stephani U. Inheritance of photosensitivity. *Neuropediatrics* 2000;31(2):82–85.

25. Watson CW, Marcus EM. The genetics and clinical significance of photogenic cerebral electrical abnormalities, myoclonus, and seizures. *Trans Am Neurol Assoc* 1962;87:251–251.

26. Claes L, Del-Favero J, Ceulemans B, et al. De novo mutations in the sodium-channel gene SCN1A cause severe myoclonic epilepsy of infancy. *Am J Hum Genet* 2001;68(6):1327–1332.

27. Baulac S, Huberfeld G, Gourfinkel-An I, et al. First genetic evidence of GABA(A) receptor dysfunction in epilepsy: A mutation in the gamma2-subunit gene. *Nat Genet* 2001;28(1):46–48.

28. Wallace RH, Marini C, Petrou S, et al. Mutant GABA(A) receptor gamma2-subunit in childhood absence epilepsy and febrile seizures. *Nat Genet* 2001;28(1):49–52.

29. Haug K, Warnstedt M, Alekov AK, et al. Mutations in CLCN2 encoding a voltage-gated chloride channel are associated with idiopathic generalized epilepsies. *Nat Genet* 2003;33(4):527–532.

30. Van Esch H, Syrrou M, Lagae L. Refractory photosensitive epilepsy associated with a complex rearrangement of chromosome 2. *Neuropediatrics* 2002;33(6):320–323.

31. Kruglyak L, Daly MJ, Reeve-Daly MP, et al. Parametric and nonparametric linkage analysis: a unified multipoint approach. *Am J Hum Genet* 1996;58(6):1347–1363.

32. Kuokkanen S, Sundvall M, Terwilliger JD, et al. A putative vulnerability locus to multiple sclerosis maps to 5p14-p12 in a region syntenic to the murine locus Eae2. *Nat Genet* 1996;13(4):477–480.

33. Satsangi J, Parkes M, Louis E, et al. Two stage genome-wide search in inflammatory bowel disease provides evidence for susceptibility loci on chromosomes 3, 7 and 12. *Nat Genet* 1996;14(2):199–202.

34. Lander E, Kruglyak L. Genetic dissection of complex traits: guidelines for interpreting and reporting linkage results. *Nat Genet* 1995;11(3):241–247.

35. Westling B, Weissbecker K, Serratosa JM, et al. Evidence for linkage of juvenile myoclonic epilepsy with absences to chromosome 1p. *Am J Hum Genet* 1996;59(S4):A1392.

36. Zara F, Labuda M, Bianchi A, et al. Evidence for a locus predisposing to idiopathic generalized epilepsies and spike-wave EEG on chromosome 3p14-p12.1. *Am J Hum Genet* 1997;61(S4):A43.

37. Sander T, Bockenkamp B, Hildmann T, et al. Refined mapping of the epilepsy susceptibility locus EJM1 on chromosome 6. *Neurology* 1997;49(3):842–847.

38. Sander T, Schulz H, Saar K, et al. (2000). Genome search for susceptibility loci of common idiopathic generalized epilepsies. *Hum Mol Genet* 2000;12;9(10):1465–1472.

39. Durner M, Zhou G, Fu D, et al. Evidence for linkage of adolescent-onset idiopathic generalized epilepsies to chromosome 8- and genetic heterogeneity. *Am J Hum Genet* 1999;64(5):1411–1419.

40. Fong GC, Shah PU, Gee MN, et al. Childhood absence epilepsy with tonic-clonic seizures and electroencephalogram 3-4-Hz spike and multispike-slow wave complexes: Linkage to chromosome 8q24. *Am J Hum Genet* 1998;63(4):1117–1129.

41. Elmslie FV, Rees M, Williamson MP, et al. Genetic mapping of a major susceptibility locus for juvenile myoclonic epilepsy on chromosome 15q. *Hum Mol Genet* 1997;6(8):1329–1334.

42. Neubauer BA, Fiedler B, Himmelein B, et al. Centrotemporal spikes in families with rolandic epilepsy: linkage to chromosome 15q14. *Neurology* 1998;51(6):1608–1612.

43. Dib C, Faure S, Fizames C, et al. A comprehensive genetic map of the human genome based on 5,264 microsatellites. *Nature* 1996;380(6570):152–154.

17

Familial Juvenile Myoclonic Epilepsy

Maria Elisa Alonso,* Marco T. Medina,[†] Iris E. Martínez-Juárez,[‡]
Reyna M. Durón,[††] Julia N. Bailey,[‡] Minerva López-Ruiz,[§]
Ricardo Ramos-Ramirez,[§] Adriana Ochoa-Morales,* Aurelio Jara-Prado,[||]
Astrid Rasmussen-Almarez,[||] Lourdes León,[¶] Gregorio Pineda,[¶]
Ignacio Pascual Castroviejo,** Sonia Khan,[††] Rene Silva,[‡‡] Lizardo Mija,[§§]
Lucio Portilla,[¶] Dongsheng Bai,[‡] Katerina Tanya Perez-Gosiengfiao,[‡]
Jesús Machado-Salas,[‡] and A.V. Delgado-Escueta[‡]

*Instituto Nacional de Neurología y Neurocirugía, Tlalpan, Mexico; [†]National Autonomous
University of Honduras, Tegucigalpa, Honduras; [‡]Comprehensive Epilepsy Program, David Geffen
School of Medicine at UCLA, Los Angeles, California; [§]Unidad de Neurología y Neurocirugía,
Hospital General de Mexico, Mexico City, Mexico; [||]Neurogenetics and Molecular Biology, Instituto
Nacional de Neurología y Neurocirugía, Tlalpan, Mexico; [¶]Department of Epilepsy, Institute of
Neurological Sciences, Lima, Peru; **Pediatric Neurology Department, University Hospital La Paz,
Madrid, Spain; [††]Neurosciences Department, Riyadh Armed Forces Hospital, Saudi Arabia;
[‡‡]Nuestra Señora de La Paz Hospital, San Miguel, El Salvador; [§§]Neurological Sciences
Institute, Lima, Peru

INTRODUCTION

Juvenile myoclonic epilepsy (JME) is a common epilepsy syndrome responsible for 4% to 11% of all epilepsies (1–8) based on hospital records and 0.00045 based on an estimate of the prevalence of JME in hospital-based studies (9). Based on population studies, the prevalence of JME is 0.003 (10). JME is genetically heterogeneous and six chromosome loci have been defined in different racial ethnic groups: 6p12-11, 6p21.3, 15q14, 6q24, 2q22-2q23, 5q34 and 3q26 (11–22) (Table 17–1). Different modes of inheritance have been described: autosomal recessive by Panayiotopoulos and Obeid in 1989 (23) autosomal dominant by Serratosa, Delgado-Escueta, Medina et al. in 1996 (12), and Cossette et al. in 2002 (20), as well as polygenic by Janz, Tsuboi and Christian in 1973 (24,25). The complexity of JME is revealed in segregation analy-

ses using small nuclear pedigrees (26). In 1988, Greenberg et al. (26) suggested a two-locus model in which one locus was inherited recessively and the other was either dominantly or recessive inherited based on segregation analysis. In 2001, Durner et al. (27) proposed an oligogenic model where a locus in chromosome 8, common to most idiopathic generalized epilepsies, is influenced by a locus on chromosome 6 to produce the JME phenotype and by a locus on chromosome 5 to produce absence seizures.

In this chapter, we describe 258 families ascertained through a proband with JME from the United States, Mexico, Honduras, Belize, El Salvador, Peru, Saudi Arabia, and Spain. We provide evidence for their subdivision into four subsyndromes based on their seizure phenotypes. We compare the seizure phenotypes in these four subsyndromes with seizure phenotypes of probands with JME in published studies that

TABLE 17–1. *Chromosomal loci for myoclonic epilepsies of adolescence*

Locus	Country/ethnic group	Number of families	Mode of inheritance	Phenotype	References
6p12-11	Los Angeles, California	22	AD	Classic JME and pCAE evolving to JME	11
	Belize	1	AD	Classic JME	12
	Mexico	31	AD	Classic JME (pyknoleptic absences excluded)	13
6p12-11	Netherlands	18	AD	JME	22
6p21.3	Los Angeles, California	24	AD	Classic JME	14
	New York	85	AD	Classic JME mixed with CAE evolving to JME	15
6p21.3	Germany	29	AD	JME	16
15q14	United Kingdom and Sweden	25	AR	JME	17
6q24	Saudi Arabia	34	AR	JME, some nonproband members with mild gait ataxia and tremors	18
2q22-2q23	Germany	1	?	Classic JME with absences Family member 3-Hz sW	19
5q34GABR1	French-Canadian	1	AD	4/8 affected family members had pCAE One epilepsy onset at 5 years	20
3q26	Germany	1	AD	Classic JME	21

identified chromosome loci for JME. We then calculate the risks of having seizures or epilepsy in relatives from families of the two most common subsyndromes, namely classic JME and childhood absence epilepsy (CAE) that evolves to JME. We discuss the implications of varying relative risks in parents, siblings, offspring, and distant relatives. We hypothesize whether one or more genes influence the heritability and expression of JME and absence.

METHODS

Patient and Family Database (Table 17–2)

During family recruitment, we encountered 293 individuals who had been diagnosed with JME by field study sites of the international consortium of GENESS (Genetic Epilepsy Studies). Of these, 258 families were ascertained through a proband with adolescent-onset myoclonias and grand-mal seizures. An extended pedigree was constructed for each family. All available affected relatives were interviewed and examined to determine their state of affectedness, clinical diagnoses, and EEGs. The number of relatives affected in nu-

clear and extended families and seizure types were registered. EEGs were also performed on asymptomatic relatives who volunteered for the procedure. Clinical diagnoses of seizure types and electroencephalographic diagnoses of affected and family members were independently verified by at least two epileptologists. Seizure types, age at onset, and evolution of seizures from infancy through adolescence and adulthood were determined. The diagnosis of seizure types and epileptic syndromes was based on the International League Against Epilepsy classification of 1981, 1985, 1989, and 1993 (28–31). Families were grouped as multiplex, multigenerational, or multiplex/multigenerational. Maternal, paternal, or bilineal transmission were determined by pedigree findings. To determine the long-term outcome, 222 patients (86%) have been followed from 1978 to 2003 in epilepsy clinics from Los Angeles (California), Mexico City (Mexico), Tegucigalpa (Honduras), Bakersfield (California), Saudi Arabia, El Salvador, Belize, Peru, and Spain. Eleven families are presently residing in the United States and were evaluated in Los Angeles, but were originally from Australia, Iran, and China.

TABLE 17–2. Characteristics of 258 probands and families with JME subsyndromes

	Classic JME n (%)	CAE evolving to JME n (%)	JME with adolescent pyknoleptic absences n (%)	JME with myoclonic astatic seizures n (%)
No. of families	186	45	18	9
No. of relatives in multiplex/ multigenerational families	1756	541	201	48
No. of relatives affected	136	91	28	5
Family structure				
Simplex	94 (51%)	13 (29%)	7 (39%)	5 (56%)
Multiplex	24 (13%)	7 (16%)	1 (5%)	—
Multigenerational	30 (16%)	12 (27%)	5 (28%)	—
Multiplex Multigenerational	38 (20%)	13 (29%)	5 (28%)	4 (44%)
Mode of transmission				
Maternal	42 (46%)	18 (57%)	4 (36%)	2 (50%)
Paternal	29 (31%)	10 (31%)	5 (45%)	2 (50%)
Bilineal	8 (9%)	1 (3%)	2 (19%)	—
Not defined (multiplex families)	13 (14%)	3 (9%)	—	—
Sex in probands				
Female	103 (55%)	29 (65%)	13 (72%)	5 (56%)
Male	83 (45%)	16 (35%)	5 (28%)	4 (44%)
Ratio of affectedness F:M	1.3:1	1.8:1	2.6:1	1.25:1
Mean age + SD (years)				
At recruitment	25.9 (14–58)	27.2 (11–62)	27.4 (17–38)	24.3 (17–36)
Onset of absences	16.8 (11–30)	6.9 (1–11)	15.8 (11–32)	15
Onset of myoclonias	15.1 (7–28)	14 (8–47)	14.3 (8–30)	16.1 (11–30)
Onset of GTCS	15.9 (8–33)	12 (2–37)	14.3 (11–20)	16.8 (8–25)
Years of follow-up	12.4 (1–41)	19.4 (5–52)	13.8 (5–26)	11.1 (3–18)

We excluded 35 patients and their families: (a) 5 with progressive myoclonic epilepsies (PME), (b) 9 with myoclonic absences (MA), (c) 4 with typical childhood absence epilepsy (CAE) that remits or persists in adolescence with or without grand-mal seizures, (d) 7 with grand-mal epilepsy only, (e) 2 with photogenic epilepsy with female preponderance, (f) 4 with early childhood myoclonic epilepsy, (g) 2 with familial adult myoclonic epilepsy, and (h) 2 whose family members had partial epilepsies that were mistaken for ME.

For genetic analysis, each class of degree relative was examined separately for history of epilepsy. First-degree relatives were parents, siblings (brothers and sisters), and offspring; second-degree relatives were uncles, aunts, nieces, and nephews, and third-degree relatives included cousins. For analysis purposes, offspring were analyzed separately from the other first-degree relatives. For risk calculations, we used the cumulative or lifetime prevalence of

having epilepsy reported from the Rochester study considering a frequency of familial history of epilepsy of 3% (32,33). An estimated prevalence of 0.00045 for JME and 0.00066 for childhood absences was used for the risk calculations (9).

RESULTS

We subdivided the 258 families into four groups according to the combination of seizure types afflicting the proband, the age of probands at onset of seizures, the results of physical, neurologic, brain-imaging examinations, and the long-term outcome after treatment with valproate (VPA) and/or the new generation of antiepileptic drugs (AEDs) (Fig. 17–1; Tables 17–2 and 17–3).

Classic JME

Classic JME accounted for 73% ($n = 186$) of all our cases, starting in adolescence as isolated

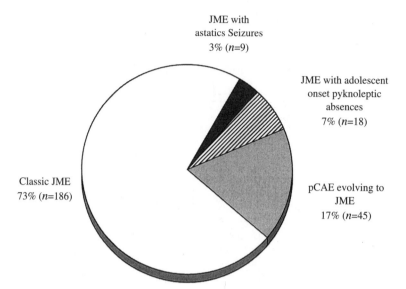

FIG. 17–1. Subsyndromes of JME in 258 probands. JME stands for juvenile myoclonic epilepsy and pCAE means pyknoleptic childhood absence.

awakening myoclonic seizures or generalized clonic–tonic–clonic seizures. Myoclonias were most often the first seizure type to appear (68% or 117/170). In 30% probands (52/170) grand-mal seizures preceded myoclonias. Almost all (95%) had tonic–clonic or clonic–tonic–clonic grand-mal seizures. Sometimes rare, isolated absence seizures (spanioleptic or sporadic absences) or rare episodes of absences appeared in clusters. In nine cases, the type of seizure at onset was not ascertained. The interictal EEG had 4- to 6-Hz spike or polyspike and slow-wave complexes, while high-voltage 12 to 30 polyspikes accompanied myoclonic seizures. Although females were numerically more common than males among probands (103 females and 83 males or 1.25 F: 1M ratio), the difference was not statistically significant ($\chi^2 = 1.078; p = 0.29$).

Figure 17–2 shows the age at onset of seizures in probands. Myoclonias started on average at 15.1 years (7 to 28 years) in 170 patients. Grand-mal seizures appeared for the first time at 15.9 years (range 8 to 33 years). Absences started at the mean age of 16.8 years (range 11 to 30 years) and were present in 33% of the patients (57/170). Absences were spanioleptic, in all cases, and were the first seizure type reported only in one case (onset at 16 years). The most

common trigger factors for seizures were sleep deprivation, stress, alcohol, noncompliance, and menses. Other less common causes of seizures were fatigue, hyperventilation, photosensitivity, and physical activity.

Of probands, 61% showed 4- to 6-Hz spike-wave or polyspike-wave complexes in a 30- to 40-min interictal EEG; 14% had 3-Hz spike-wave complexes either alone or associated with 4- to 6-Hz polyspike-wave complexes. Focal slow, sharp or spike-waves were found in 10%. Generalized bursts of 4- to 6-Hz slow waves without spikes were found in 2% and 13% of the interictal EEGs were normal. Neurologic examination was normal in all probands. Forty-nine percent (57/116) had cerebral tomography (CT), 41% (48/116) had brain magnetic resonance imaging (MRI), and 10% (11/116) had 2FDG-positron emission tomography (2FDG-PET). Almost all studies were normal except for five probands. Three had calcified neurocysticercosis, one had an asymptomatic pituitary adenoma, and one had a left temporal arachnoidal cyst.

Seizures were present in family members in 92 out of 186 cases of classic JME (49%). Of the families, 38 were both multiplex/multigenerational, 30 were multigenerational, and 24 were multiplex. Maternal inheritance

TABLE 17–3. Phenotypes of JME subsyndromes

	Classic JME (n = 186)	CAE evolving JME (n = 45)	JME with pyknoleptic absences adolescence (n = 18)	JME myoclonic-astatic (n = 9)
Age at onset of main seizure	15.1 years (7–28 years)	5 years (1–10 years)	16 years (11–32 years)	14.2 years (8–19 years)
Gender ratio	1.25 F:1 M	1.8 F:1 M	2.6 F:1 M	1.2 F:1 M
Seizure type in probands	Adolescent myoclonias, grand-mal and rare absences	Childhood pyknoleptic absences, followed by myoclonias and grand mal; 30% eyelid myoclonia + absences	Adolescent pyknoleptic absences, myoclonias and grand mal	Myoclonias, grand-mal, rare absences, and infrequent astatic seizures
EEG	4- to 6-Hz polyspike-and-slow wave complexes Photoparoxysmal response in 13%	3-Hz spike-and-slow wave complexes (1/3 mixed with 4- to 6-Hz polyspike-and-slow wave complexes) Low amplitude 15- to 25-Hz fast rhythms Photoparoxysmal response in 22%	4- to 6-Hz polyspike-and-slow wave complexes Photoparoxysmal response in 15%	4- to 6-Hz polyspike-and-slow wave complexes Photoparoxysmal response in 1/4
Family history	49%	71%	61%	5/9 probands
Main seizure type in family members	JME and tonic–clonic	Absence seizures and tonic–clonic	JME and tonic–clonic	JME and tonic–clonic
Transmission	Maternal > paternal	Maternal > paternal	Maternal = paternal	Maternal = paternal
Response to treatment	58% Seizure-free; 85% without grand mal on VPA mono- or polytherapy	7% Seizure-free; 72% without grand mal with VPA mono- or polytherapy	56% Seizure-free, on VPA mono- or polytherapy	6/8 Seizure-free
Prognosis				
Seizure breakthroughs	56% have rare to infrequent myoclonia and grand-mal breakthroughs	93% Very frequent breakthroughs	39% Rare to infrequent breakthroughs	3/8 Rare to infrequent breakthroughs
Persistent seizures	Myoclonic and tonic–clonic seizures	Absences	Absences with or without myoclonic seizures	Astatic (1/8)

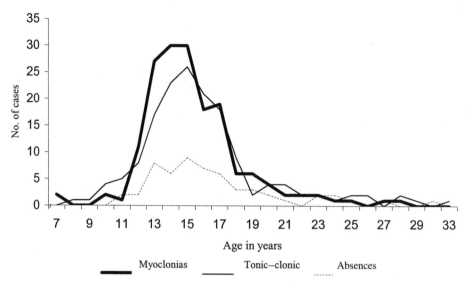

FIG. 17–2. Age at onset of each seizure type in classic JME.

was not more common (46% or 42/92) than paternal inheritance (31% or 29/92) ($\chi^2 = 1.2$; $p = 0.3$). Bilineality or epilepsy on both sides of the probands' parents was present in 9% or 8/92. Thirteen multiplex families (14%) could not provide evidence of source of epilepsy traits in either side of the family.

Epileptic seizures affected 188/1764 (11%) nonproband family members. Specific seizure types could be determined only in 136 of affected relatives. Of these members, 41% also had JME, while 40% had grand mal only, and absences were present infrequently to rarely (Fig. 17–3).

Abnormal EEGs were found in 24 asymptomatic relatives. Of these 24 relatives, 15 (63%) had 4- to 6-Hz polyspike waves, 4 (17%) had bursts of focal or diffuse slowing, 3 (12%) had 3- to 5-Hz spike-and-wave complexes, and 2 (8%) had bursts of focal or diffuse sharp waves. (Fig. 17–4). Most asymptomatic family members with EEG polyspike wave were females (10 F: 5M).

Table 17–4 shows the frequency of epileptic seizures among relatives of 79 classic JME families. Of first-degree relatives, $11\frac{1}{2}\%$ had seizures. Most common (46%) were myoclonias with or without grand mal. Rarely were absence seizures present in relatives. Only 4% of

second-degree relatives had seizures. Most common were grand-mal seizures (41.4%), followed by myoclonic seizures (28%). Because many probands were adolescent or young adults who did not have children, we only had 58 offsprings to study.

Table 17–5 shows the risks of having any seizure type in relatives of probands with classic JME compared to the risk expected in population. Parents and siblings have 69 to 136 times higher risk of having JME and 11 to 20 times of having absence compared to the general population. In contrast, parents and second degree relatives of families with CAE evolving to JME, have 15 to 36 times the risk of having classic JME compared to general population.

Pyknoleptic Childhood Absence Epilepsy Evolving to JME

A second group consisted of 45 patients who had absence epilepsy that started in childhood and persisted with myoclonic and tonic–clonic grand mal seizures into adulthood. This group accounted for 17% of all the idiopathic myoclonic epilepsies studied. Females were again numerically preponderant among probands (29 females and 16 males or 1.8F:1M ratio), but this was not

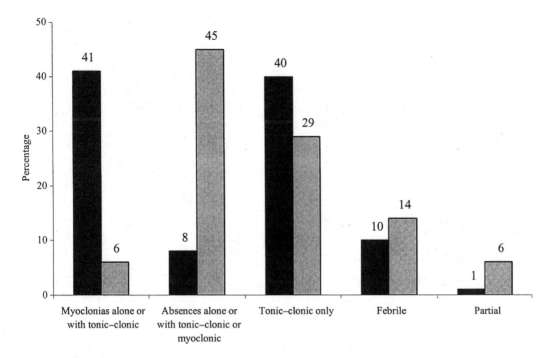

FIG. 17–3. Myoclonic and tonic–clonic seizures are more common in affected members of classic JME, while absences are more common in affected members of CAE evolving to JME: seizure types in 83 nonproband-affected family members from 32 families with CAE evolving to JME in comparison to 136 nonproband-affected family members from 92 multiplex/multigenerational families with classic JME. Of all affected nonproband family members with CAE evolving to JME, 16% had the same syndrome as proband; this group is shown in the 45% percentile.

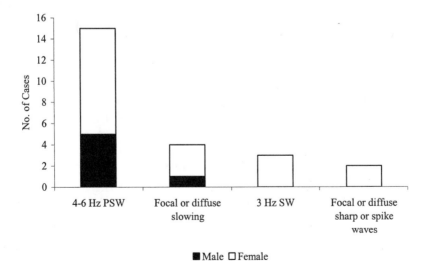

FIG. 17–4. EEG findings in 24 asymptomatic relatives of classic JME. A female preponderance was observed. PSW, polyspike-wave; SW, spike-wave.

TABLE 17–4. *Frequency of epileptic seizures among first- and second-degree relatives of probands with JME subsyndromes*

| Epilepsy syndrome and seizure types in relatives | First-degree affected | | Second-degree affected | Total n (%) |
	Parents and sibs n (%)	Offspring n (%)	Aunts, uncles, nieces, nephews n (%)	
Classic JME (92 families)				
Myoclonias with/without tonic–clonic	24 (46.2)	2 (40)	8 (27.6)	34 (39.5)
Tonic–clonic only	14 (26.9)	—	12 (41.4)	26 (30.2)
Absences with/without tonic–clonic	4 (7.7)	—	2 (6.9)	6 (7.0)
Febrile	3 (5.7)	3 (60)	3 (10.3)	9 (10.5)
Symptomatic localization related	—	—	1 (3.5)	1 (1.2)
Not validated seizure/epilepsy type	7 (13.5)	—	3 (10.3)	10 (11.6)
Total affected relatives by degree	52 (100.0)	5 (100)	29 (100.0)	86 (100.0)
Total relatives and percentage of affectedness by degree	52/454 (11.5)	5/58 (8.6)	29/705 (4.1)	86/1217 (7.0)
CAE evolving to JME (32 families)				
Myoclonias with/without tonic–clonic	1 (2.9)	—	1 (4.5)	2 (6.3)
Tonic–clonic only	8 (24.0)	1 (100)	8 (36.4)	17 (27.8)
Absences, myoclonias and tonic–clonic	19 (56.0)	—	6 (27.2)	25 (40.5)
Febrile	5 (14.7)	—	4 (18.1)	9 (15.2)
Symptomatic localization related	—	—	—	—
Not validated seizure/epilepsy type	1 (2.9)	—	3 (13.6)	4 (7.6)
Total affected relatives by degree	34 (100.0)	1 (100)	22 (100.0)	57 (100)
Total relatives and percentage of affectedness by degree	34/161 (21.1)	1/12 (8.3)	22/141 (15.6)	79/314 (25.0)

statistically significant ($\chi^2 = 1.91$; $p = 0.166$), because of the small number of cases. Childhood absence seizures were documented as the first seizure in all probands. Absences started at the average age of 6.9 years (1 to 11 years) in 41 probands (Fig. 17–5). In four probands, parents could only describe absences as starting during or before elementary school. On those with persisting seizures, absences continued to be the chief complaint in 44.4% and absences mixed with tonic–clonic or myoclonic seizures were the chief complaint in 16%. Absences occurred at least once a day (range 1 to 200 per day), namely pyknoleptic.

Myoclonias started at the mean age of 14 years (range 8 to 47 years) and most often produced sudden and involuntary jerks of shoulder and upper extremities, but sometimes also affected trunk, head, neck, and lower extremities. The most common description involved mild to moderate symmetrical, sudden lightning jerks of hands, forearms, and shoulders inward or upward often causing the individual to drop items. Myoclonic seizures preceded grand-mal convulsions

in 18%, but more often they started in adolescence simultaneously with tonic–clonic seizures (40% of patients), which appeared for the first time, on average, at 12 years (range 2 to 37 years).

All probands had the classic 3-Hz single spike-and-slow wave complexes. Of the 29 probands, 78% also had 2- to 5-Hz single spike-and-slow wave complexes. In addition, twenty individuals or 54% also had 4- to 6-Hz polyspike-wave complexes. Both single spike-wave and polyspike-waves were observed in 34% of all cases. We also found diffuse fast low-amplitude 15- to 25-Hz in 22% of cases. Bursts of 3- to 5-Hz single spike wave and/or 4- to 6-Hz polyspike wave were induced during hyperventilation in 29% of probands and during photostimulation in 22%. Background activity was normal in all cases.

Of probands (14/45), 31% had CT scan, 18% (8/45) had MRI, 7% (3/45) had both CT and MRI studies, and 18% (8) had 2FDG-PET. Neither brain CT nor MRI studies showed structural abnormalities among probands, except for one female who had an arteriovenous malformation (angioma venosum) in one frontal lobe,

TABLE 17-5. *Risk of seizures in relatives of probands with classic JME and CAE evolving to JME*

Subsyndrome	Relatives with JME			Relatives with pyknoleptic CAE			Relatives with other seizure type		
	No.	%	Relative risk[a]	No.	%	Relative risk[b]	No.	%	Relative risk[c]
Classic JME									
Parents	5/158	3.1	69	2/158	1.3	20	13/158	8.2	3
Siblings	18/296	6.1	136	2/296	0.7	11	12/296	4	1.4
Second-degree relatives	6/705	0.9	20	1/705	0.1	1.5	22/705	3	1
Offspring	2/58	3	77	0	0	0	3/58	5.8	1.7
CAE evolving to JME									
Parents	1/64	1.6	36	4/64	6.2	94	6/64	9	3.1
Siblings	0	0	0	12/97	12.4	188	11/97	11	3.8
Second-degree relatives	1/141	0.7	15	7/141	5.0	76	14/141	10	3.5
Offspring	0	0	0	1/12	8.3	126	0/12	0	0

[a] Risk of relatives to have JME in classic JME considering an estimated prevalence of 0.00045 (9).
[b] Risk of relatives to have CAE considering an estimated prevalence of childhood absences of 0.00066 (9).
[c] Risk of having other seizure type was compared to the lifetime cumulative incidence of having epilepsy in the general population (3%) according to the Rochester Study [Hauser and Hesdorffer (32)] after subtracting the risks of classic JME and CAE (0.02889).

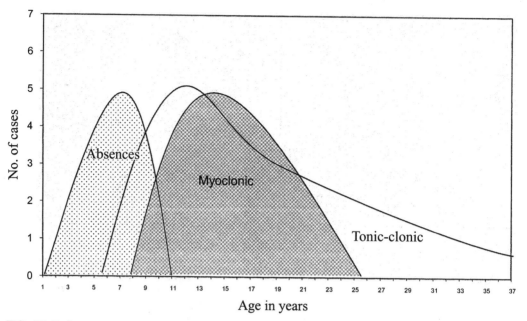

FIG. 17–5. Age at onset of each seizure type in CAE evolving to JME.

which was considered an incidental finding. Interestingly, two out of eight probands who underwent 2FDG-PET were reported to have hypometabolism in one temporal lobe. One of them was the proband who had a frontal lobe arteriovenous malformation. Neurological examinations at enrollment and during the follow-up period remained normal, but five cases (11%) had prominent jaw jerk reflexes.

Family history was positive in 32 cases (71%). Of families, 29% (13/45) were multiplex/multigenerational, twelve were multigenerational only (27%), and seven families (16%) were multiplex. Thirteen families (29%) were simplex. Maternal transmission occurred in 62% of cases vs. 38% paternal transmission, but the small number of cases prevented statistical significance ($\chi^2 = 1.16$; $p = 0.3$). There was no gender preponderance among nonproband affected members (10.6% of females vs. 9.8% males). Absence seizures most often affected nonproband family members (Fig. 17–3). Myoclonias only or myoclonias plus grand mal affected only 5 persons (6%). CAE evolving to JME was documented in 13 (16%) of nonproband affected members (8 females and 5 males).

When checking for parental affectedness in multiplex/multigenerational pedigrees, 9/32 mothers more often had had seizures (28%) than fathers (2/32 or 6%). Sixteen families (306 nonproband members) had EEG studies. Thirty members (10%) had single spike-wave or polyspike-wave complexes; 22 of these persons were asymptomatic (Fig. 17–6).

Overall, almost 20% of relatives reported seizures. Of first-degree relatives, 21% had seizures. Most common were absences (56%). Second-degree relatives commonly reported absences and tonic–clonic seizures.

Juvenile Myoclonic Epilepsy with Adolescent Onset Pyknoleptic Absence

This group accounted for 7% of all JME cases (18 families). Pyknoleptic absences started commonly at 16 years, usually between 11 to 32 years old, and were combined with myoclonia and clonic–tonic–clonic grand-mal seizures. Myoclonic seizures were the first seizure type in 61%. There was a female preponderance in probands (2.6 F:1M ratio, $\chi^2 = 1.87$; $p = 0.171$). Myoclonic seizures were the main seizure type

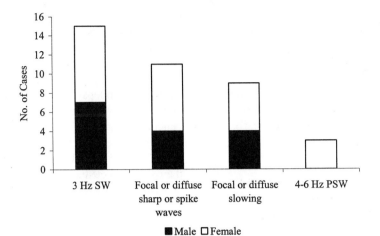

FIG. 17–6. EEG findings in 38 asymptomatic relatives of CAE evolving to JME. See Fig. 17–4 for abbreviations.

in 72% of the probands, but in eight cases with persistent seizures, absences with or without myoclonic seizures were predominant (5/8). Interictal EEG of 14 probands was available for analysis. Seven of 14 had 4- to 5-Hz spike-wave or polyspike-waves. Two showed 4- to 6-Hz polyspike-wave complexes mixed with 3-Hz spike-wave complexes. One had generalized bursts of slow waves and one had 3-Hz spike-wave complexes. Photoparoxysmal response was found in 2/14. Three probands had normal EEGs. Neurologic exam was normal in all patients. Neuroimaging studies were normal in those who had the following tests performed: CT scan was performed in 8/16, MRI in 6/16, and 2FDG-PET scan in 2/16.

Of 18 probands, 61% (11/18) had family history of epilepsy. Five families were multiplex/multigenerational families, five families were multigenerational, and one was multiplex. Maternal transmission was as common (4/11) as paternal transmission (5/11) and two families were bilineal. Mode of inheritance could not be determined in one family with monozygotic twins. Epileptic seizures affected 28 nonproband family members; 30% had JME, while 30% had grand-mal seizures only. Three nonprobands were asymptomatic, but were affected by EEG 4- to 6-Hz polyspike-wave traits. Three persons had absences only. Febrile seizures were present in

three probands and partial seizures were present in one nonproband.

Juvenile Myoclonic Epilepsy with Astatic Seizures

This group accounted for 3% of all JME cases (nine families). Aside from the adolescent-onset myoclonia and tonic–clonic or clonic–tonic–clonic grand-mal seizures, nine patients exhibited astatic seizures between 8 and 17 years, with mean age onset of 14.3 years. No gender predominance was found (5 females and 4 males). Only one of our patients had spanioleptic absences with onset also in adolescence. EEGs of four patients showed 4- to 6-Hz spike-wave or polyspike-and-slow wave complexes. One patient had the same pattern, but polyspike-waves were combined with 3-Hz spike-wave complexes. One patient's EEG consisted of generalized bursts of slow waves. General and neurologic examination was normal in all patients. Four probands had CT scans and one had a 2FDG-PET. One patient had bilateral hippocampal atrophy on MRI.

Four probands (44%) had family histories of epilepsy. One case had family history relevant not only for epilepsy but also for Huntington's Chorea. Five families were simplex and four were multiplex/multigenerational.

Maternal and paternal transmission were equally common in multiplex/multigenerational families and no bilineality was evident in this group. Among nonprobands family members, five were affected: two had JME, but one also presented astatic seizures during adolescence, one had grand mal only, one asymptomatic was affected by EEG polyspike-and-slow waves, and one with absence seizures only.

Relative Risks of Seizures in Classic Juvenile Myoclonic Epilepsy and Childhood Absence Epilepsy Evolving to JME

Tables 17–4 and 17–5 show the frequency of seizures in classic JME and CAE evolving to JME in first-, second- and third-degree relatives of probands. Examples of pedigrees with these two subsyndromes are illustrated in Figs. 17–7 and 17–8. The risk for every seizure type was compared to the risk expected in general population (3% cumulative or lifetime prevalence) (31,32). Numbers were small and not large enough to statistically compare the subsyndromes of JME with astatic seizures and JME with pyknoleptic absences during adolescence.

The risk of having seizures or epilepsy was three times higher in families with CAE evolving to JME when compared to general population. This was two to threefold increased compared to classic JME families. In CAE evolving to JME, this risk is high for all first-, second-, and third-degree relatives (3.1 to 3.8 relative risk).

Frequency of myoclonic seizures in nonproband affected members was higher in JME families when compared to frequency of myoclonic seizures in nonproband affected members of families with CAE evolving to JME (39.5% vs. 6.3%). Considering the prevalence of JME in the general population (31,32) the risk for JME in relatives was twice as high in JME compared to families with CAE evolving to JME.

In contrast to this, the frequency of absence seizures (mainly pyknoleptic) in nonproband affected members was higher in CAE evolving to JME families compared to those of classic JME families (40.5% vs. 6.8%). When the prevalence of CAE in the general population was used, the risk for absence seizures in relatives was considerably higher in CAE evolving to JME families. The risk of having tonic–clonic seizures was similar in both groups (30.2% in JME and 27.8% in CAE evolving to JME).

The risk of probands having parents with seizures or epilepsy was compared to the frequency of having family history of epilepsy in general population (31,32) The risk of having a mother with seizures was increased (1.9 in CAE evolving to JME and 1.5 in JME families), but the risk of affectedness in the father was not increased (relative risk of 1 in both syndromes).

DISCUSSION

Subsyndromes of Juvenile Myoclonic Epilepsy

Based on seizure phenotypes, JME can be divided into four groups: (a) classic JME, (b) CAE persisting with grand-mal and myoclonic seizures or CAE evolving to JME, (c) JME with adolescent onset pyknoleptic absence, and (d) JME with astatic seizures (Table 17–3). These four groups are clearly separated not only by the presence of pyknoleptic absences in the probands, but also by female preponderance (1.8:1) in CAE evolving to JME and (2.6:1) in JME with adolescent pyknoleptic absences. Maternal transmission of the epilepsy phenotype is more common than paternal transmission in the subsyndrome of absence evolving to JME. The latter syndrome also has more formed typical 3-Hz spike waves as the predominant EEG patterns. Most important, perhaps, for the patients, is the poor response of absences to VPA.

Like typical or classic CAE, (34–36) the syndrome of CAE evolving to JME is more common in females and has the characteristic 3-Hz spike-and-wave EEG pattern. During long-term follow-up, the persisting complaints of patients are absences, which are also the most common seizure type in nonproband-affected family members. For these four reasons, CAE evolving to JME is probably an absence epilepsy syndrome rather than a JME syndrome. Of interest, is the presence of low-amplitude 15- to 25-Hz rhythms found in CAE evolving to JME. The latter pattern of low-amplitude 15- to 25-Hz

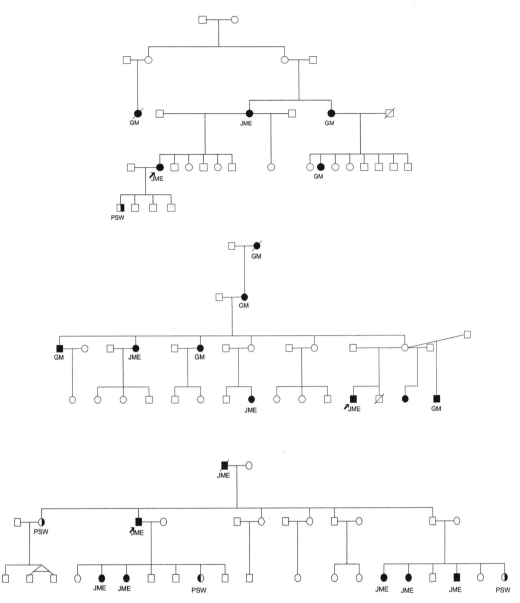

FIG. 17–7. Three examples of autosomal dominant classic JME. Solid symbols, symptomatic affected family members; half-filled symbols, asymptomatic family members affected by EEG with polyspike-wave complexes (PSW). GM, grand-mal; JME, juvenile myoclonic epilepsy.

rhythms or runs or rapid spikes has also been observed in absence epilepsies by Sato et al. (37), Gastaut et al. (38), Fakhoury and Abou-Khalil (39), and Michelucci et al. (40).

Is classic JME truly a life-long epilepsy? Perhaps. With classic JME, only 8 of 161 patients are in remission without treatment. In the other 153 patients, epilepsy is clearly lifelong. Thus,

with rare or few exceptions, classic JME is not a remitting form of epilepsy. Because we have not followed enough numbers of JME with pyknoleptic absence and JME with astatic epilepsies, we are unable to state if they are life-long disorders. In the small number of patients, however, we have not observed any patient in remission without AED treatment. For reasons

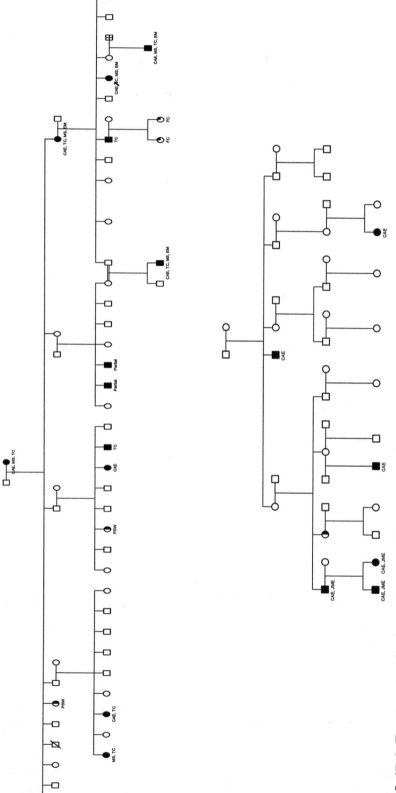

FIG. 17–8. Two examples of autosomal dominant CAE evolving to JME. MS, myoclonic seizures; EM, eyelid myoclonia; TC, tonic–clonic; FC, febrile convulsions; all other abbreviations as noted.

presently unknown, CAE evolving to JME is the hardest group to treat. Only 7% are seizure-free on VPA. Satisfaction with reduction of grand-mal seizures by VPA was reported by 72%, but 93% have frequent breakthrough absences that trouble the patients weekly, monthly, or at least every 3 months. In classic JME, 58% of patients are completely free of seizures and when breakthrough myoclonic and grand-mal seizures occur, they occur once a year to once every 5 years.

Juvenile Myoclonic Epilepsy in Published Literature

Several clinical reports on JME include probands and families with CAE evolving to JME, myoclonic absences, and juvenile absence epilepsy, and some do not specify the type and onset of absences (15,41–46). We compared seizure phenotypes in the four subsyndromes with seizure phenotypes in published material where a chromosome locus was identified for JME (Table 17–1). All authors refer to JME according to the criteria proposed by the ILAE (28–31).

In 1993, Whitehouse et al. (47) reported no significant evidence in favor of linkage to chromosome 6p. Families studied included ten absence epilepsy patients, two with pyknoleptic childhood absence, two with pyknoleptic "childhood absence with myoclonic seizures," and six with juvenile absence. Elmslie et al. used the same cohort of 34 families from the United Kingdom and Sweden and tested for linkage between JME and chromosomal regions harboring genes for nAChR subunits. They used parametric and non-parametric analysis in studying a total number of 165 members that included individuals with pyknoleptic absences only, as well as individuals with JME or tonic–clonic seizures only. There was no evidence for linkage between "nonclassic JME" or JME exhibiting pyknoleptic CAE and chromosome 15q (17).

Liu et al. showed that a JME gene is located in 6p12.11 by studying 22 families from Los Angeles and assuming an autosomal dominant model inheritance with 70% penetrance. One of the conclusions in their paper was that linkage to this locus was absent when patients with CAE

evolving to JME were included in the analysis (11).

In an attempt to replicate linkage of JME to HLA, Greenberg et al. (14) excluded probands with myoclonic absences or atonic seizures, but included 21 probands with juvenile-onset pyknoleptic absences. Escayg et al. (19) identified a mutation in the CACNB4 gene in one subject; the phenotype in the tested proband consisted of "sporadic typical absences," myoclonic, and grand-mal seizures with onset at 9 years old. In 1999, Durner et al. (48) studied linkage of all idiopathic generalized epilepsies (IGE) and proved positive LOD scores in grand mal and absences in chromosome 8 when JME was excluded.

In 2002, Cossette et al. (20) studied 14 members of a French-Canadian family with epilepsy. Eight affected family members presented similar clinical features with generalized tonic–clonic and myoclonic seizures and four presented absence seizures (two of the absence seizures started during childhood). The only exception was an individual who had an earlier onset of disease (5 years old), but with clinical features otherwise indistinguishable from other members of the family. Linkage was found in chromosome 5q34 and an Ala322-to-Asp mutation in the *GABRA1* gene was found. In this family, transmission was clearly autosomal dominant, with people affected over four generations.

Recently, Haug et al. (21) described autosomal dominant inheritance in one JME German family in which two clinically affected family members experienced frequent generalized-tonic–clonic seizures (GTC) preceded by myoclonic jerks, another with awakening grand-mal, and one asymptomatic member with EEG polyspike-wave. Affected individuals became seizure-free only when treated with high dosages of VPA in combination with other AEDs. No affected member had febrile seizures and one member with the *CLCN2* mutation had epilepsy with grand-mal seizures on awakening.

Autosomal recessive transmission in JME was originally described by Panayiotopoulos and Obeid in families from Saudi Arabia (23) and, subsequently, by Bate et al. (18). Panayiotopoulos and Obeid found parental consanguinity in 9 of 17 sibships and in 8 of the sibships more than 1 member was affected. Recently, Bate et al., (18) reported a locus for Saudi Arabia JME families in chromosome 6q24 (see Table 17–1).

Risk for Juvenile Myoclonic Epilepsy and Absence

There were not enough probands and families with the subsyndromes of JME with pyknoleptic absence and JME with astatic seizures for accurate risk calculations. Thus Tables 17–4 and 17–5 provide relative risks for seizures only in the subsyndromes of classic JME and CAE evolving to JME.

In classic JME, the relative risks for JME in parents, siblings, offspring, and second-degree relatives exhibit a genetic pattern with risks decreasing with increasing distance of relationship. The relative risk of developing JME in nuclear members is 77 to 136 that of the general population. Second-degree relatives have 20-fold more chances of developing JME as the general population. The risk of developing absence seizures in parents or siblings is 11 to 20 times more than the risk in the general population. However, the risk of developing absence seizures for second-degree relatives is not more than the risk for absence seizures in the general population. These suggest a major gene or genes for JME. These results also suggest that the genes for JME may also express as the "CAE only" phenotype in parents and siblings. Interestingly, the pattern of expression of "other seizure types" in members of classic JME families is consistent with only a mild genetic effect.

In families with CAE evolving to JME, the risk for developing absence seizures in parents, siblings, offspring, and second-degree relatives drops from 94- to 188-fold to 76-fold, compared to the general population. Notably, the risk for developing JME is 36 times the general population in parents.

The risk for developing other seizure types in families with CAE evolving to JME is increased 3 to 3.8 times the general population. Interestingly, the risk is equal in parents, siblings, and second-degree relatives, inconsistent with a genetic pattern. We cannot explain this risk pattern for "other seizures" in this subsyndrome, but the threefold increase is notable.

CONCLUSION

In conclusion, our data is consistent with the existence of four subsyndromes within the juvenile myoclonic epilepsies. Differences in electroclinical findings in probands and seizure types in relatives, familial aggregation of seizures, long-term outcome, and response to treatment help identify these subvarieties of JME. Finding specific chromosome loci and different epilepsy-causing mutations for each of the four subsyndromes will establish the existence of specific diseases causing these forms of epilepsies.

REFERENCES

1. Janz D. *Die epilepsien.* Stuttgart, Germany: George Thieme Verlag, 1969.
2. Simonsen M, Mollgaard V, Lund M. A contolled clinical and electro-encephalographic study of myoclonic epilepsy (impulsiv-petit mal). In Janz D, ed. *Epileptology.* Stuttgart, Germany: George Thieme Verlag, 1976:41–48.
3. Tsuboi T. *Primary generalized epilepsy with sporadic myoclonias of myoclonic petit mal type.* Stuttgart, Germany: George Thieme Verlag, 1977.
4. Gooses R. *Die Beziehung der fotosensibilität zu den verschiedenen epileptischen syndrmen.* Thesis. Berlin: Freie Universität Berlin, 1984.
5. Murthy JM, Yangala R, Srinivas M. The syndromic classification of the International League Against Epilepsy: a hospital-based study from South India. *Epilepsia* 1998;39:48–54.
6. Genton P, Gelisse P, Thomas P. Juvenile myoclonic epilepsy today: Current definitions and limits. In: Schmitz B, Sander T. eds. *Juvenile myoclonic epilepsy: The Janz syndrome.* Petersfield: Wrightson Biomedical, 2000:11–32.
7. Jha S, Mathur VN, Mishra VN. Pitfalls in diagnosis of epilepsy of Janz and its complications. *Neurol India* 2002;50:467–469.
8. Jain S, Tripathi M, Srivastava AK, et al. Phenotypic analysis of juvenile myoclonic epilepsy in Indian families. *Acta Neurol Scand* 2003;107:356–362.
9. Manford M, Hart YM, Sander JW, et al. The national general practice study of epilepsy. The syndromic classification of the International League Against Epilepsy applied in a general population. *Arch Neurol* 1992;49:801–808.
10. Nicoletti A, Reggio A, Bartoloni A, et al. Prevalence of epilepsy in rural Bolivia. *Neurology* 1999;53:2064–2069.
11. Lui AW, Delgado-Escueta AV, Gee MN, et al. Juvenile myoclonic epilepsy in chromosome 6p12-p11: Locus heterogeneity and recombinations. *Am J Hum Genet* 1996;63:438–446.
12. Serratosa JM, Delgado-Escueta AV, Medina MT, et al. Clinical and genetic analysis of a large pedigree with juvenile myoclonic epilepsy. *Ann Neurol* 1996;39:187–195.
13. Bai D, Alonso ME, Medina MT, et al. Juvenile myoclonic

epilepsy: Linkage to chromosome 6p12 in Mexico families. *Am J Med Genet* 2002;113:268–274.

14. Greenberg DA, Delgado-Escueta AV, Wideliz H, et al. Juvenile myoclonic epilepsy may be linked to the BF and HLA loci on human chromosome 6. *Am J Med Genet* 1988;31:185–192.

15. Greenberg DA, Durner M, Keddache M, et al. Reproducibility and complications in gene searches: linkage on chromosome 6, heterogeneity, association, and maternal inheritance in juvenile myoclonic epilepsy. *Am J Hum Genet* 2000;66:508–516.

16. Sander T, Bockenkamp B, Hildmann T, et al. Refined mapping of the epilepsy susceptibility locus EJM1 on chromosome 6. *Neurology* 1997;49:842–847.

17. Elmslie FV, Rees M, Williamson MP, et al. Genetic mapping of a major susceptibility locus for juvenile myoclonic epilepsy on chromosome 15q. *Hum Mol Genet* 1997;8:1329–1334.

18. Bate L, Mitchell W, Williamson M, et al. Molecular genetic analysis of juvenile myoclonic epilepsy in the Saudi Arabian population. *Epilepsia* 2000;41(7):72.

19. Escayg A, De Waard M, Lee DD, et al. Coding and noncoding variation of the human calcium-channel beta(4)-subunit gene CACNB4 in patients with idiopathic generalized epilepsy and episodic ataxia. *Am J Hum Genet* 2000;66:1531–1539.

20. Cossette P, Lui L, Brisebois K, et al. Mutation of GABRA1 in an autosomal dominant form of juvenile myoclonic epilepsy. *Nat Genet* 2002;31:184–189.

21. Haug K, Warnstedt M, Alekov AK, et al. Mutations in CLCN2 encoding a voltage-gated chloride channel are associated with idiopathic generalized epilepsies. *Nat Genet* 2003;33:527–532.

22. Pinto D, de Haan GJ, Janssen GAMAJ, et al. Evidence for linkage between juvenile myoclonic epilepsy-related idiopathic generalized epilepsy and 6p11-12 in Dutch families. *Epilepsia* 2004;45:211–217.

23. Panayiotopoulos, C, Obeid T. Juvenile myoclonic epilepsy: An autosomal recessive disease. *Ann Neurol* 1989;25:440–443.

24. Janz D, Durner M, Beck-Mannagetta G. Family studies on the genetics of juvenile myoclonic epilepsy (epilepsy with petit mal). In: Beck-Mannagetta G, Anderson VE, Doose H, Janz D. eds. *Genetics of the epilepsies.* Springer-Verlag, Berlin, 1989:43–52.

25. Tsuboi T, Christian W. On the genetics of primary generalized epilepsy with sporadic myoclonous of impulsive petit-mal type. *Humangenetik* 1973;19:155–182.

26. Greenberg DA, Delgado-Escueta AV, Maldonado HM, et al. Segregation analysis of juvenile myoclonic epilepsy. *Genet Epidemiol* 1988;5:81–94.

27. Durner M, Keddache MA, Tomasini L, et al. Genome scan of idiopathic generalized epilepsy: Evidence for major susceptibility gene and modifying genes influencing the seizure type. *Ann Neurol* 2001;49:328–335.

28. Commission on Classification and Terminology of the International League Against Epilepsy. Proposal for revised clinical and electrographic classification of epileptic seizures. *Epilepsia* 1981;22:489–501.

29. Commission on Classification and Terminology of the International League against Epilepsy. Proposal for classification of epilepsies and epileptic syndromes. *Epilepsia* 1985;26:268–278.

30. Commission on Classification and Terminology of the International League against Epilepsy. Proposal for revised classification of epilepsies and epileptic syndromes. *Epilepsia* 1989;30:389–399.

31. Commission on Epidemiology and Prognosis, International League Against Epilepsy. Guidelines for epidemiological studies on epilepsy. *Epilepsia* 1993;34:592–596.

32. Hauser WA, Hesdorffer DC. *Epilepsy- Frequency, causes and consequences.* Landover, Md: Demos, 1990: 1–51.

33. Annegers JF. The Epidemiology of Epilepsy. In: Wyllie E, ed. *The treatment of epilepsy. Principles and practice.* Philadelphia: Lea & Febiger, 1993:157–164.

34. Currier RD, Kooi KA, Saidman LJ. Prognosis of pure petit mal. *Neurology* 1963;13:959–967.

35. Doose H, Neubauer BA. Preponderance of female sex in the transmission of seizure liability in idiopathic generalized epilepsy. *Epilepsy Res* 2001;43:103–114.

36. Loiseau P, Panayiotopoulos CP, Hirsch E. Childhood absence epilepsy and related syndromes. In: Roger J, Bureau M, Dravet Ch, Dreifuss FE, Perret A, Wolf P. eds. *Epileptic syndromes in infancy, childhood and adolescence.* London: John Libbey, 2002:113–135.

37. Sato S, Dreifuss F, Penry J. Prognostic factors in absence seizures. *Neurology* 1976;26:788–796.

38. Gastaut H, Zifkin B, Mariani E, et al. The long term course of primary generalized epilepsy with persisting absences. *Neurology* 1986;36:1021–1028.

39. Fakhoury T, Abou-Khalil B. Generalized absence seizures with 10-15 Hz fast discharges. *Clin Neurophysiol* 1999;110:1029–1035.

40. Michelucci R, Ruboli G, Passarelli D, et al. Idiopathic generalized epilepsy with persisting absence seizures in adult life: electroclinical patterns. *J Neurol Neurosurg Psych* 1995;61:441–447.

41. Asconape J, Penry JK. Some clinical and EEG aspects of benign juvenile myoclonic epilepsy. *Epilepsia* 1984;25:108–114.

42. Panayiotopoulos CP, Obeid T, Waheed G. Absences in juvenile myoclonic epilepsy: A clinical and video-electroencephalographic study. *Ann Neurol* 1989; 25:391–397.

43. Durner M, Sander T, Greenberg DA, et al. Localization of idiopathic generalized epilepsy on chromosome 6p in families of juvenile myoclonic epilepsy patients. *Neurology* 1991;41:1651–1655.

44. Oller-Daurella L, Oller LFV. 5000 Epilépticos-Clínica y evolución. Barcelona, Spain: ESPAXS S.A. Publicaciones Médicas, 1994:169–170.

45. Mehndiratta MM, Aggarwal P. Clinical expression and EEG features of patients with juvenile myoclonic epilepsy (JME) from North India. *Seizure* 2002;11:431–436.

46. Vijai J, Cherian PJ, Sylaja PN, et al. Clinical characteristics of a South Indian cohort of juvenile myoclonic epilepsy probands. *Seizure* 2003;12:490–496.

47. Whitehouse WP, Rees M, Curtis D, et al. Linkage analysis of idiopathic generalized epilepsy (IGE) and marker loci on chromosome 6p in families of patients with juvenile myoclonic epilepsy: No evidence for an epilepsy locus in the HLA region. *Am J Hum Genet* 1993;53:652–662.

48. Durner M, Zhou G, Fu D, Abreu P, et al. Evidence for linkage of adolescent-onset idiopathic generalized epilepsies to chromosome 8-and genetic heterogeneity. *Am J Hum Genet* 1999;64:1411–1419.

18

Genetics of Juvenile Myoclonic Epilepsy: Faulty Components and Faulty Wiring?

Martina Durner,* Deb Pal,*,† and David Greenberg‡

*Division of Statistical Genetics, Department of Biostatistics, Mailman School of Public Health, Columbia University, New York, New York; †Clinical and Genetic Epidemiology Unit, New York State Psychiatric Institute, New York, New York; ‡Mailman School of Public Health and New York State Psychiatric Institute, Columbia Genome Center, Columbia–Presbyterian Medical Center, New York, New York

INTRODUCTION

Several years ago, juvenile myoclonic epilepsy (JME) was seen as the ideal model form of epilepsy to unravel the presumed genetic origins of generalized epilepsies with unknown causes, the epilepsies we called idiopathic. JME showed a strong genetic component that was similar to the genetic contribution seen in other age-dependent idiopathic generalized epilepsies (IGE). The argument, however, was that JME is the most homogenous epilepsy syndrome, easily and unambiguously identifiable through its unique clinical manifestation of myoclonic jerks experienced shortly after awakening. Nongenetic contributing factors could not be identified, and JME was therefore called the "prototype of idiopathic generalized epilepsy" (1a, Janz 1969).

Rapid progress in genetic molecular methods promised a quick success in finding "the" JME gene. In hindsight, this expectation can be seen as having been overly optimistic, underestimating the complexity of what was assumed to be a "simple" epilepsy syndrome. Subsequent research brought some successes, but also raised even more questions.

In this paper, we try to point out some of these questions. We also advocate taking a new look on how to approach the enormous challenge of not only finding the genetic basis of JME but also

other epilepsy genes, since the problems encountered in the JME work are not unique to JME and occur in other IGE syndromes as well.

ARE WE LOOKING FOR "THE" JUVENILE MYOCLONIC EPILEPSY GENE?

When gene searches for epilepsy first began, grant applications generally had as one of the specific aims "to identify *the* gene for (choose the form of epilepsy)." Almost always, a positive family history for seizures was found in many patients, otherwise there would be little justification for a genetic study. However, the fact that the overall pattern of seizures in families was not usually not consistent with a simple gene inheritance (either dominant or recessive) was largely ignored and the concept that a single gene that did not manifest itself in all gene carriers was introduced, that is, reduced penetrance. This view prevailed despite the fact that the data indicated that this concept is too simplistic and that more than one gene was likely to be involved in the explanation of the patterns seen in common JME (see below).

Another argument for questioning the concept of a single gene causing JME is the evidence for genetic heterogeneity in JME. Even though JME was chosen because it was thought to be a homogeneous, clearly defined disease, it became obvious, early on, that many patients, although they had similar clinical characteristics, did not always share the same genetic basis. Evidence for linkage was reported for several chromosomal locations and genetic heterogeneity was evident from the findings on chromosome 6q21 (1–5), 6p12 (6,7), and 15p (8–10). Cossette et al. (11) were the first to show that a mutation in a gene, *GABRA1,* encoding the alpha1 subunit of the gamma-aminobutyric acid receptor subtype A (GABA$_A$ cosegregated in a large French–Canadian family with many family members affected with JME. Sander et al. (12) found negative evidence for linkage to the location of *GABRA1* on chromosome 5q in all their JME families and we have sequenced 45 JME patients for *GABRA1* without finding any sequence variations.

To summarize, it has become clear that we have to revise our expectations of finding *the* JME gene. Most likely there are several genes that contribute to JME and many are most likely neither necessary nor sufficient to cause JME on their own. Some of these genes will be quite common in the general population, but as long as other (genetic, epigenetic or environmental) factors are not present, the disease will not manifest itself. To make matters even worse, these genes could act in several different combinations making it hard to detect their effect in different datasets due to random variation in the collection of pedigree data (13).

WHAT GENETIC MODELS MIGHT EXPLAIN THE CURRENT OBSERVATIONS IN COMMON EPILEPSIES?

Single-Gene Model

As mentioned above, the notion that we should expect to find one gene for JME persist despite the fact that the observed patterns of inheritance do not support a single-gene model for JME or other IGE. The single-gene model predicts that either one-half or one-quarter of offspring of at-risk matings will be affected with the trait. (Below, we discuss penetrance.) This is clearly not

the case in IGE. Families showing clear dominant inheritance or clear recessive inheritance are quite rare. The common epilepsy families show segregation ratios (which, crudely stated, are sibling risk ratios corrected for ascertainment bias) on the order of 0.08 to 0.12, far lower than predicted by single gene models of 0.25 or 0.50.

Would a Mixture of Cases, in Which Some Families Have a Genetic Form and Some Nongenetic (sporadic) Form, Explain the Data?

Such a model, by itself, would explain the observed segregation ratio, but little else. First, simple clustering analysis would reveal clusters of families, some with multiple affected members and some with only one affected member, if the disease showed simple inheritance. Second, under such a model, almost any linkage study would quickly reveal the cosegregation of markers and disease, even if there were heterogeneity in the data. Third, the MZ twin concordance rate would be quite low, likely 50% or less because the majority of MZ twins would have the "sporadic" form of the disease. In fact, the MZ twin rate in IGE is higher than 80%, strongly suggesting that IGE is an almost purely genetic disease in almost all of the JME cases. Thus, a single-gene model, together with some families having an environmental form, will not explain the observed data.

Would Not Reduced Penetrance Explain the Results?

For most common diseases, the simple Mendelian models can be rejected because the observed segregation ratio is far too low. Thus, the concept of reduced penetrance was invented to explain this observation. In thinking of reduced penetrance, it is tacitly assumed that there is a single gene responsible for the disease but that "other factors" play a role in the gene's expression. Usually, these factors are thought of as environmental. If the cause of reduced penetrance is environmental, then the MZ twin concordance rate should be a direct reflection of the penetrance, e.g., if the penetrance is 50%, as measured by the segregation ratio, then the MZ twin concordance rate should be 50%. However, the "other factors" could also be purely genetic; that is, other genes could play a role in the expression of the disease. If that were the case, then the segregation ratio would not be the 25% or 50% predicted by the single-gene model but would be a function of the combined segregation ratios of multiple genes and highly dependent on the gene frequencies of the genes. However, when there is no environmental influence, the model also predicts that the MZ twin concordance rate will be 100%, because MZ twins share 100% of their genes in common. This is, in fact, what is seen in IGE. The high concordance rate in MZ twins points to little environmental influence and an almost exclusive genetic basis for a "reduced penetrance." This is also confirmed by the fact that no studies have identified any environmental agents that are correlated with IGE.

Oligogenic Model

JME is one of the few examples of an epilepsy in which a formal segregation analysis was reported (14). In that case, an oligogenic model in which two specific genes must be present for disease expression (an epistatic model) was compared to the segregation ratio observed in JME families, with excellent fit. These results do not exclude the possibility of more than two genes being involved, but it is difficult to distinguish epistatic models involving two loci from those involving more loci.

Thus, the existing data strongly suggests that there is little environmental influence in IGE but that there is "reduced penetrance." These results can be best explained by an oligogenic model in which at least two genes must be present to manifest IGE.

Other Multigenic Models

One of the other models, that require multiple genes and is commonly cited, is the polygenic threshold model (PTM). The PTM assumes that many genes, each with an equal, but small, effect, contribute to disease expression. When the number of genes, out of the many possible genes, reaches a certain count, then the disease will be expressed. When this model was tested on early data on JME, it came quite close to being re-

jected (15). Finding any of these genes in a PTM model is extremely difficult because the influence of each gene is small and their combination will vary among families and patients. It means, ultimately, that everyone with the disease can have a different disease genotype.

If we modify the model so that we say that one gene predominates or provides major susceptibility but that an accumulation of other genes allows that one to act, we are back to a single-gene model, but with a so-called "polygenic background," essentially a single-gene model with reduced penetrance, but reduced penetrance that is still entirely genetic.

A pure polygenic model however, and to a lesser degree a "polygenic background" model, have become untenable through the localization of several genes via linkage analysis or, even more compellingly, the identification of specific genes. Thus, the model that appears to explain most of the currently known data is an oligogenic model in which two or more genes must be present in order for epilepsy to manifest.

SHOULD WE USE SINGLE LARGE VS. MANY SMALL FAMILIES?

The answer to this question is—it depends on what we are looking for. Heterogeneity and reduced penetrance are major problems in finding genes for common diseases. Large families were perceived to offer a way to eliminate those problems. The fact that it is one pedigree reduces the chance of heterogeneity and the fact that many members are affected means that reduced penetrance is less of a problem. This strategy has been quite successful so far in the apparent identification of ion-channel genes and neurotransmitter-related genes in epileptogenesis. However, contrary to commonly held belief, these single, large, high-density families with many affecteds that have a phenotype similar to those in families with more sparse "genetic loading" (i.e., families with low familial occurrence of seizures) did not provide us with answers for common forms of JME. These results are in line with findings in other common diseases. For example, the relevance of presenillins in common forms of Alzheimer's Disease, or parkin in common forms of Parkinson's Disease, etc., has not been established. While each of these findings provide a major step in elucidating potential pathways in these diseases and may lead to new treatment options, they have, thus far, not yet contributed to our understanding of the more common forms of disease. It appears that if we want to understand the underlying pathology of common forms of epilepsy, we have to study common families.

Even when studying large, high-density families, there are several difficulties. First, the variable phenotype in some of these families, especially the families with generalized epilepsy with febrile seizures (GEFS), point to the involvement of more genes, that together with the already discovered mutations in ion channel or GABA genes lead to the different phenotypes. Since we are limited to single rare families, each family does not have enough statistical power to detect genes that are involved in some, but not all, affected family members. Second, by requiring families to have many affected members, one is selecting for families that are more likely to have several independent disease genes segregating *within* the family, that is, families with intrafamilial heterogeneity (16). For example, in the GEFS family reported by Wallace et al. (17), several affected family members did not have a mutation in the *SCN1B* gene and were therefore labeled as "phenocopies." Fortunately, the effect of those "phenocopies" was not strong enough to mask the detection of the major contribution in this family of a *SCN1B* mutation, a biological meaningful candidate gene. It might be more difficult to dissect the genetic contributions in families with increased intrafamilial heterogeneity and disturbances in less obvious candidate genes.

WHAT PHENOTYPE ARE WE STUDYING?

Usually, genetic studies start out with a patient that is seen by a physician. A family history is then taken and family members are screened for the presence or absence of the trait under study. In families of JME patients however, a significant proportion of the family members that also have epilepsy do not have JME, but some other kind of IGE. Depending on the study, only 15% to 30% of affected family members have myoclonic jerks, 15% to 30% have absence seizures and 50% to 85% of affected family members have GTCS (18,19). On the other hand, most of the JME patients themselves also have GTCS, in addition to the myoclonic jerks; about one-third have absence seizures. This raises the question of what phenotype exactly are we studying? Are we indeed looking for a "JME" gene? Or are we looking for a more general gene that nonspecifically lowers seizure threshold? Does the same genetic disturbance underlie JME, absence epilepsy or "pure" grand-mal epilepsy and just shows variable expressivity?

This question was largely ignored until we started to question the construct of clinical epileptic syndromes that are based on a leading symptom, but also allow for additional symptoms that may or may not occur. We thought for genetic purposes, it might be better to focus on the individual symptoms, in our case, the different seizure types. We already knew that IGE is most likely caused by several genes. We postulated that there are genes common to all IGE that merely lower seizure threshold and there are specific genes that are necessary for both the manifestation of seizures and determination of specific seizure types. We analyzed our genetic data of adolescent-onset IGE, comprising of JME, juvenile absence epilepsy (JAE), and epilepsy with pure GTCS (EGTCS) according to seizure types (i.e., myoclonic seizures, absence seizures, and GTCS) and found evidence for a common gene for all these seizure types on chromosome 18, but also locations of "individual" genes for myoclonic jerks on chromosome 6 and for absence seizures on chromosome 5 (13). These findings provided support for an intriguing hypothesis and unified the observation of different seizure types in families and individual patients. Epidemiologic studies further support this notion that it is not the epilepsy syndrome, but the seizure type of myoclonic and absence seizures that have distinct genetic effects (20).

HOW CAN WE UNTANGLE GENETIC HETEROGENEITY AND IDENTIFY DIFFERENT FORMS OF JUVENILE MYOCLONIC EPILEPSY?

Disentangling genetic heterogeneity on a statistical level has proved to be rather difficult.

The statistical methods for analysis of genetic heterogeneity are limited. It would be more efficient if we could separate the genetically different forms of JME ahead of time before we analyze apples and oranges together. Some of the differentiation criteria can be applied straightforwardly, but some of them might need skilled, experienced, and observant clinicians.

For example, ethnicity seems to play a large role in different forms of JME. The locus on chromosome 6p12, identified initially by Liu et al. (6) and further discussed in this volume, is detected mostly in families of Amerindian descent. As another example, mutations in the *GABRA1* gene have been detected, so far, only in a French–Canadian family coming from a relative genetic isolate, but not in other mixed Caucasian or Indian patients (21). The locus on chromosome 6p21 does not seem to play a role in African American or Hispanic JME patients (6). Thus, another step in reducing the problem of heterogeneity is to avoid mixing populations, not only populations of different ethnicities, but even different countries. For example, we alluded above that at least some of the heterogeneity in JME may be due to ethnic differences between European and non-European populations. Even within Europe, there may be marked differences in the effect of different genes due to different population frequencies of the interacting genes. For example, in a study of autoimmune thyroid disease, families from Italy were markedly different from families from England and the United States in their linkage characteristics (22).

We also noticed, that the family with the *GABRA1* mutation identified by Cossette et al. (11) had numerous family members all affected with JME only. This is in contrast to common forms of JME families where, as mentioned above, only 15% to 30% of the family members also have JME. Perhaps, the absence of other seizure types in a family is indicative of a genetically different form of JME and future studies should differentiate between "pure" JME families and JME families/patients that exhibit other seizure types.

Obeid et al. (23) reported a sample of JME families from Saudi Arabia that showed few affected parents and concluded that JME is most likely transmitted in an autosomal recessive fashion (24). There are several caveats if one wants to generalize their finding to all JME. These families differ in their ethnic background from other studies and it is possible that Obeid et al. have identified a specific form of JME that is prominent in this region. It is also mentioned in this report that almost one-third of JME patients showed tremor, even before the commencement of antiepileptic therapy. Tremor, however, has not been recognized as a symptom associated with the JME syndrome by the International Commission on the Classification of Epilepsies and Epileptic Syndromes. It can be speculated, therefore, that this subtle clinical difference of tremor might provide clinical means to differentiate different genetic forms of JME.

The above-mentioned examples should not be taken as absolute, but are intended to illustrate possible ways to tackle the significant problem of heterogeneity. Since it is probably the biggest obstacle for finding genes for all common genetic diseases, we have to use all available resources in a concentrated effort to overcome this problem. Much of the success will depend on the quality and purity of the clinical data and the observant clinician will be the first one in line to help minimize the problem of heterogeneity.

CAN OTHER OBSERVATIONS ASSOCIATED WITH JUVENILE MYOCLONIC EPILEPSY GUIDE OUR SEARCH FOR JUVENILE MYOCLONIC EPILEPSY GENES?

Over the course of the late 20th century, the advent of new technologies, such as magnetic resonance imaging (MRI), have deepened our understanding of the symptomatic, and to some extent, the idiopathic epilepsies. In the 21st century, new experimental molecular biology tools will revolutionize our understanding of functional disturbances in the brain. The phenomenology of JME contains several unusual features, evident from neuroimaging, and electrophysiologic and pathologic studies, in addition to careful bedside observation. Each of these features may offer a clue as to the function of the genes involved in the JME trait. There are many opportunities to discover the mechanisms underlying these features by combining new experimental approaches with existing findings. Integrating these results may contribute to our understanding of genetic mechanisms.

One of the oldest questions centers on the definition of idiopathic. The term implies that there are no readily apparent causes for illness. Nonetheless, many lines of evidence suggest a disturbance involving the development of the frontal lobes in JME. This disturbance is subtle, and signs are likely to be missed in routine examination. For example, the original descriptions of Janz hint at a "frontal" personality disturbance in JME (25), and subsequent neuropsychologic research confirms deficits in frontal cortical performance in some JME patients (26,27). The neuropsychologic findings are strengthened by anatomic investigations. Detailed studies of JME autopsy brains over a number of years have shown increased neuronal density in areas of the frontal cortex (28). These findings, although disputed by other investigators (29), deserve exploration because of the consistency of evidence from other approaches pointing to disturbance in the development of the frontal cortex. Quantitative voxel-based MRI, further supports the idea of subtle abnormalities of frontal lobe development in JME, showing increased volume of frontal lobe regions in JME patients (30,31). These findings suggest that neurodevelopmental disturbances of the brain, especially the frontal lobes, may contribute to the expression of JME. Transgenic animal models may offer an opportunity to test these hypotheses, specifically whether neuronal proliferation, migration, differentiation, or apoptosis are disturbed.

A second intriguing phenomenon is the finding of possible preferential maternal inheritance in JME. "Maternal preponderance" as it used be called, has been reported in many epilepsies for many decades (32,33). In our JME family data, the risk ratio for maternal vs. paternal transmission was extraordinarily high ($RR = 12.5$) (34). Furthermore, the linkage pattern seen in our JME families that show evidence for linkage to chromosome 6p21 are consistent with patterns that one would expect when there is imprinting at

that locus (5). While other mechanisms, like sampling biases or nongenetic factors, must be considered to explain these observations of increased maternal transmission, they cannot explain our linkage results (35). Attention should, therefore, be given to imprinting in at least a part of JME families. Imprinting is a genetic phenomenon where the expression of a gene is silenced when transmitted from one sex, but not the other. The effect is that the parent whose gene is imprinted will not have affected children, although the parent transmitted the disease-associated genetic disturbance. The disease will only be seen in children of parents of the opposite sex who transmit the expressed gene.

Imprinting is not the unusual explanation for maternal inheritance in JME that it might seem. JME is a disorder that we suspect involves a developmental disturbance of the frontal lobes and one that is characterized by hallmark cortical myoclonus. There are, at least, facts which possibly connect JME directly with disturbances in cortical development. First, experiments using mouse chimera demonstrate that the telencephalon (from which the forebrain later develops) is expressed almost exclusively from paternally imprinted (silenced) genes, i.e., from the maternal alleles alone (36). In the diencephalon, the reverse holds, with the paternal alleles expressed and the maternal alleles silenced. Imprinted genes, therefore, seem to control the development of different brain regions. Second, there are two known disorders involving cortical myoclonus that show a disturbed pattern of imprinting. In Angelman syndrome, loss of expression of imprinted genes causes a severe neurodevelopmental disorder with cortical myoclonic seizures (37) and subtle changes in cortical architecture (38). Myoclonus-dystonia syndrome (MDS), in which there is cortical myoclonus, is caused by loss of function mutations in the maternally imprinted epsilon-sarcoglycan gene (SGCE) (39). Thus, not only are there precedents for a causal link between cortical myoclonus and imprinting, but there is also a developmental explanation (telencephalon growth), which links imprinting with possible frontal cortex disturbance. Nowadays, it is relatively straightforward to directly investigate imprinting. Many imprint marks are maintained by DNA or histone methylation and molecular tools can be used to find differences between methylation status in the two parental alleles. An imprinting hypothesis in JME is, therefore, testable.

The connection between JME, Angelman syndrome, and MDS prompts us to digress at this point: Is there a common pathway for epileptic cortical myoclonus? If there is, then what are the implications for the genetics of JME? There are many different clinical classifications and etiologies of myoclonus, which may be focal or generalized, or be caused by progressive metabolic, inflammatory, or other conditions. Myoclonus is classified as epileptic if it is accompanied by a spike-wave on EEG. At least two types of myoclonus, both cortical, are thought to occur in myoclonic epilepsy. First, thalamocortical (positive) myoclonus is believed to be generated by hyperexcitability of neural circuits connecting the reticular formation with the motor and somatosensory cortex. Generalized spikes produced by this hyperexcitable circuit are visible on surface EEG and are conducted through the pyramidal tract to the skeletal muscles, causing the brief myoclonic jerk. This is the probable mechanism of myoclonus in JME. Transcranial magnetic stimulation studies have shown a significant impairment in motor evoked potential inhibition in JME patients, suggesting that impaired interneuronal inhibition (rather than excessive excitation) leads to cortical hyperexcitability in JME (40). Second, negative cortical myoclonus may occur as a result of inhibition of resting muscle tone. The electrophysiologic basis of negative myoclonus is variable, but it is thought that the primary somatosensory cortex plays a generating role (41). Negative cortical myoclonus, usually seen in focal epilepsies, has not been reported in JME, but nevertheless is conceivable.

Special techniques of EEG/EMG analysis (jerk-locked backaveraging) demonstrate similarities between JME, benign myoclonic epilepsy of childhood, and the progressive myoclonic epilepsies (42). These electrophysiologic findings suggest that disorders involving cortical myoclonus of different etiology may manifest similar clinical and EEG features. We can rea-sonably hypothesize that any element in this specific thalamocortical system—cellular morphology, ion-channel function, neurotransmitter efficiency, local energy metabolism—if sufficiently deranged, may lead to the electroclinical pattern of cortical myoclonus. It, therefore, follows that various combinations and permutations of minor derangements in one or more of these elements could lead to the same clinical picture. These various permutations would be reflected in genetic heterogeneity in the population. For example, a single large derangement might be seen in an autosomal dominant pedigree, whereas several combined minor ones would give the appearance of complex inheritance.

Returning to the theme of clinical features that may give clues to underlying mechanisms, we cannot fail to ignore the impressive sex bias in JME. We found a 20:1 female to male ratio among both our community ascertained JME cases *and* their affected siblings. This extreme sex ratio among JME affecteds was not explained by the overall sex ratio in these families or by ascertainment bias. Female excess has been noted before and the pubertal age of onset in JME offers a clue that a sex-hormonal factor acts as an additional risk factor. How might this tie into a genetic explanation? Although most developmental changes in the brain occur early in childhood, some apoptotic processes are known to occur in adolescent animals, and these are perhaps influenced by hormonal factors. We can also speculate that sex hormones play a role in regulation of genes important in the integrity of the neurons in the thalamocortical loop. As with imprinting, there are molecular methods for testing the hypothesis that (say) estrogen binds and regulates a specific gene and these methods may eventually solve the puzzle of pubertal onset and female excess.

DO CHANNELOPATHIES EXPLAIN ALL OF JUVENILE MYOCLONIC EPILEPSY?

Most of the epilepsy genes discovered so far, including the *GABRA1* mutation in the French-Canadian JME family, suggest interruption of neurotransmitters or ion channels. What these genes have in common is that they have been discovered through the study of high-density pedigrees, i.e., families that have many affected family members. The high familiality of seizures seen in those families can be either due to a single-gene with simple mendelian transmission or a special accumulation of genetic effects. The mutations in those genes seem to be severe enough to either cause disease on their own or to be at least a major contributor to disease pathology. The majority of JME families, however, differ from these families in that they usually have few, if any, affected family members. Thus far, similar mutations in neurotransmitter or ion-channel genes have not been found to play a major role in those families. This suggests that in these families other mechanisms of epileptogenesis exist. It is argued that many malfunctions, perhaps ones that are subtle and remote, can lead to seizures and that excessive neuronal excitation is merely a common endpoint. However, our knowledge about the function and interaction of neuronal circuits is still limited. While the discoveries of synaptic transmission or ion channel dysfunction derived from those largely monogenic epilepsies can point to mechanisms of epileptogenesis, the viewpoint that only mutations in neurotransmitter and channel genes can lead to epilepsy seems to be overly restrictive and might prevent us from entering new avenues of finding the underlying disturbances for the more common, but also more complex epilepsies.

Our own findings in JME on chromosome 6 provide evidence for a non-ion channel pathology involved in common forms of JME. Through linkage analysis, we found evidence for a locus on chromosome 6p21 (EJM1) involved in JME, a finding that has been reproduced by several other research groups (2,4,14,43a). Obligate recombinants narrowed this locus to less than 1 cM between HLA-DQ and HLA-DP (4,5). Linkage disequilibrium mapping in these regions showed the strongest association directly at *BRD2* (RING3) (34). We identified a common variant haplotype in over one-half of JME patients from families that showed linkage to *EJM1*. This haplotype carries a high risk (odds ratio 6.5) for JME and centers on a single nucleotide polymorphism (SNP) with unknown functional sig-

nificance in the *BRD2* promoter region. Sequence analysis of the coding regions and splice sites of *BRD2* and neighboring genes failed to reveal any obvious mutations. Yet several convergent observations, including the putative biological role of *BRD2*, makes *BRD2* a credible candidate for JME. Although *BRD2* has not been studied extensively in humans, a role in regulating neuronal development is likely (43). Animal data show that *BRD2* is highly expressed in the developing mouse nervous system (44). Furthermore, *BRD2* expression is highest in the proliferating cortical zones of the mouse brain. There is also indirect evidence that *BRD2* may be involved in the regulation of genes involved in cell proliferation, because *BRD2* protein translocates from the cytoplasm to the nucleus during cell division (45). *In vitro*, *BRD2* coimmunoprecipitates with known cell cycle regulators *E2F1* and *E2F2* (46). Its location on euchromatin is consistent with its hypothesized function as a transcriptional regulator (45). The rat homolog of *BRD2* is also induced during early stages of programmed neuronal cell death in experimental conditions (47), suggesting a role in the modeling of the developing neuronal system.

While these studies are not conclusive, they offer strong circumstantial evidence that susceptibility to common JME is not caused by a critical loss or gain-of-function coding mutation. Instead, it is likely that disturbed regulation of *BRD2* leads to seizure susceptibility in JME. From our linkage data we expect that these disturbances alone will not be enough for the manifestation of JME, but that other critical factors, coded on other chromosomes, have to present.

Our findings coincide with new and exiting trends to look at the working of DNA. There are emerging insights that genes (i.e., the coding sequences of our genetic material) only tell one-half of the story. What has been called "junk" DNA is now being discovered to harbor new important elements that act on and modify distinct genes. This opens also new ways to look at disease processes. It is quite likely that disturbances in genes for ion channels or neurotransmitters present only the tip of the iceberg and we have been so successful in finding them because they are the easiest to find.

As with other electrical circuits, a malfunction can occur because of a faulty component, but sometimes all the parts are intact and the mistake is in faulty wiring. Faulty wiring is usually harder to detect because the mistake can be in any branch of the circuit. Sometimes, faulty wiring might even escape detection because the drainage on the circuit is low and only when there is an additional surge, will the circuit break down. Given the complexity of neuronal circuits, we believe that there are probably many ways that can lead to neuronal hyperexitability and faulty components, i.e., ion channels are only one out of many possibilities. We are suggesting to make use of all the observations and results from previous studies and different fields to discover many more causes for epilepsy, thus making the term "idiopathic" epilepsy a superfluous term.

REFERENCES

1. Greenberg DA, Delgado-Escueta A, Maldonado HM, et al. Segregation analysis of juvenile myoclonic epilepsy. *Genet Epidemiol* 1988;5:81–94.
1a. Janz D. Die Epilepsien. Spezielle Pathologie und Therapie. Thieme, Stuttgart, 1969.
2. Durner M, Sander T, Greenberg DA, et al. Localization of idiopathic generalized epilepsy on chromosome 6p in families of juvenile myoclonic epilepsy patients. *Neurology* 1991;41:1651–1655.
3. Whitehouse WP, Rees M, Curtis D, et al. Linkage analysis of idiopathic generalized epilepsy (IGE) and marker loci on chromosome 6p in families of patients with juvenile myoclonic epilepsy: No evidence for an epilepsy locus in the HLA region. *Am J Hum Genet* 1993;53:652–662.
4. Sander T, Bockenkamp B, Hildmann T, et al. Refined mapping of the epilepsy susceptibility locus EJM1 on chromosome 6. *Neurology* 1997;49:842–847.
5. Greenberg DA, Durner M, Keddache M, et al. Reproducibility and complications in gene searches: Linkage on chromosome 6, heterogeneity, association, and maternal inheritance in juvenile myoclonic epilepsy. *Am J Hum Genet* 2000;66:508–516.
6. Liu AW, Delgado-Escueta A, Gee MN, et al. Juvenile myoclonic epilepsy in chromosome 6p12-p11: Locus heterogeneity and recombinations. *Am J Med Genet* 1996;63:438–446.
7. Bai D, Alonso ME, Medina MT, et al. Juvenile myoclonic epilepsy: Linkage to chromosome 6p12 in Mexico families. *Am J Med Genet* 2002;113:268–274.
8. Elmslie FV, Rees M, Williamson MP, et al. Genetic mapping of a major susceptibility locus for juvenile myoclonic epilepsy on chromosome 15q. *Hum Mol Genet* 1997;6:1329–1334.
9. Sander T, Schulz H, Vieira-Saeker AM, et al. Evaluation of a putative major susceptibility locus for juvenile myoclonic epilepsy on chromosome 15q14. *Am J Med Genet* 1999;88:182–187.
10. Durner M, Shinnar S, Resor SR, et al. No evidence for a major susceptibility locus for juvenile myoclonic epilepsy on chromosome 15q. *Am J Med Genet* 2000;96:49–52.
11. Cossette P, Liu L, Brisebois K, et al. Mutation of GABRA1 in an autosomal dominant form of juvenile myoclonic epilepsy. *Nat Genet* 2002;31:184–189.
12. Sander T, Hildmann T, Janz D, et al. Exclusion of linkage between idiopathic generalized epilepsies and the GABAA receptor alpha 1 and gamma 2 subunit gene cluster on chromosome 5. *Epilepsy Res* 1996;23:235–244.
13. Durner M, Keddache MA, Tomasini L, et al. Genome scan of idiopathic generalized epilepsy: evidence for major susceptibility gene and modifying genes influencing the seizure type. *Ann Neurol* 2001;49:328–335.
14. Greenberg DA, Delgado-Escueta A, Widelitz H, et al. Juvenile myoclonic epilepsy (JME) may be linked to the BF and HLA loci on human chromosome 6. *Am J Med Genet* 1988;31:185–192.
15. Hodge SE, Greenberg DA, Durner M. Is Juvenile myoclonic epilepsy polygenic? In: Beck-Mannagetta G, Anderson VE, Doose H, Janz D. eds. *Genetics of the epilepsies.* Springer-Verlag, Berlin, 1989, 62–66.
16. Durner M, Greenberg DA, Hodge SE. Inter- and intrafamilial heterogeneity: effective sampling strategies and comparison of analysis methods. *Am J Hum Genet* 1992;51:859–870.
17. Wallace RH, Wang DW, Singh R, et al. Febrile seizures and generalized epilepsy associated with a mutation in the Na^+ channel beta1 subunit gene SCN1B. *Nat Genet* 1998;19:366–370.
18. Tsuboi T, Christian W. On the genetics of the primary generalized epilepsy with sporadic myoclonias of impulsive petit mal type. A clinical and electroencephalographic study of 399 probands. *Humangenetik* 1973;19:155–182.
19. Janz D, Durner M, Beck-Mannagetta G, Pantazis G. Family studies on the genetics of juvenile myoclonic epilepsy (epilepsy with impulsive petit mal). In: Beck-Mannagetta G, Anderson VE, Doose H, Janz D. eds. *Genetics of the epilepsies.* Springer-Verlag, Berlin, 1989; 43–52.
20. Winawer MR, Rabinowitz D, Pedley TA, et al. Genetic influences on myoclonic and absence seizures. *Neurology* 2003;61:1576–1581.
21. Kapoor A, Vijai J, Ravishankar HM, et al. Absence of GABRA1 Ala322Asp mutation in juvenile myoclonic epilepsy families from India. *J Genet* 2003;82:17–21.
22. Tomer Y, Barbesino G, Greenberg DA, et al. Mapping the major susceptibility loci for familial Graves' and Hashimoto's diseases: evidence for genetic heterogeneity and gene interactions. *J Clin Endocrinol Metab* 1999;84:4656–4664.
23. Obeid T, Panayiotopoulos CP. Juvenile myoclonic epilepsy: A study in Saudi Arabia. *Epilepsia* 1988;29:280–282.
24. Panayiotopoulos CP, Obeid T. Juvenile myoclonic epilepsy: an autosomal recessive disease. *Ann Neurol* 1989;25:440–443.

25. Janz D, Christian W. Impulsiv-petit mal. *Dtsch Z Ner-venheilk* 1957;176:348–386.
26. Swartz BE, Simpkins F, Halgren E, et al. Visual working memory in primary generalized epilepsy: an 18FDG-PET study. *Neurology* 1996;47:1203–1212.
27. Devinsky O, Gershengorn J, Brown E, et al. Frontal functions in juvenile myoclonic epilepsy. *Neuropsych Neuropsychol Behav Neurol* 1997;10:243–246.
28. Meencke HJ, Janz D. Neuropathological findings in primary generalized epilepsy: A study of eight cases. *Epilepsia* 1984;25:8–21.
29. Opeskin K, Kalnins RM, Halliday G, et al. Idiopathic generalized epilepsy: lack of significant microdysgen-esis. *Neurology* 2000;55:1101–1106.
30. Woermann FG, Free SL, Koepp MJ, et al. Abnormal cerebral structure in juvenile myoclonic epilepsy demonstrated with voxel-based analysis of MRI. *Brain* 1999;122(Pt 11):2101–2108.
31. Koepp MJ, Duncan JS. Positron emission tomography in idiopathic generalized epilepsy: imaging beyond structure. In: Schmitz B, Sander T, eds. Juvenile myoclonic epilepsy the Janz syndrome. Petersfield, UK: Wrightson Publishers, 2000:91–99.
32. Annegers JF, Hauser WA, Elveback LR, et al. Seizure disorders in offspring of parents with a history of seizures—a maternal-paternal difference? *Epilepsia* 1976;17:1–9.
33. Ottman R, Hauser WA, Susser M. Genetic and maternal influences on susceptibility to seizures. An analytic review. *Am J Epidemiol* 1985;122:923–939.
34. Pal DK, Evgrafov OV, Tabares P, et al. BRD2 (RING3) is a probable major susceptibility gene for common juvenile myoclonic epilepsy. *Am J Hum Genet* 2003;73:261–270.
35. Greenberg DA, Feenstra B, Hodge SE. Assuming independent male-female (m-f) recombination fraction (RF) can reveal imprinting. *Am J Hum Genet* 2002;71[Suppl.]:573.
36. Keverne EB, Fundele R, Narasimha M. Genomic imprinting and the differential roles of parental genomes in brain development. *Brain Res Develop Brain Res* 1996;92:91–100.
37. Guerrini R, De Lorey TM, Bonanni P, et al. Cortical myoclonus in Angelman syndrome. *Ann Neurol* 1996; 40:39–48.
38. Leonard CM, Williams CA, Nicholls RD, et al. Angelman and Prader-Willi syndrome: A magnetic resonance imaging study of differences in cerebral structure. *Am J Med Genet* 1993;46:26–33.
39. Grabowski M, Zimprich A, Lorenz-Depiereux B, et al. The epsilon-sarcoglycan gene (SGCE), mutated in myoclonus-dystonia syndrome, is maternally imprinted. *Eur J Hum Genet* 2003;11:138–144.
40. Manganotti P, Bongiovanni LG, Zanette G, et al. Early and late intracortical inhibition in juvenile myoclonic epilepsy. *Epilepsia* 2000;41:1129–1138.
41. Shibasaki H, Ikeda A, Nagamine T, et al. Cortical reflex negative myoclonus. *Brain* 1994;117(Pt 3):477–486.
42. Panzica F, Rubboli G, Franceschetti S. Cortical myoclonus in Janz syndrome. *Clin Neurophysiol* 2001;112: 1803–1809.
43. Thorpe KL, Gorman P, Thomas C, et al. Chromosomal localization, gene structure and transcription pattern of the ORFX gene, a homologue of the MHC-linked RING3 gene. *Gene* 1997;200:177–183.
43a. Weissbecker KA, Durner M, Janz D, et al. Confirmation of linkage between juvenile myoclonic epilepsy locus and the HLA region of chromosome 6. *Am J Med Genet* 1991;38:32–36.
44. Rhee K, Brunori M, Besset V, et al. Expression and potential role of Fsrg1, a murine bromodomain-containing homologue of the Drosophila gene female sterile homeotic. *J Cell Sci* 1998;111(Pt 23):3541–3550.
45. Crowley TE, Kaine EM, Yoshida M, et al. Reproductive cycle regulation of nuclear import, euchromatic localization, and association with components of Pol II mediator of a mammalian double-bromodomain protein. *Mol Endocrinol* 2002;16:1727–1737.
46. Denis GV, Vaziri C, Guo N, et al. RING3 kinase transactivates promoters of cell cycle regulatory genes through E2F. *Cell Growth Differ* 2000;11:417–424.
47. Wang S, Dibenedetto AJ, Pittman RN. Genes induced in programmed cell death of neuronal PC12 cells and developing sympathetic neurons in vivo. *Develop Biol* 1997;188:322–336.

19

Autosomal Dominant Juvenile Myoclonic Epilepsy and *GABRA1*

Patrick Cossette,* Anne Lortie,[†] Michel Vanasse,[†] Jean-Marc Saint-Hilaire,[†,*] and Guy A. Rouleau[†]

*Centre Hospitalier de l'Université de Montréal-Hôpital Notre-Dame, Montréal, Québec, Canada,
[†]Centre for Research in Neuroscience, McGill University Health Center Research Institute,
Montréal, Québec, Canada

Reports in support of hereditary factors in epilepsy date back at least to biblical times. Even a modest perusal of these reports would be a mammoth task ... The findings of the earlier as well as the more recent investigators suggest that, if hereditary factors underly some of the epilepsies, this is most likely to be demonstrated when the proband has no apparent extrinsic cause for his epilepsy. And, to hide our ignorance here, we say that the patient has idiopathic epilepsy.

Katherine and Julius Metrakos
Montreal, 1961

INTRODUCTION

In light of their pioneering genetic studies on the classical idiopathic generalized epileptic syndromes (IGE), Metrakos and Metrakos concluded that "centrencephalic type of electroencephalogram is the expression of an autosomal dominant gene, with the unusual characteristic of a very low penetrance at birth, which rises rapidly to nearly complete penetrance for ages $4\frac{1}{4}$ to $16\frac{1}{2}$ and declines gradually to almost no penetrance after the age of $40\frac{1}{2}$ years" (1,2). More than 40 years later, despite a large body of clinical evidence incriminating hereditary factors in IGE, the mode of inheritance of these syndromes remains a matter of debate, with many link-age studies providing conflicting results (3–6). These discrepancies may reflect the fact that IGE syndromes are usually not inherited in a clearly Mendelian manner, but rather show a complex inheritance pattern. Indeed, if a concordance rate in identical twins is found in up to 95% for IGE (7,8)—suggesting an almost complete genetic etiology for this syndrome—many studies have shown a relatively small increased risk of epilepsy in first- (13%) and second-degree (6%) relatives (2,9,10) for epilepsy *per se*. Based on this rapid decrease in the risk of epilepsy with each degree of relationship, many authors suggested that IGE could be caused by a multiplicative (epistatic) interaction among many contributing loci (polygenic model) (8). In addition, various environmental factors (e.g., sleep deprivation, alcohol and drug abuse, head trauma) can also increase the risk of developing epilepsy, including IGE (11). However, these epidemiologic studies probably represent a crude approximation of a very complex reality. First, because of sociocultural factors, the family history of epilepsy is often unknown to the proband and immediate family, and a systematic survey of all family members is often required to find additional affected individuals within the same family (1,2,12). In addition, these studies lumped all the IGE together, even though these syndromes

TABLE 19–1. *Genes and Loci already identified for IGE syndromes*

Phenotype	Inheritance	Methods	Locus	Gene	Reference
BNFC	AD	P	Chr. 20q13	*KCNQ2*	13
BNFC	AD	P	Chr. 8q24	*KCNQ3*	14
GEFS	AD	P	Chr. 2q24	*SCN1A*	19
GEFS	AD	P	Chr. 19q13	*SCN1B*	18
GEFS/CAE	AD	P	Chr. 5q33	*GABRG2*	28
JME	AD	P	Chr. 5q34	*GABRA1*	22
JME/JAE/EGMA	AD	P and NP	Chr. 3q26	*CLCN2*	32
CAE	AD	P	Chr. 8q24	Pending	34
BMEI	AR	P	Chr. 16p13	Pending	35
JME	AD(?)	P and NP	Chr. 6p12	Pending	36
JME	AR(?)	NP	Chr. 15q14	Pending	4
IGE	AD	P and NP	Chr. 2q36	Pending	37
IGE	AD	P and NP	Chr. 19q12	Pending	37
IGE	AD	P and NP	Chr. 14q23	Pending	37
IGE	?	NP	Chr. 8q24	Pending	8
IGE	AR	P	Chr. 18	Pending	38
IGE	AD	P	Chr. 6	Pending	38
IGE	AR	P	Chr. 5	Pending	38

BNFC, benign neonatal familial convulsions; EGMA, epilepsy with grand mal on awakening; GEFS, generalized epilepsy with febrile seizures; CAE, childhood absence epilepsy; JME, juvenile myoclonic epilepsy; JAE, juvenile absence epilepsy; BMEI, benign myoclonic epilepsy of infancy; IGE, idiopathic generalized epilepsy; AD, autosomal dominant; AR, autosomal recessive; P, parametric linkage analysis; NP, nonparametric linkage analysis; Chr, chromosome.

have been shown to be clinically, and genetically highly heterogeneous. In particular, these studies do not take into consideration the recent studies of the large kindreds with idiopathic epilepsy, where an autosomal dominant (or recessive) mode of inheritance has been demonstrated (Table 19–1). Finally, the clinical assessment itself, even by experienced clinicians, is not simple, mainly because of the variable expression of the disease during lifetime, as well as the occurrence of many intermediate phenotypes. Therefore, the current state of knowledge indicates that IGE is clearly not a single entity, but rather represents the sum of a large variety of different genetic diseases: some being clearly Mendelian traits, while others exhibiting polygenic inheritance.

DISTINCT EPILEPTIC SYNDROMES ARE CAUSED BY DEFECTS IN COMPLEMENTARY SUBUNITS OF A SAME PROTEIN COMPLEX

By taking advantage of large kindreds with many individuals affected by epilepsy, recent studies using molecular genetic approaches allowed the identification of susceptibility genes for various epileptic syndromes, including benign neonatal familial convulsion syndrome (BNFC), caused by mutations in *KCNQ2* and *KCNQ3*, encoding for two different subunits of the same potassium channel (13–15), and autosomal dominant nocturnal frontal lobe epilepsy (ADNFLE), which is caused by mutations in *CHRNA4* and *CHRNB2*, encoding for two different subunits of the ligand-gated neuronal nicotinic acetylcholine receptor (16,17).

IGE have the most significant hereditary component among all epilepsies, and represents approximately 40% of all these syndromes. However, genetic studies of IGE are hampered by the clinical heterogeneity of the syndromes and genetic heterogeneity for apparently similar syndromes. Recent studies of large kindreds provided new insights into the definition of clinical phenotypes among IGE and led to the description of a hitherto unrecognized syndrome of IGE that is associated with febrile seizure (GEFS) (12). Mutations in two different genes (*SCN1A* and *SCN1B*), encoding for two complementary subunits of the same protein complex (the $\alpha 1$ and $\beta 1$ subunits of the neuronal voltage-gated sodium channel), have been found to cause this unique epileptic syndrome (18–20). However, less than 15% of all GEFS families are explained by mutation in these genes (21). Moreover, the proportion of IGE cases meeting criteria for GEFS is currently not known. Consequently, the predisposing genes for the vast majority of sporadic and familial IGE, including those underlying the "classical" IGE syndromes [childhood absence epilepsy (CAE), juvenile absence epilepsy (JAE), juvenile myoclonic epilepsy (JME), and epilepsy with grand mal on awakening (EGMA)] remain to be determined.

GENETIC AND CLINICAL STUDY OF A LARGE FRENCH-CANADIAN FAMILY WITH IDIOPATHIC GENERALIZED EPILEPTIC SYNDROMES

We recently evaluated 14 members of a French-Canadian family segregating JME (22). In this large kindred, the transmission is clearly autosomal dominant, with affected people over four generations (Fig 19–1). Standard molecular genetic approach, including detailed clinical evaluations, allows us to identify the gene causing JME in this family. All the affected individuals from generation III and IV were followed at

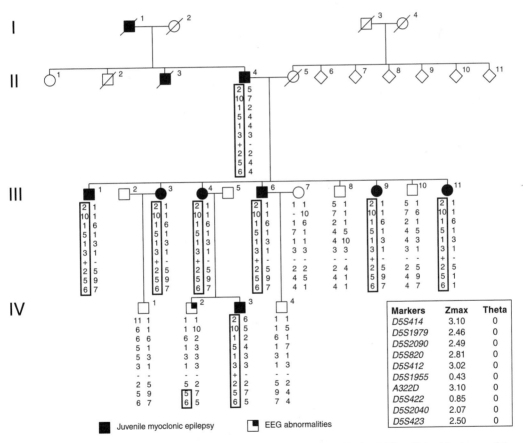

FIG. 19–1. Autosomal dominant JME in a large French-Canadian kindred. The clinical features of the epileptic syndrome remain homogeneous in all affected members of the family over four generations. The disease associated haplotype is boxed. Alleles were numbered according to their respective sizes and correspond to the CEPH genotyping database. The maximum LOD scores obtained with these markers are shown in the lower right-hand corner, including the A322D mutation in *GABRA1* gene (+).

TABLE 19–2. *Clinical manifestations of affected members of the family*

ID	Age of onset	GTCs	Absence	Myoclonus	GPSW
II-04	13	Yes	No	Yes	Yes
III-01	14	Yes	No	Yes	Yes
III-03	12	Yes	No	Yes	Yes
III-04	8	Yes	Yes	Yes	Yes
III-06	13	Yes	No	Yes	Yes
III-09	16	Yes	Yes	Yes	Yes
III-11	13	Yes	Yes	Yes	Yes
IV-03	5	Yes	Yes	Yes	Yes

GPSW, generalized polyspike-and-wave; GTCs, generalized tonic-clonic seizures.

Hôpital Ste Justine (HSJ) and Hôpital Notre-Dame (HND) from early childhood. Both affected and unaffected individuals from these generations had at least one electroencephalogram (EEG) during childhood, before treatment was initiated. All affected individuals have a similar phenotype, including generalized tonic–clonic seizures and myoclonic jerks (Table 19–2). Some patients ($n = 4$) also presented brief absence attacks with partial preservation of awareness. In affected females, all of these seizures may be trig-gered by various visual stimuli, including black-and-white linear patterns and light flickering. Unexpectedly, affected males from this kindred were unaware of this precipitating factor (see case of G.C. and M.C.). In turn, EEGs showed generalized polyspike-and-waves discharges induced by photic stimulation in all affected individuals. In three individuals, we have also found polyspike-and-wave discharges occurring spontaneously, or during hyperventilation (Fig 19–2). Seizure control was relatively easy to achieve

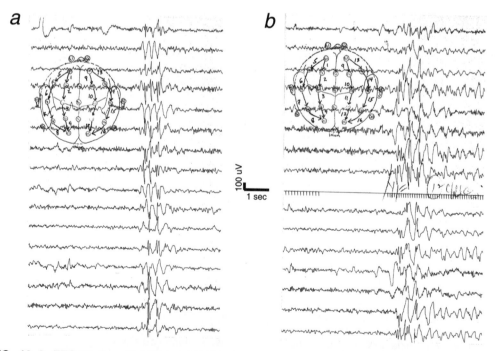

FIG. 19–2. EEG findings in affected individuals. All affected members of the family exhibit fast (>3.5-Hz) generalized polyspike-and-wave epileptic discharges that could occur spontaneously (**A**), or induced by photic stimulation (**B**). These recordings have been obtained from individual IV-03.

in affected individuals, although they all needed long-term antiepileptic drug treatment.

Case 1 (III-09)

She was born from a difficult delivery, with three turns of the umbilical cord around her neck, associated with cyanosis. She never experienced febrile seizure. She had a first generalized tonic-clonic seizure at 16 years old, while she was watching a television with blurred image. In the previous months, she experienced upper limbs myoclonus occurring in the morning, which could lead her to drop small objects. Initial EEG, neurologic examination, and intelligence appeared normal. Control EEG recordings performed at 17 years of age eventually revealed generalized polyspike-and-waves during hyperventilation and photic light stimulation. She was treated with phenytoin (PHT) 100 mg tid and phenobarbital (PB) 60 mg hs. She is now 39 years old and does not exhibit GTC seizures. However, she is still experiencing frequent, but brief, episodes of absence induced by various visual patterns, such as black and white patterns on clothing.

Case 2 (III-06)

He was born from normal pregnancy and delivery. He never experienced febrile seizures. At 9 years old, he had two EEGs because of aggressive behavior and possible episodes of loss of consciousness. Both EEG recordings revealed generalized polyspike-and-waves, exclusively during photic light stimulation. He had a first generalized tonic–clonic seizure at 13 years old, for which PB and PHT were initiated. In the previous months, he did notice myoclonic jerks occurring in the morning. He denied absence attacks or any seizure induced by environmental visual stimuli. All of the subsequent EEGs performed during treatment were normal. PHT has been replaced by clonazepam(CZP), because of persistent myoclonic jerks, and gingival hyperplasia. Sleep deprivation, as well as stressful life events, have been found to precipitate infrequent generalized tonic–clonic seizures over years. He also experienced several episodes of

depressive mood, including a suicide attempt. PB was stopped when he was 22 years old. He is now 42 and seizure-free for 18 years on CZP (2 mg hs). Recent attempts to further reduce this drug have led to the recurrence of myoclonic jerks.

Overall, affected members of the family exhibit very similar clinical features and fulfill the diagnostic criteria for JME. The only exception is individual IV-03 who had an earlier onset (5 years old), but whose clinical features remain otherwise indistinguishable from those of other members of the family. This observation is consistent with previous reports of early-onset JME syndrome and reinforces the concept of a biological continuum among classic IGE syndromes (23). We were also able to indirectly assess individuals I-01, and II-03, via individual II-04. The phenotype in these individuals appeared compatible with JME, with chronic GTCS associated with myoclonic jerks. We did not find any history of febrile seizures in this family. Finally, by doing systematic EEG during childhood in every member of this large kindred, we found a photoparoxysmal response in individual IV-02, although he denied any symptoms suggestive of a seizure disorder. Since such a response is found in up to 8.3% of the pediatric population (24,25), he was not considered as affected for the purpose of this linkage study.

LINKAGE STUDY AND *GABRA1* SCREENING

By conducting a genome scan in this family, we found evidence for linkage on chromosome 5q34 (Fig. 19–1), in a region that includes a cluster of $GABA_A$ receptor subunits [the $\beta2$ (*GABRB2*), $\alpha1$ (*GABRA1*), and $\gamma2$ (*GABRG2*) subunits]. We screened these GABA receptor genes for mutation and found a A322D mutation in the *GABRA1* gene in all affected patients ($n = 8$), and none of the unaffected members ($n = 6$) of the family. We did not find this A322D variation in control individuals, nor was it found in individual IV-02, who has only an abnormal EEG. We also did not find the A322D mutation in our cohort of 150 IGE individuals—mainly from French-Canadian origin—which included patients with JME ($n = 31$) and CAE syndromes ($n = 52$). By screening this cohort for mutation in *GABRA1*, including 30 individuals with familial IGE, we found another mutation in this gene. Interestingly, the clinical features in two affected individuals from this family were very similar to those encountered in JME, including juvenile onset of GTCS triggered by photic light stimulation (photosensitivity) [Cossette *et al.*, (26) *in preparation*]. Mutations in *GABRA1* thus appear to be a rare cause of familial IGE in the French-Canadian population, and do not seem to predispose toward so-called sporadic IGE.

MOLECULAR MECHANISM OF THE A322D MUTATION IN *GABRA1*

We investigated whether the A322D mutation found in the *GABRA1* gene altered the functional properties of GABA$_A$ receptors *in vitro* (22).

GABA$_A$ receptors are ligand-gated chloride channels mediating fast synaptic inhibition in the brain. Their molecular structure consists in a heteropentameric protein complex, assembled from different classes of subunits (α_{1-6}, β_{1-4}, γ_{1-3}, δ, ϵ, π, θ). The $\alpha1\beta2\gamma2$ combination is believed to be the most abundant in the brain (27). The optimal subunit stoichiometry and composition required to obtain functional expression of GABA$_A$ receptors exhibiting the full pharmacologic spectrum of the native receptors is also $\alpha\beta\gamma$, in a ratio of 2:2:1. To achieve this goal, we cloned the human *GABRG2*, *GABRA1*, and *GABRB2* cDNA, and introduced the A322D mutation into the *GABRA1* cDNA. Whole-cell recordings of HEK 293 cells expressing mutant GABA$_A$ receptor ($\alpha1_{A322D}\beta2\gamma2$) have a dramatic reduction in the amplitude of GABA-activated currents compared to the wild-type ($\alpha1\beta2\gamma2$) receptor,

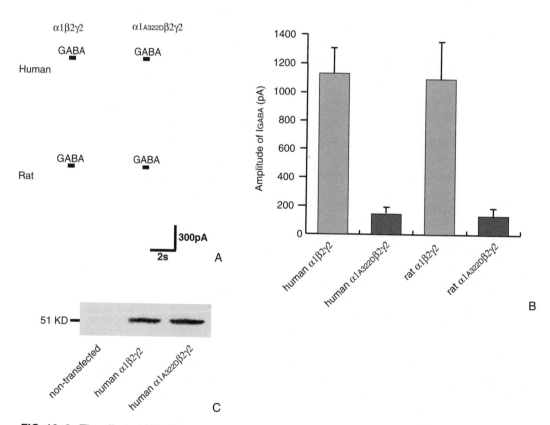

FIG. 19–3. The effect of A322D mutation on GABA-evoked currents *in vitro*. Representative individual recording trace of whole-cell currents induced by puffing GABA onto transfected HEK cells.

compatible with a loss-of-function effect of this mutation (Fig. 19–3).

COMPLEMENTARY MOLECULAR MECHANISMS UNDERLYING THE CLASSIC IDIOPATHIC GENERALIZED EPILEPTIC SYNDROMES

Interestingly, other investigators have found that mutations in GABRG2 are responsible for CAE associated with febrile seizure and GEFS in at least four different families (28–31). In addition, recent studies have shown that mutations in CLCN2 gene (voltage-gated chloride channel) can predispose toward a variety of IGE phenotypes (JME, JAE, and EGMA), in three different families. As for GABRA1 and GABRG2 genes, it appears that the frequency of mutations in CLCN2 gene is very low, even in familial cases (32).

By expressing mutant channels in vitro, these investigators have shown that mutations in GABRG2 also result in a reduction of GABA-activated currents (28,29). In addition, mutations in CLCN2 have been shown to alter chloride homeostasis, which may result in a reduction in the inhibitory function of the $GABA_A$ receptors (32). Therefore, it appears that impairment of the inhibition mechanisms mediated through the $GABA_A$ receptors is central in the pathophysiology of classic IGE.

IMPACT OF IDENTIFICATION OF EPILEPSY GENES

The treatment of the epilepsies remains symptomatic, with up to 30% of patients who continue to have intractable seizures despite adequate pharmacologic treatment. This represents considerable human and social costs. The exact mechanism by which neurons spontaneously start to fire synchronously resulting in either focal or generalized seizure is elusive. In addition, the mechanisms of action of many antiepileptic drugs (AEDs), as well as the different response rate to these drugs among individuals, are still poorly understood. We believe that the identification and the characterization of the mutated molecules involved in human epilepsies will enhance our understanding of the disease. In particular, identification of susceptibility genes for the epilepsies will allow the construction of transgenic animals that should facilitate the development of specifically targeted drugs. In addition, with a better understanding of the mode of inheritance and of the genetic etiology of the epileptic syndromes, we should be able very soon to offer better genetic counseling to the individuals with epilepsy and their family members, including DNA-based diagnostic test.

CONCLUDING REMARKS

While genetics factors have been suspected for many years to play an important role in the etiology of IGE, it is only recently that specific genes predisposing to the disease have begun to be identified. These discoveries represent significant progress in the understanding of the genetic and molecular mechanisms underlying familial IGE. Indeed, the study of rare, but distinct, epileptic syndromes identified gene defects in complementary subunits of the same voltage or ligand-gated ion-channel protein complex. More recently, genetic studies of large pedigrees segregating classic IGE phenotypes also revealed complementary molecular mechanisms. However, these epilepsy genes have been mapped and cloned in families where the inheritance pattern was clearly Mendelian. This is not the case for the vast majority of IGE, which are probably caused by an interaction between many susceptibility genes and environmental factors. Different strategies used to identify genes predisposing to complex phenotypes in humans (e.g., nonparametric linkage analysis and association studies) allowed the mapping of many loci, but these results are frequently difficult to replicate, and have rarely uncovered the predisposing gene (33–38). With these caveats, successful identification of additional genes causing familial epilepsies should provide greater insight into the pathophysiology of the disease and potentially lead to a more rational approach in the search for genes underlying common IGE phenotypes.

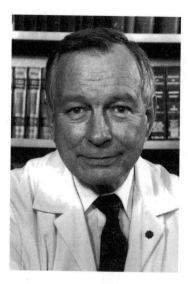

IN MEMORIAM: DR. GUY GEOFFROY
(1934–2000)

The authors are very grateful to doctor Guy Geoffroy, child neurologist and epileptologist at the Hôpital Sainte-Justine in Montreal. He was an outstanding physician and teacher, who trained and inspired many neurologists in the Province of Quebec. All the epileptic individuals from the family described here, like so many others in Montreal's area, have been diagnosed, reassured, and kindly treated by Dr. Geoffroy. While he was himself struggling with a disabling disease, he brought the family to our attention for the purpose of our genetic studies. We are indebted to him for this and numerous other lessons that he taught us.

REFERENCES

1. Metrakos JD, Metrakos K. Genetics of convulsive disorders I. Introduction, methods and base lines. *Neurology* 1960;10:228–240.
2. Metrakos JD, Metrakos K. Genetics of convulsive disorders II. Genetic and electroencephalographic studies in centrencephalic epilepsy. *Neurology* 1961;11:474–483.
3. Panayiotopoulos C, Obeid T. Juvenile myoclonic epilepsy: An autosomal recessive disease. *Ann Neurol* 1989;25:440–443.
4. Elmslie FV, Rees M, Williamson MP, et al. Genetic mapping of a major susceptibility locus for juvenile myoclonic epilepsy on chromosome 15q. *Hum Mol Genet* 1997;6:1329–1334.
5. Elmslie FV, Williamson MP, Rees M, et al. Linkage analysis of juvenile myoclonic epilepsy and microsatellite loci spanning 61 cM of human chromosome 6p in 19 nuclear pedigrees provides no evidence for a susceptibility locus in this region. *Am J Hum Genet* 1996;59:653–663.
6. Greenberg DA, Durner M, Keddache M, et al. Reproducibility and complications in gene searches: linkage on chromosome 6, heterogeneity, association, and maternal inheritance in juvenile myoclonic epilepsy. *Am J Hum Genet* 2000;66:508–516.
7. Berkovic SF, Howell RA, Hay DA, et al. Epilepsies in twins: genetics of the major epileptic syndromes. *Ann Neurol* 1998;43:435–445.
8. Zara F, Bianchi A, Avanzini G, et al. Mapping of genes predisposing to idiopathic generalized epilepsy. *Hum Mol Genet* 1995;4:1201–1207.
9. Annegers JF, Hauser WA, Anderson VE, et al. The risk of seizure disorders among relatives of patients with childhood onset epilepsy. *Neurology* 1982;32:174–179.
10. Jain S, Padma MV, Puri A, et al. Occurrence of epilepsies in family members of Indian probands with different epileptic syndromes. *Epilepsia* 1997;38:237–244.
11. Loiseau P. Seizure precipitants. In: Engel Jr J, Pedley TA. eds. *Epilepsy: A comprehensive textbook.* New York: Lippincott-Raven, 1997;93–97.
12. Scheffer IE, Berkovic SF. Generalized epilepsy with febrile seizures plus: A genetic disorder with heterogeneous clinical phenotypes. *Brain* 1997;120:479–490.
13. Biervert C, Schroeder BC, Kubisch C, et al. A potassium channel mutation in neonatal human epilepsy. *Science* 1998;279:403–406.
14. Charlier C, Singh NA, Ryan SG, et al. A pore mutation in a novel KGT-like potassium channel gene in an idiopathic epilepsy family. *Nat Genet* 1998;18:53–55.
15. Singh NA, Charlier C, Stauffer D, et al. A novel potassium channel gene, KCNQ2, is mutated in an inherited epilepsy of newborns. *Nat Genet* 1998;18:25–29.
16. Steinlein OK, Mulley JC, Propping P, et al. A missense mutation in the neuronal nicotinic acetylcholine receptor alpha 4 subunit is associated with autosomal dominant nocturnal frontal lobe epilepsy. *Nat Genet* 1995;11:201–203.
17. De Fusco M, Becchetti A, Patrignani A, et al. The nicotinic receptor beta-2 subunit is mutant in nocturnal frontal lobe epilepsy. *Nat Genet* 2000;26:275–276.
18. Wallace RH, Wang DW, Singh R, et al. Febrile seizures and generalized epilepsy associated with a mutation in the Na^+-channel beta1 subunit gene SCN1B. *Nat Genet* 1998;19:366–370.
19. Escayg A, MacDonald BT, Meisler MH, et al. Mutations of SCN1A, encoding a neuronal sodium channel, in two families with GEFS+2. *Nat Genet* 2000;24:343–345.
20. Cossette P, Loukas A, Lafrenière RG, et al. Functional characterization of the D188V mutation in SCN1A causing generalized epilepsy with febrile seizures (GEFS). *Epilepsy Res* 2003;53:107–117.
21. Wallace RH, Scheffer IE, Barnett S, et al. Neuronal sodium-channel alpha1-subunit mutations in generalized epilepsy with febrile seizures plus. *Am J Hum Genet* 2001;68:859–865.
22. Cossette P, Liu L, Brisebois K, et al. Mutation of GABRA1 in an autosomal dominant form of juvenile myoclonic epilepsy. *Nat Genet* 2002;31:184–189.

23. Berkovic SF, Andermann F, Andermann, E, et al. Concepts of absence epilepsies: Discrete syndromes or biological continuum? *Neurology* 1987;37:993–1000.

24. Doose H, Gerken H. On the genetics of EEG-abnormalities in childhood. IV. Photoconvulsive reaction. *Neuropediatrie* 1973;4:162–171.

25. Eeg-Olofsson O, Petersén I, Selldén U. The development of the electroencephalogram in normal children from the age of 1 through 15 years. *Neuropediatrie* 1971;2:375–404.

26. Cossette P, Desbiens R, Shevell M, Carmant L, and Rouleau GA. Mutation screening of *GABRA1* in idiopathic generalized epilepsy. In preparation.

27. Sieghart W, Fuchs K, Tretter V, et al. Structure and subunit composition of GABAA receptors. *Neurochem Int* 1999;34:379–385.

28. Baulac S, Huberfeld G, Gourfinkel-An I, et al. First genetic evidence of GABAA receptor dysfunction in epilepsy: a mutation in the gamma 2-subunit gene. *Nat Genet* 2001;28:46–48.

29. Wallace RH, Marini C, Petrou S, et al. Mutant GABAA receptor gamma 2-subunit in childhood absence epilepsy and febrile seizures. *Nat Genet* 2001;28:49–52.

30. Harkin LA, Bowser DN, Dibbens LM, et al. Truncation of the GABAA-receptor gamma-2 subunit in a family with generalized epilepsy with febrile seizures plus. *Am J Hum Genet* 2002;70:530–536.

31. Kananura, Haug K, Sander T, et al. A splice-site mutation in GABRG2 associated with childhood absence epilepsy and febrile convulsions. *Arch Neurol* 2002;59:1137–1141.

32. Haug K, Warnstedt M, Alekov AK, et al. Mutations in CLCN2 encoding a voltage-gated chloride channel are associated with idiopathic generalized epilepsies. *Nat Genet* 2003;33:527–532.

33. Eaves IA, Merriman TR, Barber RA, et al. The genetically isolated populations of Finland and Sardinia may not be a panacea for linkage disequilibrium mapping of common disease genes. *Nat Genet* 2000;25:320–323.

34. Fong GC, Shah PU, Gee MN, et al. Childhood absence epilepsy with tonic-clonic seizures and electroencephalogram 3-4 Hz spike and multispike-slow wave complexes: Linkage to chromosome 8q24. *Am J Hum Genet* 1998;63:1117–1129.

35. Zara F, Gennaro E, Stabile M, et al. Mapping of a locus for a familial autosomal recessive idiopathic myoclonic epilepsy of infancy to chromosome 16p13. *Am J Hum Genet* 2000;66:1552–1557.

36. Bai D, Alonso ME, Medina MT, et al. Juvenile myoclonic epilepsy: Linkage to chromosome 6p12 in Mexico families. *Am J Med Genet* 2002;113:268–274.

37. Sander T, Schulz H, Saar K, et al. Genome search for susceptibility loci of common idiopathic generalized epilepsies. *Hum Mol Genet* 2000;9:1465–1472.

38. Durner M, Keddache MA, Tomasini L, et al. Genome scan of idiopathic generalized epilepsy: evidence for major susceptibility gene and modifying genes influencing the seizure type. *Ann Neurol* 2001;49:328–335.

20

CLCN2 and Idiopathic Generalized Epilepsy

Armin Heils

Clinic of Epileptology and Institute of Human Genetics, University of Bonn, Bonn, Germany

INTRODUCTION

Epilepsy is one of the most frequent neurologic diseases affecting about 3% of the worldwide population (1). Clinical symptoms range from mild drowsiness to severe generalized convulsions and are induced by synchronous neuronal discharges due to an imbalance of inhibitory and excitatory activity in the brain. Idiopathic forms are genetically determined and account for about 40% of all epilepsies (2,3). They are defined by recurrent seizures with characteristic clinical and electroencephalographic features in the absence of any detectable brain lesion. The most frequent idiopathic form of epilepsy is idiopathic generalized epilepsy (IGE), which comprises seven clinically delineated syndromes with age-related onset (4). The most common IGE subtypes are childhood and juvenile absence epilepsy (CAE, JAE), juvenile myoclonic epilepsy (JME), and epilepsy with grand mal seizures on awakening (EGMA) (4). Absence seizures are the leading symptom of CAE and JAE, characterized by a brief loss of consciousness (usually 10–20 s) and either manifest during childhood (CAE) or adolescence (JAE). JME manifests in adolescence with bilateral myoclonic jerks of arms and shoulders (myoclonic seizures) usually occurring in the early morning without a loss of consciousness. All types of IGE can be associated with generalized tonic–clonic seizure (GTCS), which typically occur on awakening, often provoked by sleep deprivation. When this is the only seizure type, patients are diagnosed with EGMA. In all subtypes of IGE, typical electroencephalographic (EEG) features are generalized spike-wave or polyspike-wave discharges, reflecting a state of synchronized neuronal hyperexcitability.

Several genes have already been identified to cause monogenic forms of idiopathic epilepsy. Autosomal dominant nocturnal frontal lobe epilepsy (ADNFLE) has been shown to arise from mutations identified in genes encoding the α_4 or β_2 subunit of neuronal nicotinic acetylcholine receptors (*CHRNA4, CHRNB2*). Mutations in two voltage-gated potassium channel genes (*KCNQ2, KCNQ3*) are associated with benign familial neonatal convulsions (BFNC). Mutations in three different sodium channel subunits (*SCN1B, SCN1A, SCN2A*) as well as in the γ_2 subunit of the GABA$_A$ receptor (*GABRG2*) have been shown to cause generalized epilepsy with febrile seizures plus (GEFS$^+$) (see 5–7 for reviews). Thus, all genes identified in idiopathic epilepsies so far encode ion channels. Recently, autosomal dominant partial epilepsy with auditory features, an idiopathic form of temporal lobe epilepsy, has been shown to be caused by mutations in the leucine-rich, glioma-inactivated 1 gene (*LGI1*), not encoding an ion channel (8). Regarding the genetic basis of pure forms of the common IGE subtypes, thus far only one mutation in another GABA$_A$ receptor subunit gene (*GABRA1*) has been reported in a family with JME (9). A single epilepsy gene whose mutations can cause the whole spectrum of common IGE subtypes has not been identified to date.

GENOME SCAN FOR COMMON IDIOPATHIC GENERALIZED EPILEPSY LOCI

Recently, a genome wide search for chromosomal susceptibility loci of common subtypes including 130 IGE multiplex families identified a novel susceptibility locus on chromosome 3q26 (Z_{NPL} = 4.19 at *D3S3725*; P = 0.000017) (10). One of the candidate genes located in this chromosomal region is *CLCN2*, which encodes the voltage-gated chloride channel ClC-2 (11,12). ClC-2 is strongly expressed in the brain, particularly in γ-aminobutyric acid (GABA)-inhibited neurons (13,14).

Several experimental results suggest an important role of this channel in establishing and maintaining a low intracellular chloride concentration ($[Cl^-]_i$), which is necessary for an inhibitory GABA response. When hippocampal pyramidal neurons—the best studied model for GABAergic synaptic inhibition in the brain (15–17) are loaded with chloride and when K-Cl cotransport is simultaneously blocked by furosemide, a low $[Cl^-]_i$ is readjusted by activation of a chloride conductance with the physiologic and pharmacologic properties of ClC-2 (18). In hippocampal neurons, the expression of ClC-2 is correlated with the existence of a low $[Cl^-]_i$ and a hyperpolarizing GABAergic response. For example, CA1 and CA3 pyramidal neurons, which exhibit a hyperpolarizing inhibitory postsynaptic potential in response to activation of $GABA_A$ receptors, express high levels of ClC-2. In contrast, granule cells in the dentate gyrus that are depolarized by GABAergic stimulation do not express this channel (13–15,18). Furthermore, ClC-2 mRNA is upregulated postnatally in the rat hippocampus in parallel with the developmental switch of the GABA response from excitatory to inhibitory (19). Finally, experimental gene transfer of ClC-2 into dorsal root ganglion neurons that do not express this channel clamps E_{Cl} to the membrane potential and changes the GABA response of these cells from excitatory to inhibitory (20).

SCREENING FOR *CLCN2* MUTATIONS

We screened the *CLCN2* gene in index patients of 46 IGE families linked to chromosome 3q26 using single-strand conformation analysis (SSCA). Direct sequencing of aberrant bands revealed three heterozygous mutations that cosegregate with the IGE trait in three unrelated families, presenting with the typical IGE subtypes of EGMA, CAE, JAE, or JME, respectively (Fig. 20–1). None of these mutations was identified in a total of 360 control chromosomes. No further *CLCN2* mutations were found in the index patients by sequencing all coding exons and adjacent splice sites.

The leading IGE syndrome in family 1 was JME, which presented with frequent myoclonic and generalized tonic–clonic seizures (Fig. 20–1A). A single nucleotide insertion in bp-position 597 (597insG) was detected within exon 5 of individual IV:1. The 597insG mutation alters the normal translational reading frame and predicts a premature stop codon (M200fsX231) that severely truncates the protein.

Affected individuals of family 2 experienced rare GTCS on awakening (EGMA), except individual IV:4 who exclusively suffered from absence seizures (CAE) (Fig. 20–1B). An 11-bp deletion in intron 2, IVS2-14del11, was identified in this family, close to the splice acceptor site. This prompted us to search for alternative ClC-2 splice products. RT-PCR using primers located in exons 1 and 5 demonstrated the presence of a novel ClC-2 splice variant lacking exon 3 (delexon3). Skipping of exon 3 leads to an in-frame deletion of 44 amino acid residues (del74-117). Since this splice variant was also found in healthy controls, we established a quantitative competitive RT-PCR assay. In both tested patients carrying the IVS2-14del11 mutation the number of WT mRNA copies was reduced (60% and 66% of the average number found in two controls), whereas the number of delexon3 mRNA copies was increased eightfold. Accordingly, in the two control subjects, we found a delexon3:WT mRNA ratio of 5:95 and in patients carrying the intronic 11 bp deletion; the ratio was found to be 40:60.

In family 3, two affected individuals were diagnosed with JAE (Fig. 20–1C). We identified a single nucleotide exchange in bp-position 2144 (G2144A) predicting the substitution of glutamate for glycine at position 715 (G715E) located C-terminal to the last transmembrane helix.

A **Family 1: 597insG (M200fsX231)**

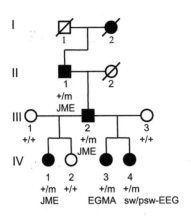

C **Family 3: G2144A (G715E)**

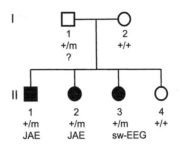

B **Family 2: IVS2-14del11 (del74-117)**

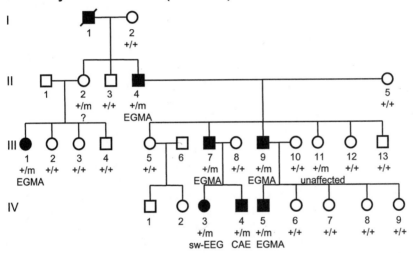

FIG. 20–1. Segregation analysis of three different *CLCN2* mutations in families with common IGE subtypes. Individuals carrying one of the mutations are denoted by +/m, whereas the absence of a mutation is denoted by +/+. Filled symbols represent individuals diagnosed with either JME, JAE, CAE, or EGMA. Three individuals were regarded as affected based on their pathologic EEG showing spontaneous generalized spike-wave and/or polyspike-wave discharges. **A:** Family 1 was ascertained through individual IV-1, who was diagnosed with JME. Segregation analyses showed perfect coseg-regation of the mutation and the affection status in this family. **B:** The index patient in family 2 (IV-4), experienced daily clusters of absence seizures during childhood (CAE). All affected family members carry the mutation, whereas the occurrence of the mutation in the unaffected individual III-11 indi-cates incomplete penetrance of this mutation. **C:** Family 3 was ascertained through the index patient II-2 whose epilepsy syndrome was classified as JAE. All affected family members were found to be heterozygous for the mutation.

PATCH CLAMP STUDIES OF EXPRESSED ClC-2 CHANNELS

To define the specific functional alterations caused by the two mutations and the splice vari-ant, we expressed WT and mutant human ClC-2 (hClC-2) channels in tsA201 cells and studied their functional properties using the whole-cell patch clamp technique. The channels were closed at positive potentials and activated slowly upon membrane hyperpolarization. The relative open probability depended not only on the membrane potential, but also on the intracellular chloride concentration ($[Cl^-]_i$). Decreasing $[Cl^-]_i$ resulted in a parallel shift of the activation curve to more hyperpolarized potentials. This particular dependence of gating on $[Cl^-]_i$ ensures that WT hClC-2 channels only open at potentials negative to the chloride reversal potential (E_{Cl}). WT hClC-2 channels thus constitute an exclusive efflux pathway for chloride ions, quite similar to that shown for native ClC-2 channels in a rat hippocampal slice preparation (18). The midpoint of activation changes in a logarithmic relationship with $[Cl^-]_i$. This behavior is compatible with a model in which the voltage dependence of channel opening arises, for the most part, from voltage-dependent binding of intracellular Cl^- (21).

The M200fsX231 mutation predicts a truncated channel protein lacking major sequence determinants of the ionic pore (22,23). As expected, heterologous expression of M200fsX231 mutant channels did not yield any detectable chloride current. However, as patients carrying this mutation are heterozygous, only a minority of ClC-2 channels will be homomeric mutant channels. ClC channels are dimeric proteins (23,24) and, therefore, channels consisting of one WT and one mutant subunit will represent the largest fraction of ClC-2 channels in heterozygous patients if the mutant is able to interact with the WT subunit. To study the functional properties of these heterodimeric channels, we expressed a concatameric construct that links one WT and one mutant allele in a single open reading frame, and, in addition, performed WT and mutant coexpression experiments. The concatamer was nonfunctional, and cotransfection with WT and mutant cDNAs in a 1:1 ratio resulted in a significantly smaller chloride current than that obtained from transfection of WT channels alone [peak current amplitude at -125 mV: 2.1 ± 0.4 nA, $n = 17$ (WT); 0.5 ± 0.3 nA, $n = 14$ (cotransfection of WT and M200fsX231), $p < 0.01$]. This dominant negative effect predicts a substantial reduction of functional ClC-2 channels in heterozygous patients.

The splice variant delexon3 predicts the deletion of helix B in the N-terminal part of the channel (del74-117) (23). Neither this mutant channel nor the concatameric proteins consisting of one WT and one del74-117 subunit were functional. Coexpression experiments revealed a dominant negative effect of del74-117 [peak current amplitude at -125 mV: 1.19 ± 0.46 nA, $n = 8$ (WT); 0.18 ± 0.05 nA, $n = 8$ (cotransfection of WT and del74-117), $p < 0.05$]. Nonfunctional homodimeric and heterodimeric mutant channels will cause a reduced number of functional ClC-2 channels in heterozygous patients carrying the IV2-14del11 mutation.

Our quantitative competitive RT-PCR assay predicted a lower expression of the del74-117 splice variant compared to that of WT. Therefore, a less pronounced effect of the IVS2-14del11 mutation on chloride current amplitudes is expected than for the 597insG mutation encoding the truncated mutant M200fsX231 (assuming a 50:50 expression of WT and mutant alleles in heterozygotes carrying the 597insG mutation). These findings are consistent with the less severe epileptic phenotype in family 2 compared to family 1.

In contrast to M200fsX231 and del74-117, G715E channels were functional, but exhibited an altered voltage-dependent gating. Neither current amplitudes (at -125 mV: WT: -2.8 ± 0.6 nA, $n = 7$; G715E: -2.8 ± 0.9 nA, $n = 6$), nor the voltage dependence of the relative open probability at a high $[Cl^-]_i$ differed significantly from WT channels. However, G715E channels displayed a distinct Cl^- dependence of channel opening. At $[Cl^-]_i$ of 4, 15, and 34 mM, the voltage dependence of activation of G715E channels was shifted to more positive potentials compared with WT channels ($p < 0.05$). As observed for WT channels, the $V_{0.5}$ of G715E channels changed in a logarithmic relationship with $[Cl^-]_i$. Assuming that the voltage dependence of channel opening arises, for the most part, from voltage-dependent binding of intracellular Cl^- (21), this dependence indicates that G715E channels exhibit a higher K_D (at 0 mV) and a steeper voltage dependence of Cl^- binding than WT channels. These alterations result in opening of mutant channels at less negative potentials than WT channels in a physiologic chloride range.

DISCUSSION

IGE is a frequent form of inherited human epilepsy. We have shown that mutations in *CLCN2*, a gene encoding the neuronal chloride channel ClC-2, can cause several common IGE subtypes. Our results demonstrate an important role of ClC-2 in the regulation of neuronal excitability in humans and explain the physiologic importance of the peculiar gating features of this ClC isoform.

WT hClC-2 channels exhibit unique gating features that allow them to act as a chloride efflux pathway well suited to establishing and maintaining a high transmembrane chloride gradient necessary for an inhibitory GABA response. Due to the coupling of channel activation to $[Cl^-]_i$ and the slow gating, they are closed under resting conditions as well as during action potentials or isolated excitatory postsynaptic potentials. WT hClC-2 channels open only with long-lasting changes of the transmembrane Cl^- gradient when E_{Cl} becomes more positive than the membrane potential, for example when $[Cl^-]_i$ is increased after intense GABAergic inhibition (16–18). As there is no voltage- and time-dependent inactivation, hClC-2 channels remain open and extrude chloride until E_{Cl} approaches the resting membrane potential.

A passive transport mechanism, such as a channel-mediated chloride flux, is, however, by itself unable to account for the large transmembrane chloride gradient of many neurons. Primary or secondary active processes are necessary to generate an E_{Cl} more negative than the resting membrane potential. It is well established that an outwardly directed coupled transport of K^+ and Cl^- by the neuron-specific KCC2 transporter plays a key role in generating the low $[Cl^-]_i$, which is essential for GABAergic synaptic inhibition (15,17,25–27). Under physiologic ionic conditions, K-Cl cotransport by KCC2 is driven by the transmembrane K^+ gradient and causes Cl^- extrusion near the resting potential (15,17). However, increases of $[K^+]_0$ affect the rate and the direction of this transport, i.e., at a low $[Cl^-]_i$ and a high $[K^+]_0$, KCC2 may operate in reverse and accumulate internal chloride (17,28,29). High-frequency activity of GABAer-

gic interneurons increases $[K^+]_0$ in the vicinity of hippocampal pyramidal neurons (30). This will cause impaired Cl^- extrusion or even inward K–Cl cotransport by KCC2 and aggravate the intracellular chloride accumulation in dendrites and somata of pyramidal neurons produced by Cl^- influx through GABA_A receptors (15–17,28,30). Under these conditions, ClC-2 appears to be the primary chloride extrusion pathway to reestablish a negative E_{Cl} crucial to the preservation of an inhibitory GABA response.

Our results in the heterologous expression system predict a substantial reduction of ClC-2 channel function in patients carrying the 597insG or the IVS2-14del11 mutation. This will impair chloride efflux and presumably result in an intracellular chloride accumulation. Consequently, the inhibitory GABA response will be reduced or might even become excitatory and thus cause epileptic seizures.

G715E hClC-2 channels express at levels similar to that of WT channels. Many functional properties are conserved in mutant channels and, therefore, no substantial alteration of chloride homeostasis is expected in the respective patients. The G715E mutation apparently causes neuronal hyperexcitability by a distinct mechanism, i.e., by conducting an enhanced chloride efflux. An efflux of negatively charged chloride ions can cause cell depolarization and thereby alter neuronal excitability. The particular chloride dependence of channel opening of WT hClC-2 channels presumably prevents substantial membrane depolarization by keeping the Cl^- efflux at a low level. In contrast, G715E channels open at less negative potentials due to their different chloride sensitivity. After intense synaptic activation causing membrane depolarization by activation of glutamate receptors and GABA_A receptor-mediated Cl^- influx, mutant channels will conduct an increased Cl^- outward current upon repolarization when E_{Cl} becomes more positive than the membrane potential. This abnormal conductance may thus induce recurrent membrane depolarization beyond action potential threshold, quite analogous to pacemaker channels in heart and brain. Such discharges can explain the initiation of epileptic seizures. The alteration of ClC-2 gating by G715E represents a gain-of-function and can explain why heterozygous patients are clinically affected.

According to our results, loss-of-function as well as gain-of-function *CLCN2* mutations can cause epilepsy in humans. In contrast, a recently reported *CLCN2* knock-out mouse model did not exhibit neuronal hyperexcitability or spontaneous seizures (31), suggesting a species-specific difference in the (patho-) physiologic role of this channel. Mouse models often differ from human diseases. For example, transgenic mice with either a knock-out or knock-in of the gene *CHRNA4*, expected to be an animal model for the human disease of autosomal dominant nocturnal frontal lobe epilepsy (ADNFLE) (6), were not reported to develop seizures (32,33). Compensatory mechanisms that are distinct in humans and mice as well as characteristic anatomic and physiologic properties may account for these phenotypic differences.

Coupling between ion permeation and gating is much tighter in ClC channels (34,35) than, for example, in voltage-gated cation channels. Our findings show that the specific effects of permeating anions on ClC gating are more than a biophysical peculiarity. They are key to the physiological function of certain ClC channels. A comparison between the two ClC isoforms expressed in excitable membranes, ClC-1 and ClC-2, illustrates the evolutionary optimization of chloride-dependent gating in ClC channels. Activation gating of ClC-1 is almost independent of $[Cl^-]_i$ (36), and this feature allows the muscle ClC isoform to provide the characteristic large resting conductance of the sarcolemma at a low $[Cl^-]_i$. A naturally occurring mutation that couples ClC-1 gating to $[Cl^-]_i$, substantially reduces the resting chloride conductance and causes myotonia congenita, a genetic disease characterized by muscle hyperexcitability (36). In contrast, ClC-2 regulates internal anion composition and does not contribute to the resting conductance. Gating of WT ClC-2 critically depends on $[Cl^-]_i$ and a genetically induced alteration of the chloride dependence of gating causes neuronal hyperexcitability.

Several genes encoding neuronal ion channels have been identified in monogenic subtypes of idiopathic epilepsy (5–7). *CLCN2* is

the first epilepsy gene, mutations of which can cause the whole spectrum of common IGE subtypes. Therefore, our results support the neurobiologic concept that the clinically different forms of this disease such as CAE, JAE, JME, and EGMA share an overlapping genetic predisposition (37). A different genetic background or unknown modifier genes might be responsible for the development of a predominant clinical phenotype, as was also observed in each of the families presented in this study.

Our findings provide further evidence for an important role of a genetically driven dysfunction of GABAergic synaptic inhibition in epileptogenesis which has often been discussed in the etiology of partial and generalized epilepsy. Recently, mutations within two different genes encoding $GABA_A$ receptor subunits have been identified in three families with GEFS$^+$ (in one family associated with frequent absence seizures) or JME (9,38,39). Attenuation of GABAergic synaptic inhibition might, therefore, evolve as a pathophysiologic concept for a significant proportion of idiopathic epilepsies. Further genetic and pathophysiologic studies of the inherited human epilepsies may open novel research directions, broaden our knowledge of the molecular mechanisms underlying epilepsy, and finally contribute to the discovery of better pharmacologic therapies.

REFERENCES

1. Hauser WA, Annegers JF, Rocca WA. Descriptive epidemiology of epilepsy: Contributions of population-based studies from Rochester, Minnesota. *Mayo Clin Proc* 1996;71:576–586.
2. Greenberg DA, Durner M, Delgado–Escueta AV. Evidence for multiple gene loci in the expression of the common generalized epilepsies. *Neurology* 1992;42:56–62.
3. Berkovic SF, Howell RA, Hay DA, et al. Epilepsies in twins: Genetics of the major epilepsy syndromes. *Ann Neurol* 1998;43:435–445.
4. Commission on Classification and Terminology of the International League Against Epilepsy. (1989). Proposal for revised classification of epilepsies and epileptic syndromes. *Epilepsia* 1989;30:389–399.
5. Steinlein OK, Noebels JL. Ion channels and epilepsy in man and mouse. *Curr Opin Genet Develop* 2000;10:286–291.
6. Berkovic SF, Scheffer IE. Genetics of the epilepsies. *Epilepsia* 2001;42[Suppl.5]:16–23.
7. Lerche H, Jurkat-Rott K, Lehmann-Horn F. Ion

channels and epilepsy. *Am J Med Genet* 2001;106:146–159.

8. Kalachikov S, Evgrafov O, Ross B, et al. Mutations in *LGI1* cause autosomal-dominant partial epilepsy with auditory features. *Nat Genet* 2002;30:335–341.

9. Cossette P, Liu L, Brisebois K, et al. Mutation of GABRA1 in an autosomal dominant form of juvenile myoclonic epilepsy. *Nat Genet* 2002;31:184–189.

10. Sander T, Schulz H, Saar K, et al. Genome search for susceptibility loci of common idiopathic generalized epilepsies. *Hum Mol Genet* 2000;9:1465–1472.

11. Thiemann A, Gründer S, Pusch M, et al. A chloride channel widely expressed in epithelial and non-epithelial cells. *Nature* 1992;365:57–60.

12. Cid LP, Montrose-Rafizadeh C, Smith DI, et al. Cloning of a putative human voltage-gated chloride channel (ClC-2) cDNA widely expressed in human tissues. *Hum Mol Genet* 1995;4:407–413.

13. Smith RL, Clayton GH, Wilcox CL, et al. Differential expression of an inwardly rectifying chloride conductance in rat brain neurons: A potential mechanism for cell-specific modulation of postsynaptic inhibition. *J Neurosci* 1995;15:4057–4067.

14. Sik A, Smith RL, Freund TF. Distribution of chloride channel-2-immunoreactive neuronal and astrocytic processes in the hippocampus. *Neuroscience* 2000;101:51–65.

15. Misgeld U, Deisz RA, Dodt HU, et al. The role of chloride transport in postsynaptic inhibition of hippocampal neurons. *Science* 1986;232:1413–1415.

16. Thompson SM, Gähwiller BH. Activity-dependent disinhibition I: Repetitive stimulation reduces IPSP driving force and conductance in the hippocampus in vitro. *J Neurophysiol* 1989;61:501–511.

17. Thompson SM, Gähwiller BH. Activity-dependent disinhibition II: Effects of extracellular potassium, furosemide, and membrane potential on E_{Cl} in hippocampal CA3 neurons. *J Neurophysiol* 1989;61:512–523.

18. Staley KJ. The role of an inwardly rectifying chloride conductance in postsynaptic inhibition. *J Neurophysiol* 1994;72:273–284.

19. Mladinic M, Becchetti A, Didelon F, et al. Low expression of the ClC-2 chloride channel during postnatal development: A mechanism for the paradoxical depolarizing action of GABA and glycine in the hippocampus. *Proc R Soc London B Biol Sci* 1999;266:1207–1213.

20. Staley KJ, Smith R, Schaack J, et al. Alteration of GABAA receptor function following gene transfer of the ClC-2 chloride channel. *Neuron* 1996;17:543–551.

21. Cui J, Cox DH, Aldrich RW. Intrinsic voltage dependence and Ca^{2+} regulation of mslo large conductance Ca^{2+}-activated K^+ channels. *J Gen Physiol* 1997;109:647–673.

21a. Fahlke C, Knittle T, Gurnett CA, et al. Subunit stoichiometry of human muscle chloride channels. *J Gen Physiol* 1997;109:93–104.

22. Fahlke C, Yu HT, Beck CL, et al. Pore-forming segments in voltage-gated chloride channels. *Nature* 1997;390:529–532.

23. Dutzler R, Campbell EB, Cadene M, et al. X-ray structure of a ClC chloride channel at 3.0 A reveals the molecular basis of anion selectivity. *Nature* 2002;415:287–294.

24. Miller C. Open-state substructure of single chloride channels from Torpedo electroplax. *Phil Trans R Soc London B Biol Sci* 1982;299:401–411.

25. Rivera C, Voipio J, Payne JA, et al. The K^+/Cl^- cotransporter KCC2 renders GABA hyperpolarizing during neuronal maturation. *Nature* 1999;397:251–255.

26. Hübner CA, Stein V, Hermans-Borgmeyer I, et al. Disruption of KCC2 reveals an essential role of K-Cl cotransport already in early synaptic inhibition. *Neuron* 2001;30:515–524.

27. Woo NS, Lu JER, McCellan R, et al. Hyperexcitability and epilepsy associated with disruption of the mouse neuronal-specific K-Cl cotransporter gene. *Hippocampus* 2002;12:258–268.

28. Payne JA. Functional characterization of the neuronal-specific K-Cl cotransporter: implications for $[K^+]_o$ regulation. *Am J Physiol* 1997;273:C1516–1525.

29. DeFazio RA, Keros S, Quick MW, et al. Potassium-coupled chloride cotransport controls intracellular chloride in rat neocortical pyramidal neurons. *J Neurosci* 2000;20:8069–8076.

30. Kaila K, Lamsa K, Smirnov S, et al. Long-lasting GABA-mediated depolarization evoked by high-frequency stimulation in pyramidal neurons of rat hippocampal slice is attributable to a network-driven, bicarbonate-dependent K^+ transient. *J Neurosci* 1997;17:7662–7672.

31. Bösl MR, Stein V, Hübner C, et al. Male germ cells and photoreceptors, both dependent on close cell-cell interactions, degenerate upon ClC-2 Cl(-) channel disruption. *EMBO J* 2001;20:1289–1299.

32. Ross SA, Wong JY, Clifford JJ, et al. Phenotypic characterization of an alpha 4 neuronal nicotinic acetylcholine receptor subunit knock-out mouse. *J Neurosci* 2000;20:6431–6441.

32a. Ma D, Zerangue N, Lin YF, et al. Role of ER export signals in controlling surface potassium channel numbers. *Science* 2001;291:316–319.

33. Labarca C, Schwarz J, Desphande P, et al. Point mutant mice with hypersensitive alpha 4 nicotinic receptors show dopaminergic deficits and increased anxiety. *Proc Natl Acad Sci USA* 2001;98:2786–2791.

34. Richard EA, Miller C. Steady-state coupling of ion-channel conformations to a transmembrane ion gradient. *Science* 1990;247:1208–1210.

35. Pusch M, Ludewig U, Rehfeldt A, et al. Gating of the voltage-dependent chloride channel ClC-0 by the permeant anion. *Nature* 1995;373:527–531.

36. Fahlke C, Rüdel R, Mitrovic N, et al. An aspartic acid residue important for voltage-dependent gating of human muscle chloride channels. *Neuron* 1995;15:463–472.

37. Reutens DC, Berkovic. Idiopathic generalized epilepsy of adolescence: Are the syndromes clinically distinct? *Neurology* 1995;45:1469–1476.

38. Baulac S, Huberfeld G, Gourfinkel-An I, et al. First genetic evidence of GABA(A) receptor dysfunction in epilepsy: A mutation in the gamma2-subunit gene. *Nat Genet* 2001;28:46–48.

39. Wallace RH, Marini C, Petrou S, et al. Mutant GABA(A) receptor gamma2-subunit in childhood absence epilepsy and febrile seizures. *Nat Genet* 2001;28:49–52.

21

Autosomal Dominant Cortical Myoclonus and Epilepsy (ADCME) with Linkage to Chromosome 2p11.1-q12.2

Renzo Guerrini,* Lucio Parmeggiani,* Carla Marini,* Paola Brovedani,* and Paolo Bonanni*

*Epilepsy, Neurophysiology and Neurogenetics Unit, Department of Child Neurology and Psychiatry, University of Pisa and Research Institute 'Stella Maris' Foundation, Pisa, Italy

INTRODUCTION

Autosomal dominant cortical myoclonus and epilepsy (ADCME) is a recently characterized nonprogressive familial syndrome that combines rhythmic cortical reflex myoclonus with focal and generalized seizures (1). In this chapter, we outline the clinical and neurophysiologic features that characterize ADCME and help to differentiate it from other conditions with similar features, such as familial adult myoclonic epilepsy (FAME).

ADCME patients present with a complex of symptoms forming a homogeneous syndromic core (Fig. 21–1), including semicontinuous rhythmic distal jerking (also termed cortical tremor), which is a particular form of cortical reflex myoclonus, generalized tonic-clonic seizures (GTCSs) that are occasionally preceded by generalized myoclonic jerks, and both generalized and focal electroencephalogram (EEG) abnormalities. Age at onset of cortical tremor and of GTCSs overlap in a given individual but vary between individuals, ranging from 12 to 50 years (1). Some patients also present with focal, intractable seizures. The pattern of inheritance is autosomal dominant with high penetrance and linkage to chromosome 2p11.1-q12.2.

CLINICAL AND GENETIC FEATURES

Clinical Neurophysiology of Cortical Tremor

The distal jerking observed in patients with ADCME has the neurophysiologic characteristics of cortical tremor (2,3). A stereotyped pattern of rhythmic, involuntary hand movements is evident during isometric muscle contraction and is accompanied by rhythmic EMG bursts at 8 to 15 Hz, involving synchronously agonist and antagonist muscles of the forearms (Fig. 21–2). Involvement of more proximal as well as facial muscles, especially the eyelids, is possible. Backaveraging and frequency analysis indicate that EEG activity is coherent with electromyography (EMG) at the frequency of the myoclonus and that time-locked EEG activity precedes EMG bursts (1,4) (Fig. 21–2). The C-reflex at rest is enhanced, somatosensory-evoked potentials (SEPs) are of high amplitude (Fig. 21–3), motor threshold at rest, obtained by transcranial magnetic stimulation, is reduced, and the silent period following motor-evoked potentials (MEP) is shortened (Fig. 21–2). Clinical and neurophysiologic characteristics suggest that myoclonic activity, in addition to a high rhythmicity, also has propensity for intra- and interhemispheric cortical spread. Intermittent photic stimulation (IPS)

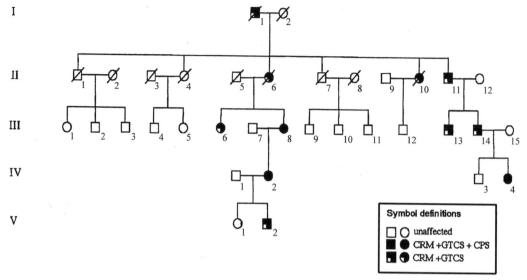

FIG. 21–1. ADCME family pedigree. CPS, complex partial seizures; CRM, cortical reflex myoclonus; GTCS, generalized tonic–clonic seizures.

at low rates evokes single occipital spikes in response to each flash and pattern-visual-evoked potentials (P-VEPs) are of very high amplitude (Fig. 21–3).

These combined findings suggest widespread cortical hyperexcitability with deficits in inhibitory cortical mechanisms (5–9). The prime origin of rhythmic motor cortex excitation is difficult to demonstrate. Rhythmic generators within cortical layers IV and V (10) might play a role. Alternatively, cortical neurons could be driven by a subcortical generator (3).

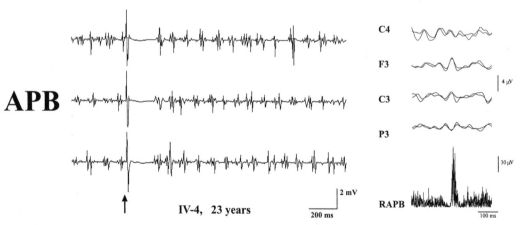

FIG. 21–2. Left: Rhythmic EMG bursts at a frequency of around 15 Hz are observed during slight muscle contraction. Transcranial magnetic stimulation administered at the time, indicated by the arrow, is followed after around 20 ms by a motor-evoked potential (MEP) that is followed by a post-MEP silent period. Rhythmic EMG bursts reappear soon after the post-MEP silent period, supporting a cortical hyperexcitability. The three traces represent three different replications. **Right:** Backaveraging from the onset of 100 rhythmic EMG bursts. A positive–negative potential, recognizable over the contralateral frontocentral electrodes, precedes the jerk by about 15–20 ms. Two traces are overlapped to show data reproducibility. RAPB, right abductor pollicis brevis.

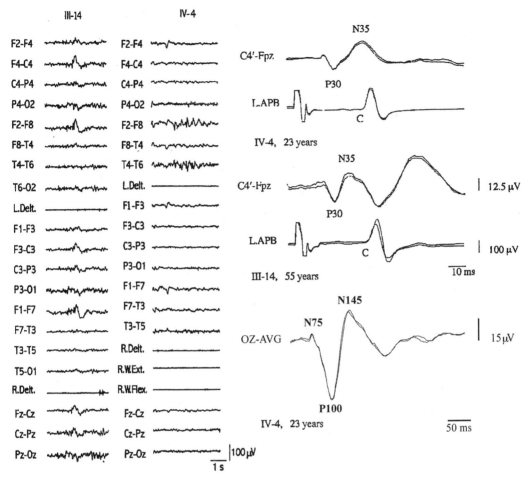

FIG. 21–3. Left: Interictal EEG–EMG recordings during relaxed wakefulness in Patients IV-4 and III-14. Interictal discharges show equipotentiality over the right frontotemporal leads. **Right, top and middle:** Cortical SEPs to electrical stimulation of the left median nerve at the wrist are recorded in the same patients whose EEG recordings are presented on the left. An enlarged N20–P30–N35 complex on right centroparietal region is followed by C-reflex in the left abductor pollicis brevis. The shock-C-reflex latency is ~45 msec. **Right, lower:** VEP in response to checkerboard stimulation in patient IV-4. An enlarged N75-P100-N145 complex is recorded. APB, abductor pollicis brevis; C, cortical reflex; Delt., deltoid muscle; Ext, extensor; Flex, flexor; L, left; R, right; W, wrist.

The corticomuscular loop underlying cortical reflex myoclonus in a highly excitable sensorimotor cortex may also play a role. Each afferent volley generated by a myoclonic jerk might, in turn, facilitate an efferent volley that sustains an ensuing myoclonic jerk, thereby sustaining a rhythmic afferent–efferent mechanism.

Cortical tremor may be observed in different clinical settings, as a consequence of multiple etiologic factors enhancing motor cortex excitability. In addition to FAME (2,9–12), it may also be observed in other genetic disorders, including a form of familial mental retardation and generalized epilepsy (13), Angelman syndrome (7), Rett syndrome (*personal observation*), and progressive myoclonus epilepsies (PME) (3), in which it may be accompanied by generalized as well as focal seizures. In addition, cortical tremor has been observed in association with focal motor seizures after ischemic brain lesions involving the sensorimotor cortex (16,17), in the presence of cortical tubers in tuberous sclerosis (18) or, as an isolated symptom after surgical removal of a frontal lobe meningioma (19), and in patients with no other neurologic abnormality (3). These observations indicate that cortical tremor is a relatively common neurologic manifestation and is often associated with epilepsy of either symptomatic or genetic etiology. It is, therefore, likely that the motor cortex has an intrinsic propensity for rhythmicity that is uncovered by different etiologic conditions having in common the ability to lower cortical inhibition, either regionally or more diffusely.

SEIZURES

All patients have rare GTCSs that are not preceded by a warning. Patients with focal seizures also have generalized seizures preceded by focal symptoms, although propensity to generalization is variable. Focal seizures are characterized by motionless stare with unresponsiveness, preceded by an epigastric aura or a nonspecific warning. These seizure patterns cannot be attributed with certainty to any specific lobar origin. A frontotemporal origin is most likely and is, in part, supported by the presence of frontal and anterior temporal interictal EEG spikes (Fig. 21–3) in all patients with focal seizures and by the finding that focal seizures are accompanied by lateralized temporal or frontotemporal ictal EEG activity (1).

However, since frontotemporal interictal EEG abnormalities are present in all patients, including those with seemingly primary GTCSs, it is also possible that pronounced cortical hyperexcitability and propensity to spread, may facilitate rapid seizure generalization, which obscurates the focal nature of epilepsy.

Since ADCME had a variable severity, it is very difficult to establish which antiepileptic drugs (AEDs) were more effective. Severity of the disorder seems to be scarcely influenced by drugs, as demonstrated by the benign seizure outcome in patients who were never treated and by drug resistance in others. In general, drugs associating antiepileptic and antimyoclonic properties such as valproic acid (VPA), phenobarbitone,

and benzodiazepines were most effective, while carbamazepine (CBZ) caused worsening of myoclonus.

NEUROPSYCHOLOGY

Patients with well-controlled seizures had low average intelligence, with normal verbal memory and difficulties in some nonverbal memory tasks. Estimated premorbid verbal intelligence was in line with the verbal intelligent quotient (VIQ), as determined using the Wechsler Adult Intelligence Scale (WAIS). Less preserved nonverbal memory in these patients, as well as the lower performance abilities on the WAIS, both requiring visuomotor integration, may be tied to continuous myoclonus. Patients with focal seizures had borderline intelligence to moderate mental retardation and global memory deficits, the latter occurring in those with intractable seizures. Premorbid estimate of verbal intelligence, using the TIB-Brief Intelligence Test (20), the Italian version of the National Adult Reading Test (NART) (21) suggested cognitive deterioration in patients with persistently intractable focal seizures, possibly as a consequence of the detrimental effect on cognition of uncontrolled seizures. On the whole, neuropsychologic evidence indicates that low IQ may not be primarily genetically determined, but may result as a consequence of long-lasting severe epilepsy. Furthermore, the memory impairment observed in patients with focal seizures may not be tied directly to selective temporal lobe dysfunction, as performance was not impaired across all long-term memory tasks and in some tasks memory performance was not compromised more than general intelligence.

GENETICS

Genome-wide linkage analysis in the index Italian family identified a critical region spanning 12.4 cM between markers D2S2161 and D2S1897 in 2p11.1-q12.2, with a maximum two-point LOD score of 3.46 at θ 0.0 for marker D2S2175. Multipoint LOD score values, reaching 3.74 around D2S2175, localize the ADCME gene to the centromeric region of chromosome 2.

Considering the putative function of the genes mapping within the 12 cM critical region of this form of epilepsy, we identified the following candidates: DREAM, downstream regulatory element antagonist modulator (22); calsenilin-KchIP3, a calcium-binding protein, which regulates voltage-gated potassium currents, and hence neuronal excitability, in response to changes in intracellular calcium (23); DREAM and calsenilin are highly homologous and are predominantly expressed in brain; the neuronal PAS domain protein 2, NPAS2 (24), a neuronal transcription factor, G protein-coupled receptor 45, GPCR45 (25), an integral membrane protein expressed in basal forebrain, caudate, and frontal cortex. In addition, several partial transcripts encoding for potential candidate genes map to the ADCME locus. However, the large chromosomal area identified by the ADCME locus renders a positional cloning strategy quite unfeasible, while new ADCME pedigrees will contribute new recombination events to narrow the candidate region.

ral EEG abnormalities and some individuals also have focal seizures starting around the same age as the other manifestations, which are either intractable or, alternatively, go into remission after several years. Linkage analysis in FAME indicates that the disease is linked to chromosome 8q23.3-q24 locus in Japanase families (12,13). The European families with a similar phenotype did not link to the same locus (29,30). In ADCME, linkage analysis identified a critical region in chromosome 2p11.1-q12.2. The two Italian families with FAME, described by de Falco and colleagues (30), showed linkage to chromosome 2p11.1-q12.2, suggesting a possible allelism with ADCME.

ADCME may be misdiagnosed as juvenile myoclonic epilepsy (JME) (31) since GTCS and proximal jerks are typical of both conditions. Focal seizures without automatisms observed in some patients with ADCME are easily confused with absence seizures. Cortical tremor is interpreted as simple tremor, a relatively frequent side effect of VPA treatment (32).

DIFFERENTIAL DIAGNOSIS

The clinical picture of ADCME shares some features with (benign) familial autosomal dominant myoclonus (FAME) (12–13), which is generally recognized as a form of autosomal dominant generalized epilepsy, with linkage on chromosome 8q23.3-q24.

FAME has been described in several families of Japanese (11–16,26–28) or European origin (29,30). Affected patients have homogeneous characteristics: (a) autosomal dominant inheritance; (b) adult onset (mean age 38 years, range: 19 to 73); (c) nonprogressive course; (d) distal, rhythmic myoclonus, enhanced during posture maintenance; (e) rare, apparently generalized seizures often preceded by worsening of myoclonus; (f) absence of other neurologic signs; (g) generalized interictal spike-and-wave discharges; (h) photoparoxysmal response; (i) giant SEPs; (j) hyperexcitability of the C-reflex; and (k) cortical EEG potential time-locked to the jerks.

ADCME patients present a similar clinical picture, but have, in addition, focal frontotempo-

CONCLUSION

Cooccurrence of focal and apparently generalized seizures has been reported on several occasions in familial epilepsy syndromes (33–35). Patients with generalized seizures only have sometimes been excluded from studies aimed at characterizing focal epilepsy phenotypes for the purpose of genotype analysis (35). However, studies on genetic epilepsies indicate that the same gene may be expressed to a different degree and with different regional predominance in different individuals. For example, patients with GEFS$^+$ may have carrier relatives with temporal lobe epilepsy (33). Some individuals with GEFS$^+$ may also present with both primary generalized and focal electroclinical features (34). In focal epilepsy with variable foci, different brain areas are involved in the same family (36).

Two phenotypes coexisted in ADCME: a core clinical syndrome, very similar to FAME, including generalized seizures and rhythmic myoclonus and a more severe phenotype that includes, in addition, difficult to treat focal seizures. We hypothesize that the responsible gene, in a unigenic model of epilepsy, causes cortical hyperexcitability that, although widespread, particularly involves frontotemporal circuits. The implication is that the genetic defect can result in regionally predominant enhancement of cortical excitability that uncovers intrinsic rhythmicity in the motor cortex and causes myoclonus and focal seizures. Spread of regional epileptogenesis may, in turn, underlie generalized seizure activity.

The motor cortex has a physiologic tendency to oscillatory discharges in the μ frequency range. The μ rhythm is present when a healthy subject is at rest and is attenuated (desynchronized) on tactile stimulation or voluntary muscle contraction (37). Nevertheless, a component of cortical activity persists in the same frequency band during isometric contraction and is coherent with EMG (38,39). It is this component that we hypothesize was exaggerated in patients with cortical tremor, as abnormal corticomuscular rhythmicity occurred in the same frequency band and under similar circumstances of isometric contraction, such as holding the arms outstretched. On the other hand, physiologic motor circuits leading to rhythmicities in the γ band (40) seem essentially spared by this condition, unlike many other myoclonic syndromes (41).

REFERENCES

1. Guerrini R, Bonanni P, Patrignani A, et al. Autosomal dominant cortical myoclonus and epilepsy (ADCME) with complex partial and generalized seizures: A newly recognized epilepsy syndrome with linkage to chromosome 2p11.1-q12.2. *Brain* 2001;124:2459–2475.
2. Ikeda A, Kakigi R, Funai N, et al. Cortical tremor: A variant of cortical reflex myoclonus. *Neurology* 1990; 40:1561–1565.
3. Toro C, Pascual-Leone A, Deuschl G, et al. Cortical tremor: A common manifestation of cortical myoclonus. *Neurology* 1993;43:2346–2353.
4. Grosse P, Guerrini R, Parmeggiani L, et al. Abnormal corticomuscular and intermuscular coupling in high-frequency rhythmic myoclonus. *Brain* 2003;126:326–342.
5. Brown P, Day BL, Rothwell JC, et al. Intrahemispheric and interhemispheric spread of cerebral cortical myoclonic activity and its relevance to epilepsy. *Brain* 1991;114:2333–2351.
6. Uozumi T, Yoichi I, Tsuji S, et al. Inhibitory period following motor potentials evoked by magnetic cortical stimulation. *Electroencephalogr Clin Neurophysiol* 1992;85:273–279.
7. Brown P, Ridding MC, Werhahn KJ, et al. Abnormalities of the balance between inhibition and excitation in the motor cortex of patients with cortical myoclonus. *Brain* 1996;119:309–318.
8. Guerrini R, DeLorey T, Bonanni P, et al. Cortical myoclonus in Angelman syndrome. *Ann Neurol* 1996;40:39–48.
9. Cicinelli P, Mattia D, Spanedda F, et al. Transcranial magnetic stimulation reveals an interhemispheric asymmetry of cortical inhibition in focal epilepsy. *Neuroreport* 2000;11:701–707.
10. Connors BW, Amitai Y. Making waves in the neocortex. *Neuron* 1997;18:347–349.
11. Yasuda T. Benign adult familial myoclous epilepsy (BAFME). *Kawasaki Med J* 1991;17:1–13.
12. Plaster NM, Uyama E, Uchino M, et al. Genetic localization of the familial adult myoclonic epilepsy (FAME) gene to chromosome 8q24. *Neurology* 1999;53:1180–1183.
13. Mikami M, Yasuda T, Terao A, et al. Localization of a gene for benign adult familial myoclonic epilepsy to chromosome 8q23.3-q24.1. *Am J Hum Genet* 1999;65:745–751.
14. Terada K, Ikeda A, Mima T, et al. Familial cortical tremor as a unique form of cortical reflex myoclonus. *Mov Disord* 1997;12:370–377.
15. Elia M, Musumeci S, Ferri R, et al. Familial cortical tremor, epilepsy, and mental retardation. *Arch Neurol* 1998;55:1569–1573.
16. Schulze-Bonhage A, Ferbert A. Cortical action tremor and focal motor seizures after parietal infarction. *Mov Disord* 1998;13:356–358.
17. Wang HC, Hsu WC, Brown P. Cortical tremor secondary to a frontal cortical lesion. *Mov Disord* 1999;14:370–374.
18. Guerrini R, Bonanni P, Rothwell J, et al. Myoclonus and Epilepsy. In: Guerrini R, Aicardi J, Andermann F, Hallett M, eds. *Epilepsy and movement disorders*. Cambridge: Cambridge University Press, 2002:165–210.
19. Botzel K, Werhahn KS. A case of myoclonic cortical tremor after extirpation of a parietal meningioma. *Mov Disord* 1999;16:1033–1035.
20. Sartori G, Colombo L, Vallar G, et al. TIB- Test di Intelligenza Breve per la valutazione del quoziente intellettivo attuale e pre-morboso [TIB- Brief Test of Intelligence for assessing present and pre-morbid intelligence]. Professione di Psicologo. Giornale dell'Ordine degli Psicologi 1995;4.
21. Nelson HE, O'Connell. A Dementia: The estimation of pre-morbid intelligence levels using the new adult reading test. *Cortex* 1978;14:234–44.
22. Carrion AM, Link WA, Ledo F, et al. DREAM is a Ca2+-regulated transcriptional repressor. *Nature* 1999;398: 80–84.
23. An WF, Bowlby MR, Betty M, et al. Modulation of A-type potassium channels by a family of calcium sensors. *Nature* 2000;403:553–556.
24. Zhou YD, Barnard M, Tian H, et al. Molecular characterization of two mammalian bHLH-PAS domain proteins selectively expressed in the central nervous system. *Proc Natl Acad Sci* USA 1997;94:713–718.
25. Marchese A, Sawzdargo M, Nguyen T, et al. Discovery of three novel orphan G-protein-coupled receptors. *Genomics* 1999;56:12–21.
26. Kuwano A, Takakubo F, Morimoto Y, et al. Benign adult familial myoclonus epilepsy (BAFME): an

autosomal dominat form not linked to the dentatorubral pallidoluysian atrophy (DRPLA) gene. *J Med Genet* 1996;33:80–81.

27. Okino S. Familial benign myoclonus epilepsy of adult onset: a previously unrecognized myoclonic disorder. *J Neurol Sci* 1997;145:113–118.

28. Okuma Y, Shimo Y, Shimura H, et al. Familial cortical tremor with epilepsy: an under-recognized familial tremor. *Clin Neurol Neurosurg* 1998;100: 75–78.

29. Labauge P, Amer LO, Simonetta-Moreau M, et al. Absence of linkage to 8q24 in a European family with familial adult myoclonic epilepsy (FAME). *Neurology* 2002;58:941–944.

30. de Falco FA, Striano P, De Falco A, et al. Benign adult familial myoclonic epilepsy: Genetic heterogeneity and allelism with ADCME. *Neurology* 2003;60:1381–1385.

31. Panayiotopoulos CP, Obeid T, Tahan AR. Juvenile myoclonic epilepsy: A 5-year prospective study. *Epilepsia* 1994;35:285–296.

32. Karas BJ, Wilder BJ, Hammond EJ, et al. Valproate tremors. *Neurology* 1982;32:428–432.

33. Singh R, Schiffer IE, Crossland F, Berkovic SF. Generalized epilepsy with febrile seizures plus (GEFS⁺): a common, childhood onset, genetic epilepsy syndrome. *Ann Neurol* 1999;45:75–81.

34. Baulac S, Gourfinkel-An I, Picard F, et al. A second locus for familial generalized epilepsy with febrile seizures plus maps to chromosome 2q21-q33. *Am J Hum Genet* 1999;65:1078–1085.

35. Picard F, Baulac S, Kahane P, et al. Dominant partial epilepsies. A clinical, electrophysiological and genetic study of 19 European families. *Brain* 2000;123:1247–1262.

36. Scheffer IE, Phillips HA, O'Brien CE, et al. Familial partial epilepsy with variable foci: A new partial epilepsy syndrome with suggestion of linkage to chromosome 2. *Ann Neurol* 1998;44:890–899.

37. Tiihonen J, Kajola M, Hari R. Magnetic mu rhythm in man. *Neuroscience* 1989;32:793–800.

38. Conway BA, Halliday DM, Farmer SF, et al. Synchronisation between motor cortex and spinal motoneuronal pool during the performance of a maintained motor task in man. *J Physiol* 1995;489:917–924.

39. Salenius S, Portin K, Kajola M, et al. Cortical control of human motoneuron firing during isometric contraction. *J Neurophysiol* 1997;77:3401–3405.

40. Brown P, Salenius S, Rothwell JC, et al. The cortical correlate of the Piper rhythm in man. *J Neurophysiol* 1998;80:2911–2917.

41. Brown P, Farmer SF, Halliday DM, et al. Coherent cortical and muscle discharge in cortical myoclonus. *Brain* 1999;122:461–472.

22

Familial Adult Myoclonic Epilepsy (FAME)

Eiichiro Uyama,* Ying-Hui Fu,† and Louis J. Ptácek†,‡

*Department of Neurology, Kumamoto University School of Medicine, Kumamoto, Japan;
†Department of Neurology, University of California San Francisco, San Francisco, California;
‡Howard Hughes Medical Institute, San Francisco, California

INTRODUCTION

The identification and characterization of genes responsible for monogenic inherited epilepsies is an exciting area of epilepsy research (1–4). It is critical for understanding the molecular basis of neuronal hyperexcitability, the etiology of epilepsy, and myoclonic jerks, and, ultimately, the development of new therapeutic agents (3). Ion channels are critical for the regulation of excitability in the central nervous system. In fact, mutations in ion channel encoding genes have been identified in a variety of epileptic disorders (2–4).

Several epilepsy disorders are characterized by combinations of symptoms such as focal or generalized and myoclonic seizures (1,2). These disorders include severe myoclonic epilepsy of infancy (SMEI) (2), progressive myoclonic epilepsy (PME) (5), juvenile myoclonic epilepsy (JME) (6), and familial adult myoclonic epilepsy (FAME) (7–9). FAME is clinically characterized by autosomal dominant inheritance, adult-onset cortical myoclonic tremor, and infrequent epileptic seizures despite constant paroxysmal discharges on electroencephalogram (EEG). JME differs from FAME with regard to age of onset (early adolescent), genetic transmission (complex), and prevalence of myoclonic jerks upon awakening.

Myoclonic epilepsy is a defining symptom in all PME syndromes, in which myoclonic seizures

seem to be generated secondarily due to neuronal degeneration rather than being a primary disorder of neuronal excitability. In contrast, myoclonic jerks in patients with JME or FAME seem to be generated from a functional abnormality of membrane excitability in neurons. In comparison with JME that is a common form of epilepsy, FAME is thought of as a rare form restricted to Japan. However, non-Japanese FAME or FAME-like families have been recently discovered around the world (10–16) and data now supports locus heterogeneity for FAME.

HISTORY

In 1984, Uyama examined the proband in Family 1 (Fig. 22–1) who showed postural finger tremulous movement mixed with myoclonic jerks from the age of 40. She had two episodes of epileptic seizures in her life. The family, originating in Kumamoto in southern Japan, included ten other patients through three generations.

Their interictal EEG always displayed epileptic discharges and cortical reflex myoclonus was implicated on somatosensory-evoked potentials (SEP). None of them revealed mental deterioration, cerebellar ataxia, progressive course, or abnormal findings on brain computed tomography (CT)/magnetic resonance imaging (MRI). Because of its unrecognized phenotype at that time, Uyama reported the details at the

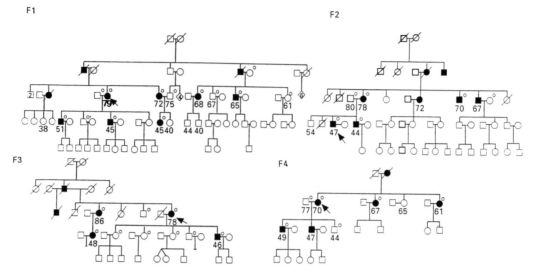

FIG. 22–1. The pedigrees of four FAME families in Kumamoto. Numbers under symbols are ages at examination. An arrow indicates the proband. The filled symbols are affected individuals. Persons with a line over their symbols are deceased. Small circles in the right upper side are subjects studied with DNA analyses.

26th Annual Meeting of Japanese Neurological Society in 1985 (7). By 1990, another three unrelated families were identified (Fig. 22–1).

Independently, Inazuki et al. (17) collected 12 similar families including 40 patients from Niigata in northern Japan. Based on clinicopathologic features, they proposed the new entity "familial essential myoclonus and epilepsy (FEME)" in a Japanese journal. Coincidentally, Ikeda et al. (18) found two familial cases in Kyoto who had similar features to Family 1. By electrophysiologic analysis, they clarified the nature of tremulous movement and defined it as "cortical tremor." Later, they presented similar families as "familial cortical myoclonic tremor (FCMT)" (19).

In another independent study, Yasuda found two Japanese families in Okayama that also shared similar features to those in Family 1. Based on electrophysiologic studies and incomplete review, excluding the report of Family 1, and one decisive articles (20), he proposed another term, "benign adult familial myoclonic epilepsy (BAFME)" instead of FEME (22). One of these BAFME families had been described as progressive myoclonic epilepsy (PME) in 1983 (23). Kuwano et al. (24) verified that four

Kumamoto families and one BAFME family in Okayama had neither DRPLA mutation nor linkage with γ-aminobutyric acid (GABA) receptor subunits, GABARβ1, GABARβ3, and GABARα6.

Regarding long-term follow-up, Uyama found that the degree of myoclonic jerks in patients increased with age but there was no degenerative components to the phenotype. However the symptoms did not resolve completely as in other benign epilepsies. He then presented the details of four families at the 121st Annual Meeting of ANA in 1996 to be established as a new phenotype of autosomal dominant myoclonic epilepsy of "familial adult myoclonic epilepsy (FAME)" (8). In 1996, efforts to map the FAME gene began with linkage analysis and the FAME locus on chromosome 8q was identified (9). In 1997, Okuma et al. (25,26) reported a similar small family as "familial cortical tremor with epilepsy (FCTE) (Table 22–1)."

Thus, manifestations of previously reported Japanese families with FEME, BAFME, FCMT, and FCTE are identical to FAME. Therefore, we will henceforth refer to all of these as FAME both for the term's simplicity and its concise description of the key elements of the diagnosis.

TABLE 22–1. *Myoclonic epilepsy gene loci with genes identified (July 2003)*

Onset	Disorders	Gene locus	Gene
Infancy	Severe myoclonic epilepsy of infancy (SMEI)	2q24	SCN1A
		5q31.1	GABRG2
Childhood	Childhood absence epilepsy type 1 (ECA1), third form	8q24	Unknown
	Dentatorubral-pallidoluysian atrophy (DRPLA)	12p13.31	DRPLA
Adolescence	Juvenile myoclonic epilepsy (JME)	5q34–q35	GABRA1
		2q22–q23	CACNB4
	Juvenile absence epilepsy (JAE) or JME or IGE	3q26	CLCN2
Adult	Familial adult myoclonic epilepsy (FAME)	8q24	Unknown
	Autosomal dominant cortical myoclonus and epilepsy (ADCME)	2p11.1-q12.2	Unknown

SCN1A, sodium channel neuronal type 1 α-subunit; *GABRG2*, gamma-aminobutyric acid receptor γ-2; *GABRA1*, gamma-aminobutyric acid receptor α-1; *CACNB4*, calcium channel-subunit 4; IGE, ideopathic generalized epilepsy.

EPIDEMIOLOGIC ASPECTS

Nationwide epidemiologic investigation of FAME has not been performed in Japan. The prevalence of FAME is uncertain, although many affected families have been identified throughout Japan (21,27–33). The data from the literature (including abstracts of meetings) indicate at least 60 FAME families, including 400 patients, have been accumulated (Fig. 22–2). To date, we have identified 7 FAME families including 54 patients in the Kumamoto Prefecture with a population of ~1.9 million inhabitants. Our estimate indicates a prevalence of ~1: 35,000.

CLINICAL CHARACTERISTICS

As suggested by cardinal features of 14 extensively evaluated patients from our four families (Table 22–2), clinical characteristics of FAME may be summarized as follows: (a) posture myoclonic jerks of the extremities accompanying fine finger tremulous movements (Fig. 22–3) become evident, usually after the third or fourth decade of life as the first symptom; (b) the occurrence of generalized tonic–clonic seizures (GTCS) is infrequent; (c) interictal EEG shows generalized spikes or multispikes and slow wave complexes (Fig. 22–4), in which photosensitivity frequently appears; (d) other neurologic signs or lesions are negative on brain MRI;

(e) SEP, visual-evoked potential (VEP), and long-loop C-reflexes indicate "cortical reflex myoclonus" (Fig. 22–5); (f) clonazepam (CZP) or sodium valproate (VPA) are usually effective; (g) lifespan appears normal; (h) no progression of findings is evident during long-term follow-up, but the degree of myoclonus seems to increase with aging (14 to 19 years follow-up), especially in patients over age 70; and (i) myoclonic episodes can be precipitated by fatigue, insomnia, and photic stimuli.

NEUROPATHOLOGIC FEATURES

To date, autopsies have been performed in three heterozygous and one homozygous FAME patients. The cause of death in these individuals was gastric cancer in case 1 at age 66 (17), pneumonia in case 2 at age 77 (34), ovarian cancer in case 3 at age 46 (35), and severe pneumonia in homozygous case 4 at age 71 (36). As expected, based on premorbid neuroradiologic studies, there were no significant neuropathologic changes in the central nervous system in any of the heterozygous cases. However, the homozygous case disclosed significant fibrous gliosis in the globus pallidus, subthalamic nuclei, thalamus, cerebellar dentate nuclei, and white matter surrounding the latter (36). In these lesions, apparent neuronal loss was not seen, although neurons seemed atrophic,

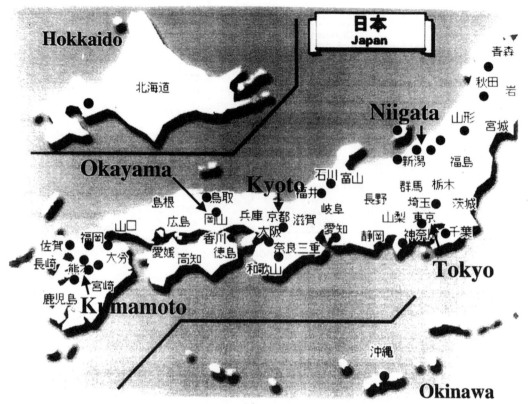

FIG. 22–2. FAME families in Japan. To date, at least 60 FAME families, including 400 affected individuals, have been found throughout Japan. The filled circles indicate locations of the reported families.

TABLE 22–2. *Summary of clinical features in index FAME patients*

Patient	Age	Sex	Onset	Myoclonus	Seizure[a]	Giant SEP	C-reflex
Family 1							
1	79	F	40	UE > LE	1G&1U	+	+
2	72	F	40	UE	3G&1U	+	+
3	68	F	38	UE	1G&2U	+	+
4	65	M	35	UE	1U	+	+
5	51	M	36	UE	2U	+	+
Family 2							
6	78	F	50	UE > LE	4G&2U	+	+
7	47	M	35	UE	3G&1U	+	+
Family 3							
8	86	F	30	UE > LE	4G&2U	NE	NE
9	78	F	20	UE > LE	3G&1U	+	+
10	48	F	38	UE	0	NE	NE
11	46	M	35	UE	3G	+	−
Family 4							
12	70	F	40	UE	4G&1U	+	+
13	67	F	28	UE	1U	+	+
14	49	M	38	UE	0	NE	NE

None of patients showed mental deterioration, cerebellar ataxia, or Babinski signs. EEGs revealed polyspike-and-wave complexes in all patients. MRI and/or CT studies were normal in all patients examined (all but #14). Treatment with CZP and/or VPA were not tried in patients 4, 13, and 14, but were effective in all others.

UE, upper extremities; LE, lower extremities; G, generalized tonic–clonic seizure; U, unconscious attack; NE, not examined.

[a] Frequency of seizure attacks before initiation of treament with CZP or VPA.

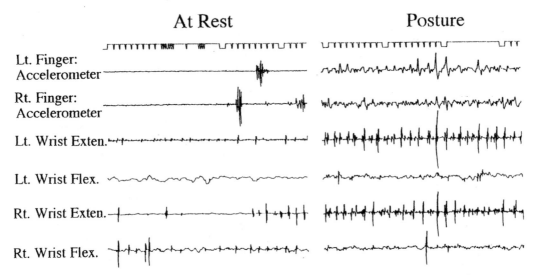

FIG. 22–3. Surface EMG in Patient 12 (Table 22–2). This patient, at age 70, was given clonazepam (1.5 mg/day). The occurrence of myoclonic jerks and tremulous movements are more prominent with posturing than at rest.

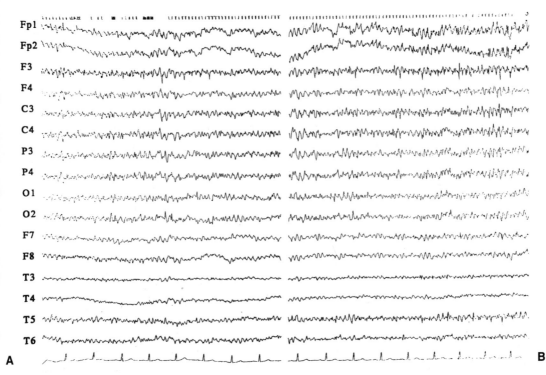

FIG. 22–4. Interictal EEG in the proband of Family 1 with FAME at age 79. **A:** Recoding during relaxed wakefulness with no stimulations shows polyspike-and-wave complexes mixed with sharp waves. **B:** Recording during relaxed wakefulness with photic stimulation shows photosensitivity.

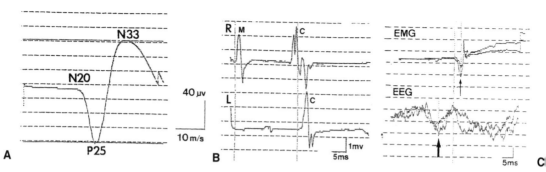

FIG. 22–5. Electrophysiological Studies. **A:** Somatosensory-evoked potentials (SEP) and **B:** C-reflex on EMG in patient 9 at age 70 from the right median nerve stimulation. The early cortical response, N20, is markedly reduced. In contrast, the amplitude of P25 and N33 are markedly increased (144 μV). The long-loop reflex (C-reflex) is recorded on not only the ipsilateral thenar muscle (38.4 msec), but also on the contralateral side (44.4 msec). **C:** Jerk-locked backaveraging in patient 6 at age 74, shows positive spike on EEG preceding myoclonus on EMG.

especially in the cerebellar cortex. There was apparent loss of Purkinje cells in the upper vermis. Furthermore, immunocytochemical study using anti-Calbindin D antibody revealed loss of dendrites in residual Purkinje cells and abundant polydendritic sprouts (cactuses) within its cytoplasm (36).

GENE LOCUS IN JAPANESE FAME FAMILIES

To clone and characterize the FAME gene, a genome-wide screen with genetic linkage analysis has been performed, using samples from 30 individuals in our initial four FAME families. In 1999, we published the locus for the FAME gene to a 4.6-cM region on chromosome 8q24 (9). Simultaneously, Mikami et al. (37) also identified the gene locus to chromosome 8q23.3-q24.1 by linkage analysis in a FAME family reported by Yasuda. Subsequently, the localization was further confirmed to chromosome 8q23.3-q24.1 by linkage study using microsatellite marker D8S555 (maximum LOD score of 3.99 at $\theta = 0$) (38). Furthermore, Ebihara et al. (39) also confirmed the causative gene locus of a large family with BAFME map to chromosome 8q23.3-q24.1. Thus, it is highly likely that FEME, BAFME, and FAME families found in Japan all result from the same mutation in a gene on chromosome 8q24. Moreover, it is also likely that a founder effect is

responsible for the relatively high frequency of FAME in Japan.

GENE LOCUS IN NON-JAPANESE

Linkage analysis in a Spanish FAME family showed absence of linkage to chromosome 8q24 (10). Additional data, based on two Italian FAME families, also disclosed negative linkage to 8q24, but positive linkage to 2p11.1-q12.2 (11), the locus of newly entertained "autosomal dominant cortical myoclonus and epilepsy (ADCME)" (12). The phenotype of these European families is extremely similar to that of FAME in Japan. Coincidental linkage analysis in a large Dutch family presenting with FAME also excluded linkage to 8q23.3-q24.1 (13). The phenotype of this Dutch family is similar to that of Japanese FAME, except for the presence of cognitive deterioration. Thus, locus heterogeneity in FAME is present, although most families with classical symptoms and signs appear to result from a single gene on chromosome 8q.

OTHER "FAME-LIKE" FAMILIES

Recently, several families presenting with a FAME-like phenotype have been found outside of Japan. Elia et al. (15) reported an Italian family including four patients presenting with the FAME phenotype. However, in contrast to

FAME, mental retardation was present in two young adult patients. The authors raised the possibility of its distinct clinical entity. Saka and Saygi (16) found a Turkish family with familial adult-onset myoclonic epilepsy associated with migraine. In the United States, Gilliam et al. (14) identified 11 cases of IGE with myoclonic jerks that began in adulthood. However, five of them were sporadic cases and the existence of absence seizures in some cases lead to the possibility of other, distinct entities. They did not report genetic screening for JME, FAME, or ADCME.

CANDIDATE GENE SCREENING

As shown in the recent identification of epilepsy genes, ion-channel genes are excellent FAME candidate genes. The FAME critical region on chromosome 8q24 includes a potassium channel, Kv8.1, but we found no mutations in our FAME patients from Kumamoto. Three years later, the same results were reported in the family in Okayama. A voltage-gated potassium channel, KCNQ3 (causative gene in benign familial neonatal convulsions type 2, BFNC2), is located on chromosome 8q24. As expected, based on phenotypic differences between BFNC and FAME, sequencing of entire coding region of KCNQ3 in FAME/BAFME individuals did not identify any mutations (40).

We have constructed a physical map of the FAME region and genes that reside within the boundaries determined by obligate recombinants are being examined for FAME-causing mutations in DNA from affected individuals. Discovery and characterization of the FAME gene will provide further insight into the molecular basis of epilepsy and neuroexcitability that results in myoclonic jerks.

REFERENCES

1. Adams RD, Victor M, Ropper AH. Epilepsy and other seizure disorders. *Principles of neurology.* 6th ed. New York: McGraw-Hill, 1997.
2. Delgado–Escueta AV, Medina MT, Bai DS, et al. Genetics of idiopathic myoclonic epilepsies: An overview. *Adv Neurol* 2002;89:161–184.
3. Ptacek LJ, Fu Y-H. Channelopathies: Episodic disorders of the nervous system. *Epilepsia* 2001;42:35–43.
4. Ptacek LJ, Fu YH. What's new in epilepsy genetics? *Mol Psych* 2003;8:463–465.
5. Koskiniemi M. Progressive myoclonus epilepsies. In: Vinken PJ, Bruyn GW, Meinardi H, eds. *Handbook of clinical neurology.* Vol. 73, Amsterdam, Elsevier, 2000: 293–306.
6. Schmitz B and Sander T, eds. Juvenile myoclonic epilepsy: The Janz syndrome. Petersfield: Wrightson Biomedical, 2000.
7. Uyama E, Kumamoto T, Ikeda T, et al. A family of familial myoclonic epilepsy characterized by middle-adult onset presenting with finger tremulous involuntary movements and benign course. *Clin Neurol* (Jpn) 1985;25:1491–1492.
8. Uyama E, Tokunaga M, Murakami T, et al. Familial adult myoclonus epilepsy: A new phenotype of autosomal dominant myoclonus epilepsy. *Ann Neurol* 1996;40:505.
9. Plaster N, Uyama E, Uchino M, et al. Genetic localization of the familial adult myoclonic epilepsy (FAME) gene to chromosome 8q24. *Neurology* 1999;53:1180–1183.
10. Labauge P, Amer LO, Simonetta-Moreau M, et al. Absence of linkage to 8q24 in a European family with familial adult myoclonic epilepsy (FAME). *Neurology* 2002;58:941–944.
11. De Falco FA, Striano P, De Falco A, et al. Benign adult familial myoclonic epilepsy: genetic heterogeneity and allelism with ADCME. *Neurology* 2003;60:1381–1385.
12. Guerrini R, Bonanni P, Patrignani A, et al. Autosomal dominant cortical myoclonus and epilepsy (ADCME) with complex partial and generalized seizures: A newly recognized epilepsy syndrome with linkage to chromosome 2p11.1-q12.2. *Brain* 2001;124:2459–2475.
13. van Rootselaar F, Callenbach PM, Hottenga JJ, et al. A Dutch family with familial cortical tremor with epilepsy: Clinical characteristics and exclusion of linkage to chromosome 8q23.3-q24.1. *J Neurol* 2002;249:829–834.
14. Saka E, Saygi S. Familial adult onset myoclonic epilepsy associated with migraine. *Seizure* 2000;9:344–346.
15. Elia M, Musumeci SA, Ferri R, et al. Familiar cortical tremor, epilepsy, and mental retardation: a distinct clinical entity? *Arch Neurol* 1998;55:1569–1573.
16. Gilliam F, Steinhoff BJ, Bittermann H-J, et al. Adult myoclonic epilepsy: A distinct syndrome of idiopathic generalized epilepsy. *Neurology* 2000;55:1030–1033.
17. Inazuki G, Naito H, Ohama E, et al. A clinical study and neuropathological findings of a familial disease with myoclonus and epilepsy—the nosological place of familial essential myoclonus and epilepsy (FEME). *Psych Neurol Jpn* (Jpn) 1990;92:1–21.
18. Ikeda A, Kakigi R, Funai N, et al. Cortical tremor: A variant of cortical reflex myoclonus. *Neurology* 1990:1561–1565.
19. Terada K, Ikeda A, Mima T, et al. Familial cortical myoclonic tremor as a unique form of cortical reflex myoclonus. *Mov Disord* 1997;12:370–377.
20. Inoue S. On a pegidree of the hereditary tremor with epileptiform seizures. *Psych Neurol Jpn* (Jpn) 1951;53:33–37.
21. Wakeno M. A family with heredofamilial tremor associated with epileptic disorders. *Psych Neurol Jpn* (Jpn) 1975;77:1–18.

22. Yasuda T. Benign adult familial myoclonic epilepsy (BAFME). *Kawasaki Med J* 1991;17:1–13.
23. Yasuda T, Morimoto K, Terao A. C-response: Its clinical application for progressive myoclonic epilepsy. *Neurol Med* 1983;18:189–191.
24. Kuwano A, Takakubo F, Morimoto Y, et al. Benign adult familial myoclonus epilepsy (BAFME): An autosomal dominant form not linked to the dentatorubral pallidoluysian atrophy (DRPLA) gene. *J Med Genet* 1996;33:80–81.
25. Okuma Y, Shimo Y, Hatori K, et al. Familial cortical tremor with epilepsy. *Parkinsonism Rel Disord* 1997;3: 83–87.
26. Okuma Y, Shimo Y, Shimura H, et al. Familial cortical tremor with epilepsy: an under-recognized familial tremor. *Clinic Neurol Neurosurg* 1998;100:75–78.
27. Sekino Y, Imamura L, Yamaguchi T. Clinical features in myoclonus epilepsy. *Psych Neurol Jpn* (Jpn) 1958;60:617–632.
28. Kawase Y. Electrophysiological studies in patients with benign familial myoclonic epilepsy. In: Miyatake T. eds. *Myoclonus epilepsy: Recent advances.* [Niigata symposium series on neurology No.12]. Tokyo: Kagakuhyoronsha, (Jpn) 1994:19–36.
29. Hashimoto O, Honda M, Niwa S, et al. Linkage analysis between familial myoclonus epilepsy and short arm of chromosome 6 using HLA phenotype as genetic marker. *Jpn J Psych Neurol* 1993;47:275–277.
30. Okino S. Familial benign myoclonus epilepsy of adult onset: A previously unrecognized myoclonic disorder. *J Neurol Sci* 1997;145:113–118.
31. Nagayama S, Kishikawa H, Yukitake M, et al. A case of familial myoclonus showing extremely benign clinical course. *Clinic Neurol* (Jpn) 1998;38:430–434.
32. Kato M, Onuma T. A clinical study of benign adult familial myoclonus epilepsy. *Ann Rep Jpn Res Found* 1999;11:99–108.
33. Manabe Y, Narai H, Warita H, et al. Benign adult familial myoclonic epilepsy (BAFME) with night blindness. *Seizure* 2002;11:266–268.
34. Oyanagi S, Masaharu T, Naito A, et al. A neuropathological study of 8 autopsy cases of degenerative type of myoclonus epilesy: With special reference to latent combination of degeneration of the pallido-luysian system. *Adv Neurol Sci* (Jpn) 1976;20: 410–424.
35. Tokiguchi S, Nagano Y. An autopsy case of form of myoclonus epilepsy. *Neurol Med* (Jpn) 1984;21:464–468.
36. Hayashi M, Endo K, Suzuki T, et al. Benign adult familial myoclonic epilepsy: An autopsy case of homozygous affected individual. *Neuropathology* (Jpn) 2001;21[Suppl.]:106.
37. Mikami M, Yasuda T, Terao A, et al. Localization of a gene for benign adult familial myoclonic epilepsy to chromosome 8q23.3-q24.1. *Am J Hum Genet* 1999;65:745–751.
38. Kobayashi H, Suzuki T, Tsuji S, et al. Linkage analysis in families with familial essential myoclonus epilepsy (FEME). *Abstr Ann Rep Res Nervous Mental Dis* (Jpn) 1999:9.
39. Ebihara M, Ohba N, Ohkubo Y, et al. Linkage analysis in a family with benign adult familial myoclonic epilepsy. *Abstr 15th Ann Rep Jpn Res Found* (Jpn) 2003: 11–12.
40. Sano A, Mikami M, Nakamura M, et al. Positional candidate approach for the gene responsible for benign adult familial myoclonic epilepsy. *Epilepsia* 2002;43 [Suppl 9]:26–31.

23

Treatment of Myoclonic Epilepsies in Infancy and Early Childhood

Raman Sankar,* James W. Wheless,† Charlotte Dravet,‡ Renzo Guerrini,§
Marco T. Medina,¶,‖ Michelle Bureau,‡ Pierre Genton,‡ and
Antonio V. Delgado–Escueta¶

*Departments of Neurology and Pediatrics, David Geffen School of Medicine at UCLA and Mattel
Children's Hospital at UCLA, Los Angeles, California; †Departments of Neurology and Pediatrics,
University of Texas School of Medicine, Houston, Texas; ‡Centre Saint-Paul- Hôpital Henri Gastaut,
Marseille, France; §Epilepsy, Neurophysiology, Neurogenetics Unit, Department of Child Neurology
and Psychiatry, University of Pisa and Research Institute 'Stella Maris' Foundation, Pisa Italy,
‖National Autonomous University of Honduras, Tegucigalpa, Honduras; ¶Comprehensive Epilepsy
Program and Epilepsy Center of Excellence at VA GLAHS, David Geffen School of Medicine at
UCLA, Los Angeles, California

INTRODUCTION

As described amply in the many chapters of this book, the myoclonic epilepsies comprise a very broad spectrum of clinical disorders in which myoclonus is an important epileptic manifestation. Their etiologies can range from the so-called idiopathic varieties (many of which are now revealing themselves to be channelopathies, receptoropathies, and modulators/sensors of ion channels) to others with neurodegenerative features—these latter again comprising a heterogeneous group. While this book addresses itself to the idiopathic myoclonic epilepsies, the medications used to treat myoclonic seizures do not distinguish between idiopathic and symptomatic myoclonic syndromes. In traditional thinking, idiopathic epilepsies have been thought of as genetic epilepsies without a structural and metabolic basis, and generally not associated with major neurologic deficits. There are now beginning to be attributed to altered excitability resulting from mutations of ion channels receptors or sensors/modulators of ion channels. An epilepsy that is accompanied by severe, medically refractory seizures and mental retardation was classified as cryptogenic, rather than idiopathic, if no structural or metabolic etiology is identified according to the International League Against Epilepsy. The discovery of different germ line missense mutations of *SCNA1A* to be associated with GEFS+ and *de novo* somatic "stop" mutations of *SCNA1* in Dravet syndrome certainly challenges our traditional use of the term cryptogenic. Regardless of such semantic diversions, there is a need for screening strategies to facilitate drug discovery for the symptomatic treatment of myoclonic seizures. Ultimately, development of drugs designed against specific genetic mutations or specific epilepsy syndromes will need to be pursued.

Animal models of myoclonic seizures have played a role in evaluating the possible efficacy of drug therapy for treatment of human myoclonic seizures. Animal models can be classified as those involving provoked seizures and those involving genetic models. Provocation of seizures in the former is commonly accomplished by chemical or electrical means, although other means, such as hypoxia and intermittent light stimulation, have also been used. Classic pharmacologic screening involving rodents, as used by the Anticonvulsant Screening Project of the National Institute of Neurologic Disorders and Stroke, has produced inconsistent information for predicting the efficacy of potential therapeutic agents against myoclonus. With earlier-generation antiepileptic drugs (AEDs), the models used were only somewhat predictive of efficacy. Only clonazepam (CZP) and valproic acid (VPA) have demonstrated efficacy in animal models for protection against all three seizure provocations involving subcutaneous (sc) pentylenetetrazole, bicuculline, and picrotoxin (1). Ethosuximide, which was only marginally active against bicuculline, has been shown not to be a useful antimyoclonic AED (1,2). Phenytoin (PHT) and carbamazepine (CBZ) clearly distinguished themselves as agents that were mainly active in the maximal electroshock model (3). Among new-generation AEDs, felbamate has shown clinical utility in a variety of myoclonic seizures and was also active in protecting rats against sc pentylenetetrazole, sc bicuculline, and sc picrotoxin (4). Gabapentin (GBP), the next agent to arrive on the United States market, has been shown to be ineffective in sc bicuculline and picrotoxin provocations in the rodent (5) and appears to be clinically useful only for partial and secondarily generalized seizures (6). Vigabatrin (VGB), like GBP, has not demonstrated significant activity against sc bicuculline or picrotoxin challenge, and is not a clinically useful agent for most syndromes involving myoclonic seizures (7). Experience with GBP highlights another difficulty in the use of animal models for screening compounds to treat myoclonus. Kanthasamy et al. (8) found GBP to be antimyoclonic in a posthypoxic rodent model, but not for myoclonus induced by administration of p,p'-DDT [1,1,1-trichloro-2,2-bis(p-chlorophenyl)ethane].

Experience with other new-generation AEDs has also revealed many inconsistencies. Lamotrigine (LTG), which has an animal testing profile resembling that of PHT (9), has demonstrated clinical utility for treating some patients with juvenile myoclonic epilepsy (JME) (10). Paradoxically, LTG is also known to exacerbate myoclonus in some patients (11–13). Topiramate (TPM), another new-generation agent, has been shown to be ineffective in blocking chemically induced seizures (14). Nevertheless, this medication may be of value in treating a variety of syndromes that involve myoclonus, as is discussed later in this chapter.

The most extensively described genetic model of epilepsy involves *Papio papio*, the photosensitive baboon. Killiam et al. (15) first reported that when these animals were subjected to intermittent photic stimulation (IPS), paroxysmal discharges in the form of spikes and waves or polyspikes and waves resulted. Behaviorally, bilateral and synchronous myoclonic jerks appeared and were followed by generalized convulsive seizures. The involvement of the GABAergic system in this model was described in detail by Meldrum and Wilkins (16). This model correctly predicted lack of efficacy of GBP in human myoclonic epilepsies (17). It also predicted efficacy of ethosuximide at high doses in myoclonic epilepsies (18,19). However, vigabatrin (VGB), was shown to be effective in blocking photically induced epileptic activity in the baboon (18), suggesting that the baboon model also has limitations in its ability to predict the clinical utility of test AEDs. This model is apparently not routinely employed in screening and many of the new-generation AEDs have no published literature describing their use in this model.

Another well-characterized genetic model involves the tottering mouse. The *tg* locus causes a delayed-onset recessive neurologic disorder in the mouse, featuring a stereotyped triad of ataxia, intermittent absence seizures, and bursts of generalized 6- to 7-Hz spike waves. This model has not been routinely used in screening for AEDs; hence, its reliability for this purpose is unknown. Other genetic models of inherited myoclonus include a disorder of the inhibitory glycine receptor that results in spontaneous and stimulus-sensitive myoclonus in Polled Hereford calves (19) and spontaneous and photically induced myoclonus in a mutant strain of Fayoumi chickens (20). The possible importance of the glycine receptor in some myoclonic disorders is highlighted by the recent development of a transgenic mouse model of hypereklexia, which involves a mutation in the gene for the $\alpha 1$ subunit of the glycine receptor (21). However, the cost and inconsistent availability of these animals precludes their routine use for developing highly specific antimyoclonic drugs. Economic forces continue to drive the development of AEDs for partial seizures, with subsequent adoption of some AEDs to treat myoclonic seizures based on clinical experience.

TREATMENT OPTIONS FOR SPECIFIC EPILEPSY SYNDROMES WITH MYOCLONIC SEIZURES IN EARLY INFANCY

Wheless and Sankar, recently reviewed this topic in detail (22). In this chapter, we limit our discussion to the treatment of those disorders that generally have their onset in the first 5 years or so of life. Detailed discussion of the pharmacokinetic and pharmacodynamic properties are not considered within the scope of this discussion. We have preferred to indicate the available choice of therapeutic agents and provide the literature citations to support the basis for that choice. Detailed and specific guidelines on the use of specific medications can be obtained elsewhere.

The information provided in this chapter on the treatment options for clinical syndromes involving myoclonus as a prominent feature (with the exception of the stiripentol trial) is not derived from controlled clinical trials. It remains difficult to quantify myoclonic seizures accurately to assess the effect of treatment precisely. Fortunately, myoclonic seizures are often associated with more easily quantified seizures such as astatic drop attacks, absence seizures, generalized clonic and generalized tonic–clonic seizures (GTCS). Further, many of these syndromes are relatively less common, compared to localization-related partial epilepsies with or without secondary generalization. In this chapter, we provide the guidelines in the management of the relatively more common epilepsies of infancy and early childhood, the Dravet syndrome of SMEI (Fig. 23–1) and genetic form of myoclonic-astatic epilepsy (MAE) (Fig. 23–2). Much of the information in these algorithms are obtained from what the American Academy

of Neurology Quality Standards Subcommittee practice guidelines (23) would categorize as Class II (case-controlled and cohort studies) and Class III (case series, case reports, and expert opinions) evidence, rather than Class I (controlled clinical trials) evidence.

The algorithms represent practice habits of the experts who have the most extensive experience in these syndromes, these practice habits should be put to a test by controlled clinical trials.

Early Myoclonic Encephalopathy

Massive bilateral or axial myoclonias are the myoclonic features of early myoclonic encephalopathy. This rare syndrome has its onset during the first month of life and is often fatal by 1 year of age. The electroencephalogram (EEG) in patients with this condition reveals a burst-suppression pattern and may evolve toward typical hypsarrhythmia (24). No controlled clinical trials have investigated the treatment of early myoclonic encephalopathy. Treatment options are all based on anecdotal reports, and although drug therapy has demonstrated some efficacy, response to treatment is typically poor, and seizure freedom is rarely achieved. None of the conventional AEDs, adrenocorticotropic hormone (ACTH) gel, prednisone, or pyridoxine has been effective in treating this syndrome (25). The myoclonias of this syndrome gradually decrease with age. However, the overall prognosis is poor, and patients evolve towards West syndrome and eventually towards Lennox–Gastaut syndrome (24).

Infantile Spasms—West Syndrome

The treatment of IS is based on the underlying etiology of the spasms (25,26). With respect to both seizure control and developmental outcome, infants who have underlying focal cortical dysplasia, porencephalic cysts, or (rarely) a brain tumor may show the best response to epilepsy surgery. At UCLA such surgery is undertaken early in the course of the syndrome with the goal of maximizing the developmental outcome. Both anecdotal and controlled trial data indicate that vigabatrin is the treatment of choice for IS associated with tuberous sclerosis complex (28–32).

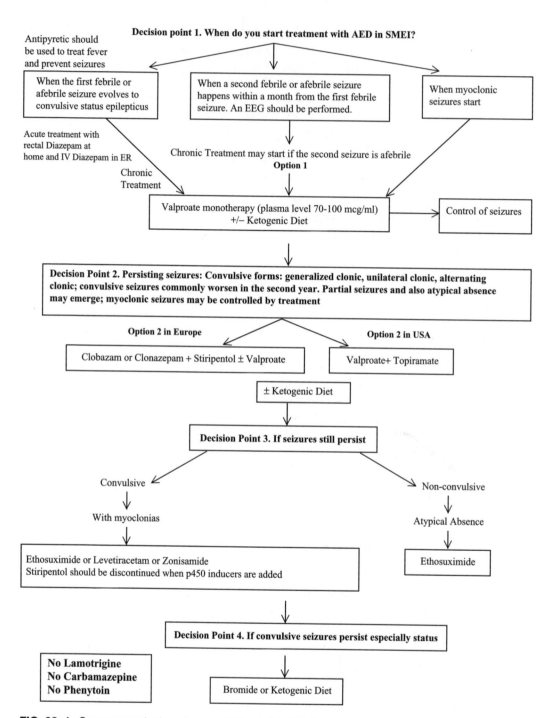

FIG. 23–1. Severe myoclonic epilepsy of infancy (Dravet Syndrome).

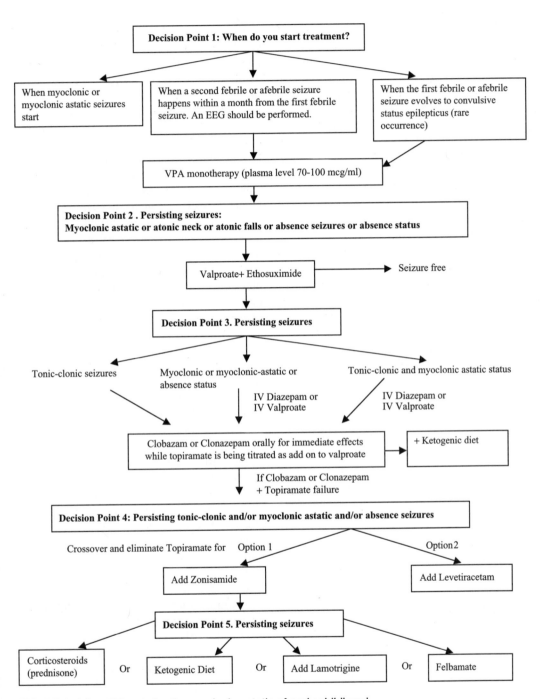

FIG. 23–2. Idiopathic or genetic myoclonic-astatic of early childhood.

Children with cryptogenic IS show the best response to ACTH in clinical trials (27,33). Use of VGB (27–30,34) and nitrazepam (35) to treat cryptogenic IS has also been evaluated in clinical trials. In Japan, pyridoxine is typically administered as initial therapy, but has a low response rate (36–38). Other treatment options that have been pursued in case series include VPA, prednisone, felbamate, LTG, TPM, and zonisamide (ZNS) (33,34,39,40). The ketogenic diet has recently shown success in children with refractory IS (cryptogenic and symptomatic etiologies) (41). Children with symptomatic etiologies are often treated with the same medications, but the response rate is much lower than in children with a cryptogenic etiology (27,33,34,39). As such, in patients with symptomatic etiologies, a risk/benefit assessment must be made for each therapeutic option and discussed with the child's parents.

Severe Myoclonic Epilepsy of Infancy (SMEI)—Dravet Syndrome

Figure 23-1 illustrates decision points and treatment options in the Dravet syndrome, SMEI. The first step is to decide when to start treatment with an AED. Severe myoclonic epilepsy in infancy (Dravet syndrome) begins with unilateral or generalized, often prolonged, febrile seizures in normal infants before 1 year of age. The diagnosis of Dravet syndrome cannot be affirmed at this stage. Treatment should be started when the first febrile or afebrile seizures evolve to convulsive status or when a second febrile or afebrile seizure appear within a month of the first febrile seizure. An EEG should be performed at this time. Myoclonus rarely appears before 1 year and more often occurs between the ages of 1 and 4 years. When myoclonic seizures appear after a febrile seizure, treatment is obligatory, VPA monotherapy is recommended as option 1. Children typically progress to experience multiple seizure types in their second year, generalized or unilateral or alternating clonic or partial seizures, atypical absences, and worsening myoclonic seizures compel addition of a second antiepileptic drug. Because psychomotor development becomes retarded after the second year of life, an aggressive treatment plan should be carried out in the latter months of the first year

and early during the second year. Two options can be pursued. Option 2 in Europe is stiripentol plus CLB and VPA. Option 2 in USA is VPA plus TPM. One placebo-controlled, multicenter study in the treatment of severe myoclonic epilepsy in infancy (Dravet syndrome) assessed efficacy of stiripentol* (42,43). In this study by Chiron et al. (42), 41 children enrolled were typically treated with VPA and CLB during the baseline phase. They were then randomized to treatment with stiripentol or placebo for 8 weeks. Subsequently, patients entered an open-label phase, during which they were treated with stiripentol at dosages of 50 to 100 mg/kg per day. Responder rates (i.e., proportions of patients experiencing a >50% decrease in seizure frequency) were significantly greater for the stiripentol group (71%) than for the placebo group (5%). The proportion of patients who were free from generalized clonic and GTCS during the study was also significantly greater in the stiripentol group (43%) than in the placebo group (0%). The same authors (78) retrospectively studied 46 patients treated with stiripentol, clobazam and valproate for a mean period of 2.9 years. Sixty five percent were still improved (>50% seizure reduction). Most striking was disappearance of convulsive states. Prior to these trials, treatment of severe myoclonic epilepsy in infancy was based on anecdotal evidence for the efficacy of drugs, such as VPA, CZP, methsuximide, TPM, and intravenous gammaglobulin. Because treatment results with topiramate are supported only by 2 open studies (not blinded or randomized), Europeans favor the use of the stiripentol, clobazam, valproate trio as a choice option 2 after valproate monotherapy. Lamotrigine, carbamazepine and phenytoin are reported to exacerbate seizures in this condition and should not be used (11). If seizures do not respond to treatment between 2 and 3 years of age, bromide has been used by Oguni et al, with success (see chapter 8). Ketogenic diet can also be instituted. Two separate studies albeit open and not randomized, from Japan and Argentina report startling and favorable responses to ketogenic diet (see chapters by Oguni and by Fejerman) (Figure 22-2).

---

*Stiripentol is not available in the United States and not approved by the Food & Drug Administration (FDA).

Benign Myoclonic Epilepsy of Infancy

Benign myoclonic epilepsy of infancy (BMEI) is the only epilepsy syndrome associated with myoclonic seizures in infancy or childhood that can have a favorable prognosis. Seizures are characterized by symmetric myoclonus, and these are the only seizure type associated with this syndrome (with the exception of occasional febrile convulsions). GTCS may develop later during adolescence. The EEG background for individuals with this syndrome is normal and the myoclonus is accompanied by a generalized spike or polyspike-and-slow wave complex. Almost all publications confirm efficacy of VPA monotherapy. If pharmacoresistance develops, diagnosis must be questioned. Anecdotal evidence suggests that TPM, LTG, and CZP are effective (44). Some children may require relatively brief therapy (i.e., 1 to 2 years), while others may require longer-term therapy.

Lennox–Gastaut Syndrome

We include treatment of Lennox-Gastaut syndrome (LGS) in this chapter because severe myoclonic epilepsy of Dravet and idiopathic myoclonic-astatic epilepsy (MAE) are often mistaken for this syndrome. The ability of a drug to effectively treat LGS was considered the gold standard for declaring an AED to have broad-spectrum efficacy in childhood epilepsy. VPA has been used to treat LGS for 25 years and there is a wealth of clinical evidence indicating its efficacy in open-label trials, although no double-blind trials have been performed (26,45–49). It was not until approximately 15 years after the introduction of valproate in the United States that a successful controlled clinical trial was conducted to investigate the treatment of LGS; felbamate was the first drug to show efficacy in this manner (50,51). Unfortunately, potential side effects of felbamate have limited its use, but the drug is still recommended as a third- or fourth-line agent. Felbamate is particularly efficacious in controlling the drop attacks associated with LGS. Two other drugs, specifically, LTG and TPM, have also emerged as broad-spectrum AEDs with demonstrated efficacy in the treatment of LGS in controlled clinical trials (52–58). It should be pointed out that myoclonic seizures *per se* and strictly speaking are not an essential component of LGS, were not one of the efficacy variable in these studies. Rather, drop attacks were considered as one endpoint of the studies. The availability of these two drugs has been a major asset to pediatric neurologists who previously had only VPA available. In addition, there have been anecdotal reports of success in treating this syndrome with CLB, ZNS, steroids, CZP, MSM, and nitrazepam (46). Nonpharmacologic treatments can also be of benefit. Both the ketogenic diet and vagus nerve stimulation may be particularly useful in the treatment of drop attacks associated with this condition (59–64). Vagus nerve stimulation has been so efficacious in the treatment of drop attacks that corpus callosotomies are seldom performed. However, when such procedures are performed, there appears to be a synergistic effect in patients who had previously received vagus nerve stimulation (65). Interestingly, GABAergic drugs, such as GBP and VGB, may exacerbate the myoclonic seizures rarely associated with LGS (66,67). Epileptic myoclonus in Lennox-Gastaut syndrome originates from a stable generator in the frontal cortex and spreads to other cortical areas, whereas the myoclonus in Doose syndrome (myoclonic-astatic epilepsy of early childhood) appears to be a primary generalized epileptic phenomenon (68).

Myoclonic-Astatic Epilepsy–Doose Syndrome

Epileptologists now agree that the "true Doose syndrome" is the idiopathic (genetic) form of myoclonic-astatic epilepsy (MAE). Still, treatment outcome varies from well-controlled patients to drug-resistant forms. Doose syndrome occurs in children between 2 and 5 years of age. In 60%, febrile or afebrile convulsions herald onset of this syndrome. Some weeks later, myoclonic and/or myoclonic-astatic seizures appear in abundance, frequently with absences. Treatment with valproate is obligatory at this stage. The jerks associated with this syndrome, followed by atonia, often lead to abrupt falling and injury although no formal clinical trials have documented the efficacy of AEDs in treating

Doose syndrome, information regarding its treatment is based on anecdotal experience, VPA is still the first drug used by most epileptologists (option 1). When seizures persist, option 2 is to add ethosuximide to valproate. When drop attacks, absences or absence status recurr, clonazepam or clobazam are option 3 as topiramate is instituted gradually. Results of Fejerman's group from Argentina suggest early treatment with ketogenic diet (see Chapter 29).

Antiepileptic drugs for option 4 include zonizamide and lamotrigine (69–72). Vagus nerve stimulation has been used as nonpharmacologic agents for treatment of intractable drop attacks sometimes associated with this condition. Exacerbation of myoclonic-astatic seizures has been reported in patients treated with PHT, CBZ, and VGB (73). We had mentioned earlier the exacerbation of myoclonus in some patients caused by LTG (11–13) and this is certainly a possibility with Doose syndrome as well, and patients should be carefully observed for this possibility.

There is one case report of felbamate use in the treatment of Doose syndrome (74). However, felbamate-induced aplastic anemia in 1/3000 to 1/5000 per year and hepatic failure in 1,64/10,000 limit its use. The profile of patients at risk for felbamate-related aplastic anemia is: a person more than 17 years of age, female, concomitant antiepileptic drugs, and history of prior cytopenia and immune disease. If a trial in this syndrome of early childhood should involve felbamate, 2-phenylpropenal should be measured in 24 hours urine to monitor potential risk for felbamate toxicity. Twenty standard deviations predict neutropenia (75,76,77).

REFERENCES

1. White HS, Woodhead JH, Franklin MR, et al. Experimental selection, quantification, and evaluation of antiepileptic drugs. In: Levy RH, Mattson RH, Meldrum BS, eds. *Antiepileptic drugs.* 4th ed. New York: Raven Press, 1995:99–122.
2. Ferrendelli JA, Holland KD, McKeon AC, et al. Comparison of the anticonvulsant activities of ethosuximide, valproate, and a new anticonvulsant, thiobutyrolactone. *Epilepsia* 1989;30:617–622.
3. Rho JM, Sankar R. The pharmacologic basis of antiepileptic drug action. *Epilepsia* 1999;40:1471–1483.
4. Swinyard EA, Sofia RD, Kupferberg HJ. Comparative anticonvulsant activity and neurotoxicity of felbamate and four prototype antiepileptic drugs in mice and rats. *Epilepsia* 1986;27:27–34.
5. Taylor CP. Gabapentin: mechanism of action. In: Levy RH, Mattson RH, Meldrum BS, eds. *Antiepileptic drugs.* 4th ed. New York: Raven Press, 1995:829–841.
6. Holmes GL, Pearl PL. Gabapentin. In: Pellock JM, Dodson WE, Bourgeois BFD, eds. *Pediatric epilepsy: Diagnosis and therapy.* 2nd ed. New York: Demos Medical, 2001:453–459.
7. Sankar R, Derdiarian AT. Vigabatrin. *CNS Drug Rev* 1998;4:260–274.
8. Kanthasamy AG, Vu TQ, Yun RJ, et al. Antimyoclonic effect of gabapentin in a posthypoxic animal model of myoclonus. *Eur J Pharmacol* 1996;297:219–224.
9. Miller AA, Wheatley P, Sawyer DA, et al. Pharmacological studies on lamotrigine, a novel potential antiepileptic drug: 1. Anticonvulsant profile in mice and rats. *Epilepsia* 1986;27:483–489.
10. Buchanan N. The use of lamotrigine in juvenile myoclonic epilepsy. *Seizure* 1996;5:149–151.
11. Guerrini R, Dravet C, Genton C, et al. Lamotrigine and seizure aggravation in severe myoclonic epilepsy. *Epilepsia* 1998;39:508–512.
12. Guerrini R, Belmonte A, Parmeggiani L, et al. Myoclonic status epilepticus following high-dosage lamotrigine therapy. *Brain Develop* 1999;21:420–424.
13. Janszky J, Rasonyi G, Halasz P, et al. Disabling erratic myoclonus during lamotrigine therapy with high serum level: Report of two cases. *Clin Neuropharmacol* 2000;23:86–89.
14. Shank RP, Gardocki JF, Vaught JL, et al. Topiramate: preclinical evaluation of a structurally novel anticonvulsant. *Epilepsia* 1994;35:450–460.
15. Killiam KF, Killiam EK, Naquet R. Mise en evidence chez certains singes d'un syndrome myoclonique. *CR Acad Sci (Paris)* (Fr.) 1966;262:1010–1012.
16. Meldrum B, Wilkins AJ. Photosensitive epilepsy in man and the baboon: integration of pharmacological and psychosocial evidence. In: Schwartzkroin PA, Wheal HV, eds. *Electrophysiology of epilepsy.* London: Academic Press, 1984:51–77.
17. McLean MJ. Gabapentin. In: Wiley E, ed. The treatment of epilepsy: Principles and practice. 2nd ed. Baltimore: Williams & Wilkins, 1997:884–898.
18. Meldrum BS, Horton R. Blockade of epileptic responses in the photosensitive baboon, Papio papio, by two irreversible inhibitors of GABA-transaminase, gamma-acetylenic GABA (4-amino-hex-5-ynoic acid) and gamma-vinyl GABA (4-amino-hex-5-enoic acid). *Psychopharmacology* 1978;59:47–50.
19. Gundlach AL. Disorder of the inhibitory glycine receptor: Inherited myoclonus in Poll Hereford calves. *FASEB J* 1990;4:2761–2766.
20. Avanzini G, Fariello R. Animal models of epilepsies. In: Avanzini G, Regesta G, Tanganelli P, Avoli M, eds. Molecular and cellular targets for anti-epileptic drugs. London: John Libbey, 1997:91–109.
21. Becker L, von Wegerer J, Schenkel J, et al. Disease-specific human glycine receptor alpha1 subunit causes hyperekplexia phenotype and impaired glycine- and GABAA-receptor transmission in transgenic mice. *J Neurosci* 2002;22:2505–2512.
22. Wheless JW, Sankar R. Treatment strategies for myoclonic seizures and epilepsy syndromes with myoclonic seizures. *Epilepsia* 2003;44(Suppl 11):27–37.

23. AAN Practice Guidelines. American Academy of Neurology Web site. Available at: http//www.aan.com/professionals/practice/index.cfm. Accessed January 6, 2003.

24. Yamatogi Y, Ohtahara S. Age-dependent epileptic encephalopathy: a longitudinal study. *Folia Psych Neurol Jpn* 1981;35:321–332.

25. Ohtahara S, Yamatogi Y. Severe encephalopathic epilepsy in early infancy. In: Pellock J, Dodson WE, Bourgeois BFD, eds. *Pediatric epilepsy: Diagnosis and therapy*. 2nd ed. New York: Demos, 2001:193–199.

26. Trevathan E. Infantile spasms and Lennox-Gastaut syndrome. *J Child Neurol* 2002;17(Suppl 2):2S9–2S22.

27. Mackay M, Weiss S, Snead OC, III. Treatment of infantile spasms: An evidence-based approach. *Int Rev Neurobiol* 2002;49:157–184.

28. Dulac O, Chiron C, Luna D, et al. Vigabatrin in childhood epilepsy. *J Child Neurol* 1991;6(Suppl):2S30–32S37.

29. Luna D, Dulac O, Pajot N, et al. Vigabatrin in the treatment of childhood epilepsies: A single-blind placebo-controlled study. *Epilepsia* 1989;30:430–437.

30. Elterman RD, Shields WD, Mansfield KA, et al. Randomized trial of vigabatrin in patients with infantile spasms. *Neurology* 2001;57:1416–1421.

31. Curatolo P, Seri S, Verdecchia M, et al. Infantile spasms in tuberous sclerosis complex. *Brain Develop* 2001;23:502–507.

32. Curatolo P, Verdecchia M, Bombardieri R. Vigabatrin for tuberous sclerosis complex. *Brain Develop* 2001;23:649–653.

33. Hancock E, Osborne JP, Milner P. The treatment of West syndrome: A Cochrane review of the literature to December 2000. *Brain Develop* 2001;23:624–634.

34. Mikati MA, Lepejian GA, Holmes GL. Medical treatment of patients with infantile spasms. *Clin Neuropharmacol* 2002;25:61–70.

35. Dreifuss F, Farwell J, Holmes G, et al. Infantile spasms. Comparative trial of nitrazepam and corticotropin. *Arch Neurol* 1986;43:1107–1110.

36. Toribe Y. High-dose vitamin B6 treatment in West syndrome. *Brain Develop*. 2001;23:654–657.

37. Gospe SM. Pyridoxine-dependent seizures: findings from recent studies pose new questions. *Pediatr Neurol* 2002;26:181–185.

38. Baxter P. Pyridoxine-dependent and pyridoxine-responsive seizures. *Develop Med Child Neurol* 2001;43:416–420.

39. Nabbout R. A risk-benefit assessment of treatments for infantile spasms. *Drug Safety* 2001;24:813–828.

40. Suzuki Y, Imai K, Toribe Y, et al. Long-term response to zonisamide in patients with West syndrome. *Neurology* 2002;58:1556–1559.

41. Kossoff EH, Pyzik PL, McGrogan JR, et al. Efficacy of the ketogenic diet for infantile spasms. *Pediatrics* 2002;109:780–783.

42. Chiron C, Marchand MC, Tran A, et al. Stiripentol in severe myoclonic epilepsy in infancy: a randomized placebo-controlled syndrome-dedicated trial. STICLO study group. *Lancet* 2000;356:1638–1642.

43. Perez J, Chiron C, Musial C, et al. Stiripentol: Efficacy and tolerability in children with epilepsy. *Epilepsia* 1999;40:1618–1626.

44. Todt H, Muller D. The therapy of benign myoclonic epilepsy in infants. *Epilepsy Res Suppl* 1992;6:137–139.

45. Clancy RR. Valproate: An update—the challenge of modern pediatric seizure management. *Curr Prob Pediatr* 1990;20:161–233.

46. Wheless JW, Constantinou JE. Lennox-Gastaut syndrome. *Pediatr Neurol* 1997;17:203–211.

47. Jeavons PM, Clark JE. Sodium valproate in treatment of epilepsy. *BMJ* 1974;2:584–586.

48. Covanis A, Gupta AK, Jeavons PM. Sodium valproate monotherapy and polytherapy. *Epilepsia* 1982;23:693–720.

49. Henriksen O, Johannessen SI. Clinical and pharmacokinetic observations on sodium valproate: A 5-year follow-up study in 100 children with epilepsy. *Acta Neurol Scand* 1982;65:504–523.

50. The Felbamate Study Group in Lennox-Gastaut Syndrome. Efficacy of felbamate in childhood epileptic encephalopathy (Lennox-Gastaut syndrome). *N Engl J Med* 1993;328:29–33.

51. Siegel H, Kelley K, Stertz B, et al. The efficacy of felbamate as add-on therapy to valproic acid in Lennox-Gastaut syndrome. *Epilepsy Res* 1999;34:91–97.

52. Motte J, Trevathan E, Arvidsson JF, et al. Lamotrigine for generalized seizures associated with the Lennox-Gastaut syndrome. Lamictal Lennox-Gastaut Study Group [published correction appears in *N Engl J Med*. 1998;339:851–852]. *N Engl J Med* 1997;337:1807–1812.

53. Donaldson JA, Glauser TA, Olberding LS. Lamotrigine adjunctive therapy in childhood epileptic encephalopathy (the Lennox Gastaut syndrome). *Epilepsia* 1997;38:68–73.

54. Glauser TA, Levisohn PM, Ritter F, et al. Topiramate in Lennox-Gastaut syndrome: open-label treatment of patients completing a randomized controlled trial. Topiramate YL Study Group. *Epilepsia* 2000;41(Suppl 1):S86–S90.

55. Glauser TA. Topiramate in the catastrophic epilepsies of childhood. *J Child Neurol* 2000;15:S14–S21.

56. Wheless JW. Use of topiramate in childhood generalized seizure disorders. *J Child Neurol* 2000;15(Suppl 1):S7–S13.

57. Sachdeo RC, Glauser TA, Ritter F, et al. A double-blind, randomized trial of topiramate in Lennox-Gastaut syndrome. Topiramate YL Study Group. *Neurology* 1999;52:1882–1887.

58. Coppola G, Caliendo G, Veggiotti P, et al. Topiramate as add-on drug in children, adolescents and young adults with Lennox-Gastaut syndrome: An Italian multicentric study. *Epilepsy Res* 2002;51:147–153.

59. Vining EP. Clinical efficacy of the ketogenic diet. *Epilepsy Res* 1999;37:181–190.

60. Wheless JW, Baumgartner J, Ghanbari C. Vagus nerve stimulation and the ketogenic diet. *Neurol Clin* 2001;19:371–407.

61. Parker AP, Polkey CE, Binnie CD, et al. Vagal nerve stimulation in epileptic encephalopathies. *Pediatrics* 1999;103:778–782.

62. Frost M, Gates J, Helmers SL, et al. Vagus nerve stimulation in children with refractory seizures associated with Lennox-Gastaut syndrome. *Epilepsia* 2001;42:1148–1152.

63. Wheless JW. Vagus nerve stimulation. In: Wyllie E, ed. The treatment of epilepsy: Principles and practice. 3rd ed. Baltimore: Lippincott, Williams and Wilkins, 2001:1007–1015.

64. Majoie HJ, Berfelo MW, Aldenkamp AP, et al. Vagus

nerve stimulation in children with therapy-resistant epilepsy diagnosed as Lennox-Gastaut syndrome: Clinical results, neuropsychological effects, and cost-effectiveness. *J Clin Neurophysiol.* 2001;18:419–428.

65. Helmers SL, Wheless JW, Frost M, et al. Vagus nerve stimulation therapy in pediatric patients with refractory epilepsy: Retrospective study. *J Child Neurol* 2001;16: 843–848.

66. Vossler DG. Exacerbation of seizures in Lennox-Gastaut syndrome by gabapentin. *Neurology* 1996;46: 852–853.

67. Lortie A, Chiron C, Mumford J, et al. The potential for increasing seizure frequency, relapse, and appearance of new seizure types with vigabatrin. *Neurology* 1993;43(Suppl 5):S24–S27.

68. Bonanni P, Parmeggiani L, Guerrini R. Different neurophysiologic patterns of myoclonus characterize Lennox-Gastaut syndrome and myoclonic astatic epilepsy. *Epilepsia* 2002;43:609–615.

69. Wallace SJ. Myoclonus and epilepsy in childhood: a review of treatment with valproate, ethosuximide, lamotrigine and zonisamide. *Epilepsy Res* 1998;29:147–154.

70. Arzimanoglou A. Treatment options in pediatric epilepsy syndromes. *Epileptic Disord* 2002;4:217–225.

71. Oguni H, Tanaka T, Hayashi K, et al. Treatment and long-term prognosis of myoclonic-astatic epilepsy of early childhood. *Neuropediatrics* 2002;33:122–132.

72. Dulac O, Kaminska A. Use of lamotrigine in Lennox-Gastaut and related epilepsy syndromes. *J Child Neurol* 1997;12(Suppl 1):S23–S28.

73. Perucca E, Gram L, Avanzini G, Antiepileptic drugs as a cause of worsening seizures. Epilepsia 1998;39:5–17. *Neurology* 2001;57:1518–1519.

74. Szczepanik E, Pakszys M, Rusek G. Positive effect of felbamate therapy in a boy with refractory epilepsy. *Neurol Neurochir Pol* 2000;33(Suppl 1):195–201.

75. Pellock JM. Felbamate in epilepsy therapy: evaluating the risks. *Drug Safety* 1999;21:225–239.

76. Kaufman DW, Kelly JP, Anderson T, et al. Evaluation of case reports of aplastic anemia among patients treated with felbamate. *Epilepsia* 1997;38:1265–1269.

77. Thompson CD, Barthen MT, Hopper DW, et al. Quantification in patient urine samples of felbamate and three metabolites: Acid carbamate and two mercapturic acids. *Epilepsia* 1999;40:769–776.

78. Than TN, Chiron C, Dellatolas G, et al. Long term efficacy and tolerance of stiripentol in severe myoclonic epilepsy of infancy (Dravet's Syndrome). *Arch Pediatr* 2002;11:1120–1127.

24

Ketogenic Diet in Patients with Dravet Syndrome and Myoclonic Epilepsies in Infancy and Early Childhood

Natalio Fejerman,* Roberto Caraballo,* and Ricardo Cersosimo*

*Department of Neurology, Hospital de Pediatria Juan P. Garrahan, Buenos Aires, Argentina

INTRODUCTION

The ketogenic diet has been used as a therapeutic alternative to antiepileptic drugs for refractory epilepsy (1–3). The diet consists of an intake of three or four times as much fat as carbohydrates and protein combined (1–4).

Fasting has long since been believed to be a cure for epilepsy. Hippocrates used fasting as a specific treatment for patients with epilepsy in the 5th century BC and in the Bible Jesus suggests fasting after an epilepsy attack (New Testament: Saint Mark 9; 14–29).

In 1921, Wilder (5), formulated the ketogenic diet to induce the metabolic effects of fasting for the management of seizures. In spite of its effectiveness, the diet was replaced by the new antiepileptic drugs (AEDs). Phenobarbital (PB), the first AED, was introduced in 1912 and between 1935 and 1968, 16 additional AEDs became available. The ketogenic diet was reserved for use in selected patients and at selected treatment centers. A variant of the classical diet using medium-chain triglycerides was introduced in the 1970s (6), but, in the last decade, most of the centers adopted the classic diet in a 4:1 ratio of fat to combined proteins and carbohydrates. The group of Johns Hopkins Hospital and Health System in Baltimore was the most enthusiastic in advising the ketogenic diet; they were able to reach public recognition through a movie and a very practical little book entitled "The Epilepsy Diet Treatment" (1). Furthermore, the popularity of the Atkins diet as a weight-loss diet in the United States helped the development of many food products that are also "Keto-compatible," increasing the tolerability of this diet (7).

MECHANISMS OF ACTION

No mechanism of action of the diet has been defined. Its efficacy has been ascribed to acidosis, cellular and extracellular dehydration, the direct action of acetoacetate or β-hydroxybutyrate, and changes in the source or utilization of energy within the brain (8).

Ketones are induced within the first 24 to 36 hours. Ketones are lower in cerebrospinal fluid than in plasma and do not accumulate in the brain. Although there is a metabolic acidosis resulting from accumulation of ketones and decreased bicarbonate, plasma pH normalizes because of a reduction of both bicarbonate and partial pressure of carbon dioxide. Recent neuroimaging data suggest that there is an increase in brain ketones and the phosphocreatine/organic phosphate ratio (9–11).

Alternative mechanisms for the action of the ketogenic diet are an increase in brain gamma-aminobutyric acid (an inhibitory central nervous system neurotransmitter) (12). Whether ketones themselves have GABAergic effects on the brain and serve as direct neuroinhibitors remains uncertain (13). The proposed enhancement of a gamma-aminobutyric acid shunt has also been suggested (14). The potential effects of changes in water and electrolytes have also been indicated as antiepileptic mediators (3). There are decreased Na^+, K^+, and Mg^{2+} stores, with an increased Ca^+ turnover. It is unclear what the direct consequences of these ionic alterations are within the central nervous system. As of yet, a predictable and definite effect on brain tissue concentrations of these plasma ionic alterations (Na^+, K^+, and Cl^-) has not been demonstrated.

REPORTED SERIES

Recent reports of series of patients after 1 year on the diet show an overall efficacy ranging from 15% to 50% in terms of patients becoming seizure-free or having a 50% to 90% reduction in seizures (2–4,15–19). Use of ketogenic diet was generally advised for children between 2 and 6 to 8 years of age. A retrospective review of 32 infants treated with ketogenic diet (14 of whom started treatment at ages ≤ 12 months) showed that 71% were able to maintain strong ketosis, 19.4% became seizure free, and an additional 35.5% had > 50% reduction in seizure frequency. The diet was most effective for infants with infantile spasms or myoclonic seizures and overall effectiveness in infants was similar to that reported for older children (20). The largest prospective study done between 1994 and 1996 enrolled 150 consecutive children aged 1 to 16 years having a minimum of two seizures per week, despite the appropriate use of at least two anticonvulsant medications. Children were followed for a minimum of 1 year or until diet discontinuation. At 12 months, 55% remained on the diet and 27% had a >90% decrease in seizure frequency. Comparing efficacy in different seizure types after 6 months of diet, 5 of 13 children with infantile spasms (IS), 13 of 28 with myoclonic seizures, 9 of 17 with atonic seizures/drops, 4 of 11 with clonic seizures, and 5 of 11 with partial seizures achieved ≥90% seizure control or became seizure-free (21). A recent retrospective study of ketogenic diet in 45 adolescents between

the ages of 12 and 19 years showed that 20 of them were still on the diet at 12 months of diet duration with >90% efficacy in 6 patients and 50% to 90% efficacy in 7. The authors concluded that ketogenic diet is as well tolerated and efficacious for adolescents with epilepsy as for the general childhood population (22). A prospective study of ketogenic diet in 11 adults with intractable epilepsy was presented not long ago. At the 8 months follow-up, seven remained on the diet with a >90% seizure reduction in three, 50% to 89% reduction in three, and <50% reduction in seizure activity in one (23).

ADVERSE EFFECTS

Adverse effects or complications of ketogenic diet occurring during the initial hospital stay included: hypoglycemia, dehydration, vomiting, diarrhea, and refusal to eat, which may lead parents to early drop out (1). Long-term complications appear after several weeks of treatment and comprise metabolic derangements such as hyperuricemia, hypocalcemia, hypoproteinemia, carnitine deficiency, metabolic acidosis, hyperlipemia, and hypercholesterolemia. Some of these complications are seen during the course of intercurrent infections. The risk of hyperlipemia and hypercholesterolemia is obviously the first thought and it is reported in 25% to 65% of the cases (24,25). When successful in controlling the seizures, the diet should not be stopped because of lipid abnormalities, as adjustment of the diet ratio will bring the lipids levels toward normal. Ballaban–Gil et al. (26) prospectively monitored 52 children with ketogenic diet, aged 8 months to 16.5 years, looking for complications: five of their patients had serious adverse effects and the authors pointed out that four were receiving, at the same time, valproic acid (VPA).

Overall tolerability of the diet is good for both children and their parents (27). Parents may believe that their children do not grow as well on the diet, but mistake the lack of weight gain for lack of linear growth (14). The diet should be calculated and adjusted carefully so that children gain weight only in proportion to the increase in their height. Children grow on the diet, and there are indications that this linear growth may occur at a lower—but still normal—rate (28). Compared with the problems posed by the seizures and the medications, growth is considered by parents to be the lesser problem (26).

Kidney stones occur in approximately 10% of children who are on the diet and can be treated and perhaps even prevented by providing adequate fluid intake and alkalinization of the urine (29,30). Occasionally, patients need lithotripsy or surgical removal of the stones. The occurrence of stones has not been a reason for discontinuing the diet in children whose seizures have been improved.

Cardiomyopathy was reported in patients on the ketogenic diet. Prolonged QT interval in three patients and cardiac chamber enlargement in other three were found in a series of 20 pediatric patients on this diet (31). Hyperlipidemia and subsequent atherosclerosis have caused concerns (24). Research needs to be conducted to assess the long-term effects of the diet on the cardiovascular system.

Two particular situations in relation to ketogenic diet were recently reported. In 14 children cotreated with ketogenic diet and topiramate, a decrease in bicarbonate level occurred, mostly at the time of ketogenic diet induction when added to prior topiramate (TPM) therapy. The authors recommended to give bicarbonate supplements (32). Nine children on ketogenic diet safely underwent general anesthesia for surgical procedures, although there was an increased risk of metabolic acidosis (33).

DIET IN PRACTICE

The Johns Hopkins protocol for ketogenic diet is now widely accepted. Children begin fasting after dinner the night before admission, although parents are advised to decrease carbohydrates 2 days before admission. Fasting is maintained in the hospital with monitoring of blood sugar (every 4 hours) until the child becomes deeply ketotic. The diet is then introduced gradually. Hospitalizations last 4 to 7 days and parents are instructed to monitor urinary ketones and to avoid potential sources of glucose. The recommended allowance of protein should be strictly maintained for children at a minimum of 1 gr/kg

per day, while carbohydrates are kept to a minimum. In practical terms, the fat requirements of the diet are given through heavy cream, oils, and other dietary fats. Starchy fruits or vegetables, breads, cookies, pasta or grains and sources of simple sugars are not allowed; neither are medications in syrup forms. The prohibition of even minimal amount of candies, cookies, and common beverages renders the management of the diet quite difficult, but, in general, it ends up to be fairly well accepted. In the past, we had serious difficulties in acceptance on the part of the families and we might say that ketogenic diet was not easy to implement in Latin American countries. We had the example of an Italian origin family in Argentina in which the grandmother of a little girl hit the nurse during admission because she took away a cookie from the hands of the child. At the end, the most important task is to gain acceptance and conviction of parents regarding its possible benefits.

EXPERIENCE WITH THE KETOGENIC DIET IN PATIENTS WITH DRAVET SYNDROME AND MYOCLONIC EPILEPSIES IN INFANCY AND EARLY CHILDHOOD

On the occasion of the meeting held in Seattle in December 2002 in honor of Dr. Charlotte Dravet, we reviewed our patient population seen from 1990 to 2002 to identify the nosology of idiopathic or cryptogenic myoclonic epilepsy syndromes in infancy and early childhood (34). Children with symptomatic myoclonic epilepsies, severe myoclonic epilepsy in infancy (SMEI) or Dravet syndrome, and cryptogenic Lennox–Gastaut syndrome (LGS) were excluded. We collected 62 children fulfilling inclusion criteria. Twenty-six children were diagnosed with benign myoclonic epilepsy in infancy (BMEI), eight with reflex myoclonic epilepsy in infancy (35,36), and 28 with epilepsy with myoclonic-astatic seizures (EMAS) (37). During the same period, we saw about 3000 children between 3 months and 6 years of age with epilepsy, excluding febrile seizures (FS). Careful analysis of seizure evolution and intellectual development lead us to distinguish BMEI and three subgroups

TABLE 24–1. *Nosology of idiopathic or cryptogenic myoclonic epilepsies in infancy and early childhood (excluding severe myoclonic epilepsy in infancy or Dravet syndrome)[a,b]*

Epilepsy syndrome[c]	Number of cases	Sex	Mean age of onset (m)	Mean time of follow-up (y)
BMEI	26	Male: 15 Female: 11	12	3.5
RMI	8	Male: 5 Female: 3	10	6
EMAS (variants in relation to evolution)				
Seizure free and normal IQ	9	Male: 6 Female: 3	36	3
Persistent seizures and normal IQ	9	Male: 6 Female: 3	36	4
Persistent seizures and mental retardation	10	Male: 4 Female: 6	18	5.5

[a] Presentation of 62 patients.

[b] Patients seen between 1990 and 2002 diagnosed in accordance to the list of syndromes proposed by ILAE's Task Force on Classification (43).

[c] BMEI, benign myoclonic epilepsy in infancy; RMEI, reflex myoclonic epilepsy in infancy; EMAS, epilepsy with myoclonic astatic seizures.

of EMAS, divided by severity of outcome. Patients with BMEI can resemble those with a favorable outcome subgroup of EMAS, although seizures in BMEI are only myoclonic, whereas seizures in EMAS usually display head drops or falls due to myoclonic-atonic seizures causing astasia (Table 24–1). We excluded from the mentioned series of patients the cases with SMEI (38) because it has been recognized that this syndrome may present or not myoclonic components. Therefore, the term "Dravet syndrome" is welcome as a distinction from the true myoclonic epilepsies (39). The use of Ketogenic diet in patients with Dravet syndrome and true myoclonic epilepsies include the following:

1. We have been following 43 children with diagnosis of Dravet Syndrome for 2 to 11 years. Of these, 17 (11 boys and 6 girls) were treated with ketogenic diet as an add-on to previous use of one to three AEDs. Ages at onset of ketogenic diet were 3 to 9 years (mean 6 years). Two of the children had to interrupt the diet due to intolerance (vomiting, diarrhea, etc.) and six dropped out between 2 and 3 months after onset because no significant improvement was achieved. The diet was maintained for 14 to 36 months (mean 24 months) in nine children. The results were: seven children achieved 75% to 100% control of seizures, four are still on diet, but one began to

have more seizures again after 12 months. The other three patients are off the diet for more than 2 years. One of them is seizure-free, one has sporadic seizures, and one relapsed and abandoned the diet after 2 years adherence. In two patients, seizure control was 50% to 74% during 2 years and one of them is now off the diet, still with VPA + clobazam (CLB) and in the same category of seizure control.

Because of the severity and intractability of seizures in patients with Dravet syndrome, the fact that 9 of the 15 children that maintained the diet had a significant reduction in number of seizures shows that ketogenic diet is, at present, the best therapeutic alternative. Even in the cases in which the reduction in seizures was not dramatic, there was an improvement in quality of life. In all patients, the AEDs were lowered to one or two. One of these patients did not show further mental deterioration. The youngest child on ketogenic diet in our series of patients with Dravet syndrome was 3 years old, which is due, in part, to the difficulties we had in the past to clearly define this diagnosis and to the time necessary to elapse while trying AEDs. We think that children with Dravet syndrome should be offered a ketogenic diet as early as possible.

2. We have followed the 28 patients with variants of idiopathic or cryptogenic myoclonic epilepsies in infancy and early childhood for 3 to

13 years. Eleven children with EMAS, of whom seven were boys, received ketogenic diet due to failure of appropriately selected AED treatment. In each case, the ketogenic diet was added to one or two AEDs. One patient interrupted the diet due to early adverse effects and four did not show any significant reduction in the number of seizures. The other six children were kept on the diet between 18 and 48 months (mean 26 months); the follow-up showed a 75% to 100% control of seizures in four. Two patients remained on the diet for more than 24 months and two have been off the diet for several years, remaining seizure-free and without AEDs. From the mentioned six patients, two achieved a 50% to 75% control of seizures and we were able to reduce medication to only one AED; both are enjoying a better quality of life.

The fact of having significant improvement in quality of life and reduction of seizure frequency in 6 out of 11 children with refractory idiopathic or cryptogenic myoclonic epilepsies shows that this therapeutic alternative is quite useful. We want to emphasize that in the follow-up of our series of 28 children with this syndrome and its variants, being free of seizures was synonymous to normal mental development. Mental retardation was evident in one-half of the two thirds of cases who showed persistent seizures, despite AEDs and/or ketogenic diet treatment.

3. Our criteria to diagnose BMEI was: onset of myoclonic seizures before 3 years of age in otherwise normal infants. Including our eight cases of reflex myoclonic epilepsy in infancy, we have been following 34 children having myoclonic seizures (not myoclonic-atonic or astatic) with typical polyspike–wave discharges in EEGs for 3 to 7 years. Even when most of the patients with BMEI present a good response to treatment with VPA, in all reported series, a few cases show persistence of seizures and/or impairment in neuropsychologic development (40,41). Two girls and one boy with BMEI, tried the ketogenic diet; one of the girls and the boy had a very good response and have been on the diet for 20 and 40 months.

DISCUSSION

Our experience with the ketogenic diet in 17 children with Dravet syndrome, 11 with EMAS in infancy and early childhood, and 3 with (not so benign) BMEI shows an overall good response in terms of seizure frequency and quality of life (Table 24–2).

To our knowledge, this is the first description of ketogenic diet treatment evaluated in specific epilepsy syndromes. Previous studies of a specific epilepsy syndrome were reported mainly in infants with West syndrome (20). In some way, our results confirm the general assumption that the ketogenic diet is effective in patients with myoclonic seizures. We do think that the recognition of epilepsy syndromes includes the possibility of ascribing particular prognosis in each case and that this concept should be applied to every therapeutic trial in epilepsies. When idiopathic and symptomatic focal seizures, for instance, are considered together in evaluating efficacy of AEDs, results may be false and erroneous since children with benign focal epilepsies respond well to AEDs. Another

TABLE 24–2. *Ketogenic diet in 31 patients with particular epilepsy syndromes*

Epilepsy syndrome[a]	Number of cases	Adverse effects (AE) or no response (NR)	Significant response (50%–100% control of seizures)	Follow-up since onset of ketogenic diet (Mean in m)	Significant decline in efficacy	Patients without diet and still good control
SMEI (or) DS	17	AE: 2 NR: 6	9	24	2	4
EMAS	11	AE: 1 NR: 4	6	26	—	2
BMEI	3	NR: 1	2	30	—	—

[a]Severe myoclonic epilepsy in infancy (SMEI) or Dravet syndrome (DS), epilepsy with myoclonic-astatic seizures (EMAS), and benign myoclonic epilepsy in infancy (BMEI).

consideration is the length of follow-up of trials. Results at 3 or 6 months are of no real value in evaluating AEDs, ketogenic diet, or even surgical treatments.

It has been reported that a clear diminution in seizure control occurs with ketogenic diet over time (21,42). The significant decline in efficacy after 9–12 months of treatment with a ketogenic diet in patients with refractory symptomatic and cryptogenic partial or generalized epilepsies found in one study may have been due to the inclusion of various etiologies for epilepsies (42).

Finally, the selection of families able to follow this type of dietary treatment has to be very strict in order to reduce the number of failures.

REFERENCES

1. Freeman JM., Kelly MT, Freeman JB. *The epilepsy diet treatment.* New York: Demos, 1994.
2. Lefevre F, Aronson N. Ketogenic diet for the treatment of refractory epilepsy in children: A systematic review of efficacy. *Pediatrics* 2000;105(4):E46.
3. Phelps SJ, Hovinga CA, Rose DF, et al. The ketogenic diet in pediatric epilepsy. *Nutr Clin Pract* 1998;13:267–282.
4. Di Mario FJ, Holland J. The ketogenic diet: A review of the experience at Connecticut children's medical center. *Pediatr Neurol* 2002;26:288–292.
5. Wilder RM. The effect of ketogenemia on the course of epilepsy. *Mayo Clin Bull* 1921;2:307–314.
6. Huttenlocher PR, Wilbourn AJ, Signore JM. Medium-chain triglycerides as a therapy for intractable childhood epilepsy. *Neurology* 1971;21:1097–1103.
7. Thiele EA. Assessing the efficacy of antiepileptic treatments: The ketogenic diet. *Epilepsia* 2003;44[Suppl 7]:30–37.
8. Vining EP. Ketogenic diet. In Engel J, Pedley TA. *Epilepsy: A comprehensive textbook.* Philadelphia: Lippincontt-Raven Publishers, 1997;1339–1344.
9. Seymour KJ, Bluml S, Sutherling W, et al. Identification of cerebral acetone by IH-MRS in patients with epilepsy controlled by ketogenic diet. *MAGNA* 1999;8:33–42.
10. Pan JW, Bebin BM, Chu WJ, et al. Ketosis and epilepsy: 31P spectroscopic imaging at 4.IT. *Epilepsia* 1999;40:703–707.
11. Shen J, Novotny EJ, Rothman DL. In vivo lactate and beta-hydroxybutyrate editing using a pure-phase refocusing pulse train. *Magn Reson Med* 1998;40:783–788.
12. Daikhin Y, Yudkoff M. Ketone bodies and brain glutamate and GABA metabolism. *Develop Neurosci* 1998;20:358–364.
13. Thio LL, Wong M, Yamada KA. Ketone bodies do not directly alter excitatory or inhibitory hippocampal synaptic transmission. *Neurology* 2000;54:325–331.
14. Nordli DR, De Vivo DC. The ketogenic diet revisited: Back to the future. *Epilepsia* 1997;38:743–749.
15. Schwartz RH, Eaton J, Bower BD, et al. Ketogenic diets in the treatment of epilepsy: Short-term clinical effects. *Develop Med Child Neurol* 1989;31:145–151.
16. Schwartz RH, Boyes S, Aynsley-Green A. Metabolic effects of three ketogenic diets in the treatment of severe epilepsy. *Develop Med Child Neurol* 1989;31:152–160.
17. Kinsman SL, Vining EPG, Quaskey A, et al. Efficacy of the ketogenic diet for intractable seizure disorders: Review of 58 cases. *Epilepsia* 1992;33:1132–1136.
18. Swink TD, Vining EPG, Freeman JM. The ketogenic diet. Barnes LA, ed. *Advances in pediatrics.* Vol. 44. St. Louis, MO: Mosby, 1997:297–329.
19. Vining EPG, Freeman JM, Ballaban-Gil K, et al. A multicenter study of the efficacy of ketogenic diet. *Arch Neurol* 1998;55:1433–1437.
20. Nordli DR, Kuroda MM, Carroll J, et al. Experience with the ketogenic diet in infants. *Pediatrics* 2001;108:129–133.
21. Freeman J, Vining E, Pillas D, et al. The efficacy of the ketogenic diet—1998:A prospective evaluation of intervention in 150 children. *Pediatrics* 1998;102(6):1358–1363.
22. Mady MA., Kossoff EH, McGregor AL. The ketogenic diet: adolescents can do it, too. *Epilepsia* 2003;44(6):847–851.
23. Sirven J, Whedon B, Caplan D, et al. The ketogenic diet for intractable epilepsy in adults: Preliminary results. *Epilepsia* 1999;40:1721–1726.
24. Vining EPG, Freeman JM, Kwiterovitch P Jr, et al. The ketogenic diet induces dyslipidemia. *Epilepsia* 1999;40[Suppl 7]:122.
25. Rios VG, Panico LR, Demartini MG, Carniello MA. Complications of treatment of epilepsy by a ketogenic diet. *Rev Neurol* 2001;33(10):909–915.
26. Ballaban-Gil K, Callahan C, O'Dell C, et al. Complications of the ketogenic diet. *Epilepsia* 1998;39:744–748.
27. Caraballo R, Tripoli J, Escobal L, et al. Ketogenic diet: efficacy and tolerability in childhood intractable epilepsy. *Rev Neurol* 1998;26(149):61–64.
28. Hemingway C, Freeman J, Pillas D, et al. The ketogenic diet: A 3 to 6 year follow-up of 150 children enrolled prospectively. *Pediatrics* 2001;4:898–905.
29. Vining EPG, Casey JC, McGrogan JR, et al. Children grow on the ketogenic diet [abstract]. *Epilepsia* 1998;[Suppl. 6]:168.
30. Furth SL, Casey JC, Pyzik PL et al. Risk factors for urolithiasis in children on the ketogenic diet. *Pediatr Nephrol* 2000;15:126–128.
31. Best TH, Franz DN, Gilbert DL, et al. Cardiac complications in pediatric patients on the ketogenic diet. *Neurology* 2000;54:2328–2330.
32. Takeoka M, Riviello J, Pfeifer H, et al. Concomitant treatment with topiramate and ketogenic diet in pediatric epilepsy. *Epilepsia* 2002;43(9):1072–1075.
33. Valencia I, Pfeifer H, Thiele EA. General anesthesia and the ketogenic diet: Clinical experience in nine patients. *Epilepsia* 2002;43(5):525–529.
34. Dulac O, Plouin P, Shewmon A. Myoclonus and epilepsy in childhood. 1996 Royaumont meeting. *Epilepsy Res* 1998;30:91–106.
35. Ricci S, Cusmai R, Fusco L, et al. Reflex myoclonic epilepsy in infancy: A new age-dependent idiopathic

epileptic syndrome related to startle reaction. *Epilepsia* 1995;36(4):342–348.

36. Caraballo R, Cassar L, Monges S, et al. Reflex myoclonic epilepsy in infancy: a new reflex epilepsy syndrome or a variant of benign myoclonic epilepsy in infancy. *Rev Neurol* 2003;36:429–432 (Spanish).

37. Oguni H, Fukuyama Y, Tanaka T, et al. Myoclonic-astatic epilepsy of early childhood—clinical and EEG analysis of myoclonic-astatic seizures, and discussions on the nosology of the syndrome. *Brain Develop* 2001;23(7):757–764.

38. Dravet C, Bureau M, Oguni H, et al. Severe myoclonic epilepsy in infancy (Dravet syndrome). In: Roger J, Bureau M, Dravet C, Genton P, Tassinari CA, Wolf P, eds. *Epileptic syndromes in infancy, childhood and adolescence.* 3rd ed. London: John Libbey, 2002:81–103.

39. Fejerman N. Severe myoclonic epilepsy in infancy (Dravet Syndrome). In: Wallace S, Farrell K, eds. *Epilepsy in children.* 2nd ed. London: Arnold, 2004:157–160.

40. Dravet C, Bureau M. Benign myoclonic epilepsy in infancy. In: Roger J, Bureau M, Dravet C, Genton P, Tassinari CA, Wolf P, eds. *Epileptic syndromes in infancy, childhood and adolescence.* 3rd ed. London: John Libbey, 2002:69–79.

41. Fejerman N. Benign myoclonic epilepsy in infancy. In: Wallace S, Farrell K, eds. *Epilepsy in children.* 2nd ed. London: Arnold, 2004:153–156.

42. Coppola G, Veggiotti P, Cusmai R, et al. The ketogenic diet in children, adolescents and young adults with refractory epilepsy: an Italian multicentric experience. *Epilepsy Res* 2002;48(3):221–227.

43. Engel J. A proposed diagnostic scheme for people with epileptic seizures and with epilepsy: Report of the ILAE Task Force on Classification and Terminology. *Epilepsia* 2001;42(6):796–803.

25

Treatment of Myoclonic Epilepsies of Childhood, Adolescence, and Adulthood

Marco T. Medina,* Iris E. Martínez-Juárez,† Reyna M. Durón,*,†
Pierre Genton,‡ Renzo Guerrini,§ Charlotte Dravet,‡ Michelle Bureau,‡
Katerina Tanya Perez-Gosiengfiao,† Claudia Amador,* Julia N. Bailey,†
Franz Chaves-Sell,‖ Antonio V. Delgado-Escueta†

*National Autonomous University of Honduras, Tegucigalpa, Honduras; †California Comprehensive
Epilepsy Program, David Geffen School of Medicine at UCLA, Los Angeles, California; ‡ Centre
Saint-Paul-Hôpital Henri Gastaut, Marseille, France; §Epilepsy, Neurophysiology, and
Neurogenetics Unit, Department of Child Neurology and Psychiatry, University of Pisa and Research
Institute 'Stella Maris' Foundation, Pisa, Itlay; ‖Hospital Clinica Biblica, San José, Costa Rica

INTRODUCTION

Myoclonic epilepsies are still often misdiagnosed, treated with undue delay, or treated with inappropriate drugs. Difficulties in choosing the right treatment in these epilepsies have been discussed in recent reviews (1–3). New antiepileptic agents have opened new possibilities, but have also increased risks of paradoxical aggravation of myoclonic epilepsies. Specific treatment strategies of the different forms of idiopathic myoclonic epilepsies have been discussed in various chapters of this book and the reader can refer to them. However, a summary of this complex field would be useful for the clinician.

No Class I study, which implies a controlled and randomized study, has been performed regarding the myoclonic epilepsies. Most of the literature is based on uncontrolled comparisons, such as groups of patients or case studies. Some randomized trials have been conducted that include myoclonic epilepsies together with other primary generalized epilepsies.

In this chapter, we first describe the results of a long-term follow-up in 222 patients with juvenile myoclonic epilepsy (JME), subdivided into its subsyndromes. We analyze the responses to antiepileptic drug (AED) treatment based on the constellation of seizure types, common trigger factors, seizure types that persist after antiepileptic drug treatment, frequency of breakthroughs, and side effects of antiepileptic, during more than 10 years of follow-up. We next describe AEDs reported in literature used in the management of myoclonic absence epilepsy, eyelid myoclonic epilepsy, JME and familial adult myoclonic epilepsy (FAME). Finally, we provide an algorithm for treatment of JME based on our 222 patients and the Marseille/Nice cohort on JME. This algorithm also considers opinions of experts and available information from recent published studies.

JUVENILE MYOCLONIC EPILEPSY CONSORTIUM OF GENESS: TREATMENT RESULTS AND LONG-TERM OUTCOME IN 222 PATIENTS

Classic Juvenile Myoclonic Epilepsy

At the time we initially evaluated 161 classic JME patients (91F:60M), 60% (96/161) had myoclonic and tonic–clonic seizures, 34% (54/161) had myoclonic, tonic–clonic, and spanioleptic absence seizures, 6% (10/161) had myoclonic seizures only, and 1% (1/161) had both myoclonic and absence seizures. We were able to follow these 161 patients for a mean period of 11.6 years (range 1 to 41 years) (Fig. 25–1); 57% were female (91/161) and 43% were male (70/161).

In evaluating the results of this long-term follow-up, we first asked how many patients were completely free of tonic–clonic grand-mal convulsions (Table 25–1). Eighty-five percent (137/161) were free from tonic–clonic seizures, most often because of AED treatment. We then asked how many patients were completely free of all type of seizures due to AED treatment. Of the 161 patients, 72 (54%) were seizure-free and did not suffer any breakthrough seizures during the follow-up period of 10.1 years (range 1 to 41 years).

We also asked how many patients had uncontrolled seizures in spite of treatment and the reason why. At the initial portion of the follow-up period, there were 89/161 patients who identified various trigger factors as responsible for breakthrough seizures (Table 25–2). In subsequent months and years of follow-up, some patients were able to correct trigger factors, such as sleep deprivation and noncompliance, thereby increasing the number of patients whose seizures completely ceased from 72 to 93. When analyzed separately, these 93 patients achieved complete freedom from seizures for a mean period of 34 months. Among them were 17 patients who were in remission from seizures for 4 to 11 years (Fig. 25–2).

Next, we turned our attention to the 68 patients who habitually suffered breakthrough seizures in spite of recognizing the responsible trigger factors (Table 25–2). Thirty-one of these patients only had myoclonic seizures more often on awakening. Five other patients had myoclonic and absence seizures, while 9 had breakthrough tonic–clonic grand-mal convulsions.

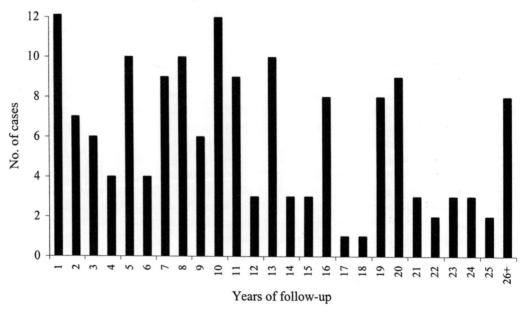

FIG. 25–1. Years of follow-up in 161 patients with classic JME.

TABLE 25–1. *Long-term follow-up and outcome of juvenile myoclonic epilepsy subsyndromes*

	Classic JME	CAE evolving to JME	JME with adolescent pyknolepsy absence	JME with myoclonic astatic
Grand mal controlled	137/161 (85%)	26/35 (74%)	17/18 (94.4%)	6/8 (75%)
Persisting myoclonic seizures	31/161 (19%)	4/35 (11%)	2/18 (11%)	0
Persisting MS + ABS	5/161 (3%)	0	5/18 (28%)	0
Persisting grand mal	9/161 (5.5%)	6/35 (17%)	1/18 (6%)	1/8 (12.5%)
Persisting ABS only	0	16/35 (46%)	0	0
Persisting myoclonic astatic	0	0	0	1/8 (12.5%)

MS, myoclonic seizures; ABS, absence seizures.

We next asked what AEDs patients were receiving, how long the patients remained seizure-free, and what were the adverse effects of AEDs. Of the 93 patients who were completely seizure-free, 85 were receiving AEDs. 60 patients (65%) were on valproate (VPA) monotherapy. They were seizure-free as long as 22 years, the mean interval of seizure-free period being 36 months.

Of seizure-free patients 11% (10/93) were receiving VPA plus one or more other AEDs. Some 15% (14/93) were taking AEDs other than VPA either as mono- or polytherapy.

Interestingly, there were eight patients (9%) who were seizure-free, but were not on any AEDs (Fig. 25–3). Among them was one patient who had been seizure-free for 11 years.

The most common side effects in 150 patients taking AEDs were weight gain (12 patients), tremors (6 patients), hair loss (5 patients), nausea and vomiting (3 patients), polycystic ovary (2 patients), gastritis (1 patient), diarrhea (1 patient), hepatotoxicity (1 patient) and memory problems (1 patient). All side effects were observed in the group of patients taking VPA either as mono- or polytherapy. Tremor was found in one patient taking topiramate (TPM) monotherapy. Weight gain was reported also in one patient taking primidone (PRM) monotherapy.

It seemed that the more combinations of seizure types, the harder to control seizures with AEDs. Among patients presenting with myoclonic seizures only, 80% (8/10) were seizure-free. Of patients presenting myoclonic and tonic–clonic seizures, 63% (60/96) were seizure-free. On the other hand, only 46% (25/54) of patients with myoclonic, tonic–clonic, and absence seizures were seizure-free. The sole patient who had myoclonic and absence seizures had not achieved seizure control.

Among 68 patients who had recurrent seizures, 3 patients chose not to take any medication. Two were planning to get pregnant; they suffered mainly from myoclonic seizures and rare tonic–clonic convulsions. Among these 68 patients, 25 reported dissatisfaction with AED treatment because seizure frequency did not change.

Episodes of convulsive tonic–clonic *status epilepticus* (two patients) and myoclonic and absence status (one patient) were uncommon and were reported in only three patients. We did not observe any significant difference regarding response to treatment among women and men. Of women, 57 were seizure-free (61%), compared to 36 men (52%) who were seizure-free.

We also reviewed what AEDs patients were receiving at the time they were initially referred to our service. Among the 161 classic JME patients, 104 (64%) received carbamazepine (CBZ)

TABLE 25–2. *Trigger factors for seizures (mainly myoclonic seizures) in 161 patients with classic JME*

Trigger factors	No. of cases	%
Sleep deprivation	71	44
Awakening	61	38
Stress	32	20
Alcohol	26	16
Noncompliance	23	15
Menses	17	10
Fatigue	16	10
Light (TV, video games, strobe)	14	9
Physical activity	3	3
Cognitive tasks (e.g., reading)	3	3
Anger	1	1
Hunger (hypoglycemia)	1	1

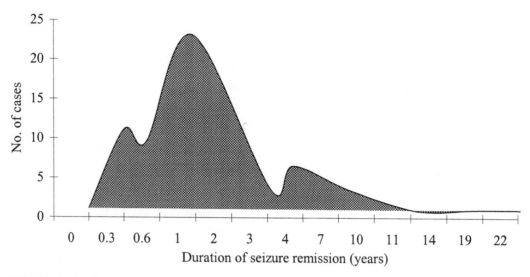

FIG. 25–2. Remission of seizures (years) in 93 patients with classic JME.

and/or phenytoin (PHT) prior to referral to our service. Only 14% reported some improvement of seizures. In contrast, 14 of 21 (66%) blamed CBZ monotherapy for increasing frequencies of tonic–clonic grand mal, absence, and myoclonic seizures. PHT in combination with VPA phenobarbital (PB) or CBZ increased seizure frequency even more [18/23 or 78% of patients receiving PHT]. PHT monotherapy also aggravated seizures of nine out of 21 patients (42%). PHT in combination with VPA, PB or PRM aggravated seizures in fewer patients (8/25 or 32%). Overall, CBZ and/or PHT increased seizure frequency in 50 of 104 patients (48%). In two patients, this drug combination could have triggered the first appearance of absence seizures. Genton et al. (1) described similar results. (Table 25–3)

Childhood Absence Epilepsy Evolving to Juvenile Myoclonic Epilepsy

We followed 35 patients with childhood absence epilepsy (CAE) evolving to juvenile myoclonic epilepsy (JME) for a mean period of 19.8 years (range 1 to 47 years) (Fig. 25–4). When initially seen, 32 had pyknoleptic absences, tonic–clonic and myoclonic seizure, and only one patient had absence and myoclonic seizures only;

66% were female (23/35) and 44% were male (12/35).

During the long period of follow-up, 3 patients among the 35 original cohort achieved complete seizure control from 2 to 40 years (Table 25–1). Even though 32 patients had persisting seizures, VPA mono- (27 patients) or polytherapy [5 patients: combination with lamotrigine (LTG) or PB or zonisamide (ZNS) with levetiracetam (LEV)] completely suppressed tonic–clonic seizures in 23 patients (72%). Thus 26 patients out of a total number of 35, had satisfactory seizure control because grand-mal seizures had ceased. In this syndrome, absence seizures comprised the most common phenotype that persisted (16/35 patients). Rarely, breakthrough tonic–clonic (6/35 patients) and myoclonic seizures (4/35 patients) were observed.

Of three patients (3/35) who were completely free of seizures, one was taking PB and mephenytoin, another was on LEV and TPM, while one was on VPA monotherapy.

Juvenile Myoclonic Epilepsy with Adolescent-Onset Pyknoleptic Absence

We followed 18 patients with adolescent-onset pyknoleptic absence mixed with JME for a mean period of 13.4 years (range 5 to 26 years). A majority of patients were female (13/18 or 72%).

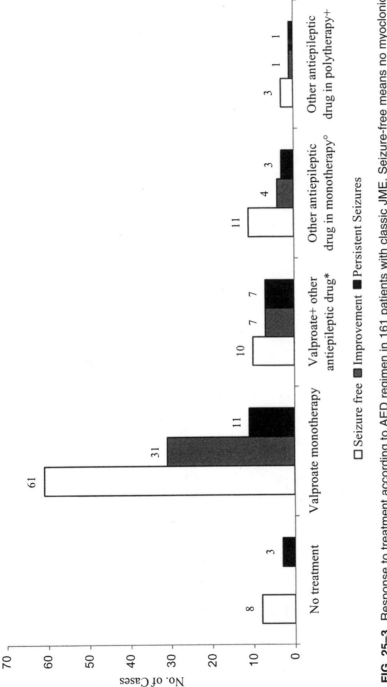

FIG. 25–3. Response to treatment according to AED regimen in 161 patients with classic JME. Seizure-free means no myoclonic, tonic–clonic, or absence seizures. Improvement means either 50% reduction in seizures or the persistence of breakthrough myoclonic or rare tonic–clonic seizures when trigger factors appear. Persistent seizures means no change in seizure pattern and frequencies. *, Other AEDs include: carbamazepine (CBZ), phenytoin (PHT), lamotrigine (LTG), clonazepam (CZP), ethosuximide (ESM), methsuximide (MSM), and lorazepam. One patient was seizure-free on valproate (VPA) + carbamazepine (CBZ), one patient on valproate (VPA) + phenytoin (PHT), five patients on valproate (VPA) + lamotrigine (LTG), one patient on valproate (VPA) + clonazepam (CZP), one patient on valproate (VPA) + topiramate (TPM), and one patient on valproate (VPA) + lorazepam. °, Other AEDs in monotherapy included lamotrigine (LTG), carbamazepine (CBZ), topiramate (TPM), phenobarbital (PB), primidone (PRM), and levetiracetam (LEV). Three patients were seizure-free on carbamazepine (CBZ), two patients on lamotrigine (LTG), two patients on phenobarbital (PB), two patients on levetiracetam (LEV), one patient on topiramate (TPM), and one patient on primidone (PRM). +, One patient was seizure-free on topiramate (TPM) + lamotrigine (LTG) and one patient on phenobarbital (PB) + clonazepam (CZ).

TABLE 25–3. *Response to treatment with traditional AEDs in patients with myoclonic epilepsies of adolescence*

Treatment	Patients from Marseille/Nice (n = 40)				Patients from GENESS consortium (n = 104)			
	No.	Aggravated	No change	Improved	No.	Aggravated	No change	Improved
CBZ								
Monotherapy	13	10	1	2	21	14	5	2
+ PHT					12	10	2	
+ VPA	5	1	3	1	3	2	1	
+ PB	6	5	1					
+ PB + VPA	1			1				
+ PHT + VPA	1	1						
+ PHT + PB	1	1			8	6	2	
+ PB + VGB + CLB	1	1						
Without PHT, n (%)	26	17 (65)	5 (20)	4 (15)	24	16 (67)	6 (25)	2 (8)
All, including those treated in polytherapy with PHT n (%)	**28**	**19 (68)**	**5 (18)**	**4 (14)**	**44**	**32 (73)**	**10 (22)**	**2 (5)**
PHT								
Monotherapy	4	1	2	1	21	9	8	4
+ VPA	1	1		1	6	2	3	1
+ PB	7	2	4	1	12	5	6	1
+ PRM					3	1	2	
+ CLB	1		1					
+ PB + VPA	1		1					
+ PB + CLZ					1		1	
+ CLZ					2		2	
+ ZNS					1			1
Without CBZ, n (%)	14	4 (29)	8 (57)	2 (14)	46	17 (37)	22 (48)	7 (15)
All, including those treated in polytherapy with CBZ n (%)	**16**	**6 (38)**	**8 (50)**	**2 (12)**	**66**	**33 (50)**	**26 (39)**	**7 (11)**
PB or PRM[a]								
Monotherapy					12	1	7	4
+ CLZ					2			2
+ CBZ	7	6	1					
+ PHT	8	2	5	1	13	5	7	1
+ PHT + CBZ	1	1			8	6	2	
All with PB/PRM alone or in polytherapy	**16**	**9 (56)**	**6 (38)**	**1 (6)**	**35**	**12 (34)**	**16 (46)**	**7 (20)**
Total patients, n (%)	**40**	**23 (57)**	**11 (28)**	**6 (15)**	**104**	**50 (48)**	**39 (38)**	**15 (14)**

Data taken from 40/172 patients from Marseille/Nice (23%) and 104/254 (41%) patients from the GENESS Consortium.

[a]Only 3 with PRM in the GENESS group.

Myoclonic, tonic–clonic, and absence seizures were present in 15/18, while 3/18 had myoclonic and absence seizures only.

Ten patients (56%) were seizure-free, while eight (44%) still had seizures. However, 7 of these 8 patients had no persisting tonic–clonic seizures, bringing a total of 17 out of 18 patients who were satisfied with seizure control because grand-mal convulsions stopped. The mean time that patients were seizure-free was 33 months.

Characteristically, absences with or without myoclonic seizures persisted in 5/8. Myoclonic seizures persisted in 2/8 and tonic–clonic in one.

Seventy percent (7/10) were seizure-free on VPA monotherapy while 30% (3/10) were seizure-free on VPA associated with LTG, TPM, or LEV. Seven patients decreased seizure frequency, but in one, seizures persisted.

Side effects associated with AEDs were weight gain (three patients), depression (one

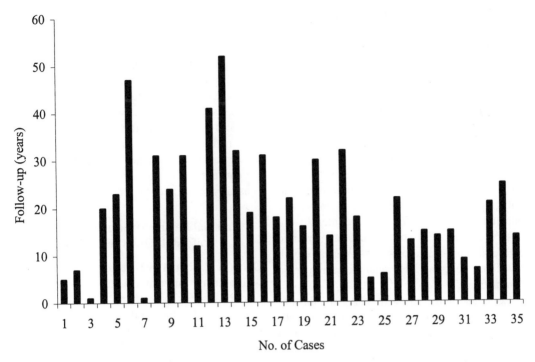

FIG. 25–4. Long-term follow-up in a cohort of 35 patients with CAE evolving to JME.

patient), hair loss (one patient), hirsutism (one patient), and tremor (one patient).

PHT, CZP, PB, PRM, and ZNS had been previously used in 11/18 (61%) of the probands, but were changed due to increase in myoclonic, tonic–clonic, and absence seizures. In one patient, absence seizures appeared at 15 years of age while taking PHT and CBZ.

Juvenile Myoclonic Epilepsy with Astatic Seizures during Adolescence

Eight patients who had astatic seizures during adolescence were followed up for a mean period of 11.1 years (range 3–18 years). Four were female and four men. Myoclonias with or without tonic–clonic and astatic seizures were present in all patients; only one reported spanioleptic absences.

Six patients were seizure-free (6/8). One had persistent astatic seizures, while another one had breakthrough tonic–clonic seizures when carba-

mazepine (CBZ) levels decreased. Mean time without seizures was 20 months.

Trigger factors for seizures were awakening (four patients), noncompliance (three patients), fatigue (two patients), alcohol (one patient), light (one patient), menses (one patient), sleep deprivation (one patient), and monetary problems leading to noncompliance (one patient).

Four out of the seven patients that were seizure-free were on VPA monotherapy; of the other two, one was taking VPA plus CBZ the other was on VPA plus LTG. Reported side effects were weight gain (two patients), hair loss (one patient), and tremor (one patient).

In one patient, the previous use of CBZ and PHT was related to the appearance of the myoclonic-astatic seizures. One patient previously treated with PHT had daily astatic seizures; this patient remained seizure-free after VPA monotherapy was started. Finally, one patient with PHT and PRM had persistent tonic–clonic seizures that stopped with VPA monotherapy.

TREATMENT OF SPECIFIC MYOCLONIC EPILEPSIES ACCORDING TO LITERATURE (TABLES 25–4 to 25–6)

Myoclonic Absence Epilepsy

Few studies have been done regarding treatment of myoclonic-absence seizures. Myoclonic absence epilepsy originally described by Tassinari et al. (4), starts during childhood (mean age 7 years) and is characterized by a specific seizure type, i.e., myoclonic absences, the diagnosis of which rests on clinical observation and polygraphic recording. Clinically rhythmic and bilateral myoclonic jerks of severe intensity are observed. The EEG shows bilateral rhythmic 3-Hz spike-and-wave complexes associated with myoclonic jerks at 3-Hz and increasing tonic contraction (5).

Combination therapy with VPA and ethosuximide (ESM) suppress myoclonic absences in almost 50% of patients. VPA in combination with other AEDs, such as clobazam (CLB) or clonazepam (CZP), can lead to good seizure control. Trials with the new generation of drugs, such as LEV, LTG, or TPM would be appropriate.

Gabapentin (GBP) and felbamate were considered to have no place in the treatment of absence seizures based on the evidence available (6). CBZ, oxcarbazepine (OXC), and vigabatrin (VGB) may worsen absence seizures. Tiagabine (TGB) as mentioned previously was reported to induce absence status (7).

Eyelid Myoclonia with Absences

Patients with this seizure type remain difficult to treat and no satisfactory drug trials have been conducted. Regarding eyelid myoclonia with absences, in the European Congress of Epileptology at Oporto, Portugal in 1994, Covanis et al. (8) reported 25 patients with eyelid myoclonia with absences or tonic–clonic seizures. Monotherapy with VPA was successful in 14, of whom 7 discontinued treatment after a mean period of 5 ± 1.3 years of treatment and all relapsed. Three patients who were not controlled with VPA responded to lamotrigine (LTG). Covanis et al. describe the utility of VPA in this group of patients in Chapter 14.

Giannakodimos et al. (9) reported a prevalence of 2.7% for eyelid myoclonia with absences in a hospital-based population study. In their series of 11 patients, 8 were treated with VPA alone or in combination with ESM, CZP, and PRM. One case was treated with CLB monotherapy and two cases were not treated with AEDs. Although absences improved in all patients taking AEDs, none had tonic–clonic seizures and eyelid myoclonia continued in nine. This finding supports the concept that eyelid myoclonia with absence is usually resistant to treatment.

Familial Benign Myoclonus Epilepsy of Adult Onset (FAME)

Okino et al. (10) in 1997 featured three families with an adult onset myoclonia. Movement and emotional stress intensify myoclonus and onset is between the third and fifth decades. Symptoms gradually worsen with age in some cases, but are not associated with dementia that distinguishes this condition from progressive myoclonus epilepsy (PME). In two of their patients clonazepam (CZP) and VPA were effective in relieving the myoclonus.

No trials on treatment for this type of epilepsy have been conducted.

TREATMENT ALGORITHM FOR JUVENILE MYOCLONIC EPILEPSY

Choice of Anticonvulsants in Juvenile Myoclonic Epilepsy: Pros and Cons

In their description of JME in 1957, Janz and Christian (11) pointed out the superior efficacy of PB compared to that of PHT. They specified the varying efficacy of AEDs and the potential for aggravation of myoclonus. In clinical practice, the treatment of myoclonic epilepsies is dominated by two facts: (a) VPA has become the standard drug, but many problems persist when efficiency is insufficient and side effects occur; (b) various AEDs clearly aggravate myoclonic seizures. Some AEDs systematically aggravate myoclonias in varying epileptic syndromes, while some aggravate myoclonic seizures of specific epilepsy syndromes. It is thus useful to provide here an

TABLE 25–4. Commonly used antiepileptic drugs in myoclonic epilepsies

Antiepileptic drugs (AEDs)	Usual adult daily doses[a]	Usual child daily doses[a]	Time required to reach steady state (days)	Blood level[b]	Elimination half-life (h)[c]	Protein binding (%)	Side effects
First- and second-generation AEDs							
Clobazam (CLB)[d]	10–30 mg (divided)	2.5 mg/kg/day	—	Not established	10–30	85	Sedation, ataxia, behavioral changes, increase salivation
Clonazepam (CZP)	1–10 mg (divided)	0.1–0.2 mg/kg/day	—	10–70 ng/ml	20–40	45	Sedation, ataxia, behavioral changes, increase salivation
Ethosuximide (ESM)	1000 mg (divided)	20–30 mg/kg/day	7–10	50–100 μg/ml	20–60	None	Nausea, fatigue, gastrointestinal irritation, behavioral changes
Methsuximide (MSM)	300–1200 mg (divided)	20 mg/kg/day	8–16	10–40 mg/l	30–80	Low	Somnolence, ataxia, headache, behavioral changes, nausea, vomiting
Valproate (VPA)	1000–3000 mg (divided)	15–60 mg/kg/day	1–2	40–150 μg/ml	6–15	80–95	Nausea, vomiting, somnolence, weight gain, gastrointestinal irritation, tremor, transient alopecia, hepatotoxicity, thrombocytopenia, hyperammonemia
Third generation AEDs							
Lamotrigine (LTG)	100–500 mg (divided)	2–8 mg/kg/day (monotherapy) 1–5 mg/kg/day (polytherapy)	7–10	1–10 μg/ml	29(14–60)	55	Headache, nausea, dizziness, diplopia, rash, ataxia, Stevens-Johnson syndrome, toxic epidermal necrolysis
Levetiracetam (LEV)	1000–3000 mg (divided)	40 mg/kg/day	2	5–40 mg/l	6–8	None	Behavioral changes
Topiramate (TPM)	100–400 mg (divided)	6–15 mg/kg/day	5	4–10 mg/l	19–23	9–17	Lethargy, paresthesias, ataxia, poor concentration, renal lithiasis, acute-angle closure glaucoma, weight loss
Zonisamide (ZNS)	200–400 mg (divided)	4–20 mg/kg/day	14	15–40 mg/l	50–70	40–60	Fatigue, somnolence, behavioral changes, anorexia, renal lithiasis

[a]This is a maintenance dose; a lower dose is necessary when initiating therapy.
[b]Therapeutic levels may change with multiple drugs.
[c]Half-life may also change with multiple drugs. Half-life is given for adult dosages. Steady state is reached in four half-lives.
[d]Not FDA approved.

TABLE 25–5. *Effect of first- and second-generation antiepileptic drugs on myoclonic epilepsies based on class III and IV evidence*

Seizure type	First- and second-generation AEDs						
	PB/PRM	PHT	MSM	CZP	CLB	CBZ	VPA
Myoclonic astatic	↑	↑	+	+/↑	+	↑	+
Myoclonic		↑		+	+	↑	+
Absences	↑	↑	+	+		↑	+
Clonic		↑		+		↑	+
Tonic–clonic and clonic–tonic–clonic	+	+		+	0	+/↑	+

+, decreases seizures; ↑, aggravates seizures; 0, no effect on seizures.
PB, Phenobarbital; PRM, primidone; PHT, phenytoin; MSM, methsuximide; CZP, clonazepam, CLB, clobazam; CBZ, carbamazepine; VPA, valproic acid.

algorithm for the treatment of JME based on the accumulated experience of the editors. The treatment results from the two largest JME cohorts, namely, the Marseille/Nice experience (12) and GENESS JME (13) consortium as well as recent published literature.

Decision Point 1. When Do You Start Treatment with Antiepileptic Drugs in Juvenile Myoclonic Epilepsy? (Fig. 25–5)

Treatment is started when "myoclonic seizures only" are present with EEG (electroencephalogram) polyspike-and-slow wave complexes or when the patient with "myoclonic seizures only" is known to belong to a family afflicted with JME. This is the usual clinical presentation of 68% of JME patients, whose first seizures consist of "myoclonic seizures only" (13).

Treatment is obligatory when JME starts with a single tonic–clonic seizure associated with EEG polyspike-and-slow wave complexes or when JME is initiated by two tonic–clonic or clonic–tonic–clonic grand-mal seizures. Treatment is also obligatory when JME starts with myoclonic seizures associated with absence seizures.

When myoclonic seizures are recurrent and the EEG is normal, prolonged EEG recordings especially in the awakening hours either as an outpatient or inpatient should be performed.

Decision Point 2. What Are the Treatment Options for Juvenile Myoclonic Epilepsy?

Among the various AEDs, VPA has historically been considered the drug of choice for JME. Jeavons et al. (14,15) first reported the effectiveness of VPA in patients who fit the

TABLE 25–6. *Effect of third-generation drugs on myoclonic epilepsies based on class III and IV evidence*

Seizure type	Third-generation AEDs							
	GBP	LTG	VGB	ZNS	OXC	TGB	TPM	LEV
Myoclonic/astatic		+/↑	↑					+
Myoclonic		+/↑	↑	+	↑	↑	+	+
Absences	↑	+		↑	↑	↑	0	+/↑
Clonic		+/↑	+					−
Tonic–clonic and clonic–tonic–clonic		+	+				+	+

+, decreases seizures; ↑, aggravates seizures; 0, no effect on seizures.
GBP, gabapentin; LTG, lamotrigine; VGB, vigabatrin; ZNS, zonisamide; OXC, oxcarbacepine; TGB, tiagabine; TPM, topiramate; LEV, levetiracetam.

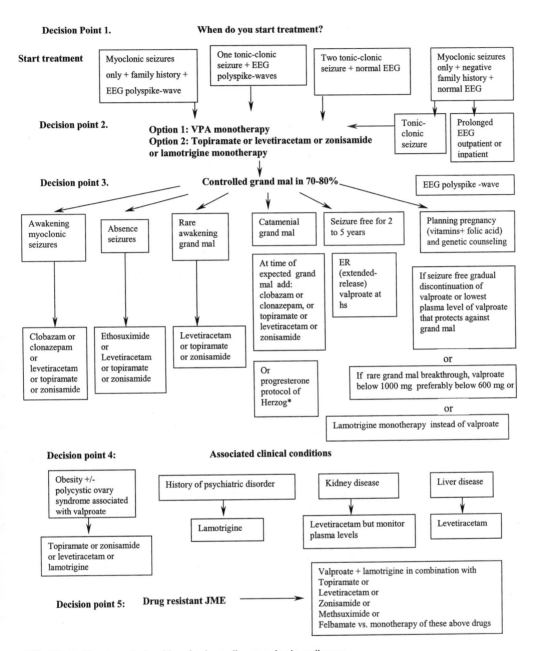

FIG. 25–5. Treatment algorithm for juvenile myoclonic epilepsy.

diagnosis of JME listed under the aegis of generalized epilepsies of childhood and adolescence. Delgado-Escueta and Enrile-Bacsal (16) in their series of 43 JME patients, observed as high as 86% of patients were either seizure-free or satisfactorily controlled on VPA as mono- or poly-therapy. Since then, various authors have reported VPA to be effective in 25% to 95% of JME patients depending on the series (12,17–24). In our study of 161 classic JME patients, VPA completely suppressed all forms of seizures in 56% (71/127) of patients and tonic–clonic or clonic–tonic–clonic grand-mal seizures in 85% of patients that had been followed up from a mean period of 10.1 years (range 1 to 41 years) (13).

However, pharmacoresistance in some, the risk of weight gain, and polycystic ovarian syndrome and the potential for teratogenesis during pregnancy can make VPA an unacceptable choice, especially for women in their childbearing years.

Topiramate, LEV, ZNS, and LTG as single-entry drugs are options, based on small series that show promising results. Earlier studies assessed TPM in primary generalized epilepsies in randomized double-blind studies, but few JME patients were included (25,26). Kellett et al. (27) reported one case of "refractory juvenile myoclonic epilepsy" in which addition of 100 mg of TPM to current dose of VPA and LTG resulted in remission of seizures. Prasad et al. (28) retrospectively studied 72 patients with JME. They reported that seizure outcome did not differ in JME patients receiving VPA mono- (36 patients) or polytherapy (22 patients) compared to those receiving LTG mono- (14 patients) or polytherapy (21 patients). No differences were found in patients that used VPA polytherapy (22 patients) vs. TPM polytherapy (15 patients) ($p > 0.05$ for all). Prasad et al. (28) concluded that "lamotrigine and topiramate offered advantages with regard to improved myoclonic seizure control."

Lamotrigine use in myoclonic epilepsies, however, is controversial. Although effective against absences and tonic–clonic seizures, LTG has been reported to exacerbate myoclonic seizures or even to produce nonconvulsive *status epilepticus* (29–31). It, nevertheless, has also been reported to be effective as monotherapy in JME (32–37).

Although studied in small cohorts, LEV and ZNS also show promise as monotherapy agents in JME. Greenhill et al., in a report at the American Epilepsy Society Meeting in 2002, studied 37 JME patients who had been on levetiracetam (LEV) for at least 6 months to as long as 5 years; 60% were seizure free. They remark that it "seems even more effective for patients with JME than partial onset epilepsy…" (38). Mullin

et al. reported 9 patients with poorly controlled JME who were placed on zonisamide (ZNS) as adjunctive treatment. Among 9 patients who received this drug, eight had marked improvement (>50% reduction in seizure frequency) and four were seizure-free on monotherapy. One patient developed a rash (39).

Nicolson et al. (40,41) studied 726 patients from Liverpool, England with idiopathic generalized epilepsies and estimated overall remission rates. Kaplan–Meier analyses showed similar retention rates for VPA, LTG, and TPM "reflecting similar equivalence in combined measures of efficacy and tolerability." However, when 1-year period of remission rates were compared, VPA monotherapy was superior (52%), with lower rates for LTG (16.7%) and TPM (35%). Nicolson et al. concluded that "valproate may be the most effective antiepileptic drug in the treatment of the IGEs." Trinka et al. (42) reached similar conclusions after studying 126 JME patients from Innsbruck, Austria, who received VPA, LTG, PRM, CZP, and ESM was found to be most effective for achieving complete freedom from seizures; 66% of seizure-free patients were on this AED. Only 4% of patients who were prescribed an agent other than VPA as their first agent were seizure-free.

Because of the reports of Nicolson et al. (40,41) and Trinka et al. (42) and because of our long-term experience with VPA we still prefer to start treatment of JME with this drug in the absence of pregnancy plans and weight gain.

Decision Point 3. Breakthrough Awakening: Myoclonic or Myoclonic Plus Absence Seizures

Valproate monotherapy completely suppressed tonic–clonic and clonic–tonic–clonic seizures in 85% of patients with classic JME, in 74% of childhood absence epilepsy evolving to JME, in 94% of JME with adolescent pyknoleptic absences, and 75% of JME with astatic seizures. Myoclonic and absence seizures can breakthrough in classic JME during awakening hours (21/103 or 20% of VPA monotherapy in classic JME patients). European neurologists usually prescribe 10 mg CLB or 0.5 mg CZP at the hour of sleep as add-on therapy.

In a retrospective study on CLB in Canada, frequencies of myoclonic seizure dropped more than 50% in approximately one-half of the patients, while complete control was achieved in approximately 20%. The study did not specify the type of epileptic syndrome, but only the seizure types. In this study, CLB was not effective in stopping tonic–clonic seizures. Somnolence was reported as the most common side effect (43).

Two patients with JME were included in an open–labeled trial evaluating CLB in 26 cases of drug-naïve adult patients with epilepsy. Overall results reported 64% of the 26 cases became seizure-free. The most common side effect was sedation (44). Obeid and Panayiotopoulos (45) prospectively studied CZP in 17 JME patients. It was given alone or in combination with VPA, CBZ, or PHT. It reduced myoclonic seizures but not generalized tonic–clonic seizures.

Because CLB is not approved by the FDA (Food and Drug Administration) and because it does not reduce tonic–clonic convulsions, we prefer to add LEV, TPM, or ZNS. Avoidance of sleep deprivation, alcohol, extreme fatigue, and other trigger factors (Table 25–2) should also be part of the treatment in JME.

When absence seizures break through as the sole phenotype in the subsyndromes of childhood absence evolving to JME and pyknoleptic adolescent absence with JME, ESM can be added to VPA.

Rare Breakthrough Awakening Tonic–Clonic Grand-Mal Seizures

As in awakening myoclonic or myoclonic and absence seizures, a change in life style is recommended to diminish effects of trigger factors (Table 25–2). LEV 500 mg bid or TPM 50 mg bid or ZNS 100 mg in the morning and 200 mg at night as add-on therapy to VPA can reduce breakthrough tonic–clonic seizures.

Catamenial Exacerbation of Tonic–Clonic Grand-Mal Seizures

Grand-mal seizures can breakthrough 2 days before, during, or 2 days after menses (menstruation phase) or during ovulatory phase (46). CLB, CZP, TPM, LEV, or ZNS can be added, as suggested above, during the expected time of breakthrough grand-mal seizures. When these additions fail, the use of progesterone, according to Herzog's protocol (47), may be recommended, or progesterone may be used according to the Herzog's protocol.

Seizure-Free for 6 Months to 5 Years

Once JME patients have been seizure-free for 6 months, the dosage of VPA can be reduced to prevent chronic side effects, such as obesity and polycystic ovary syndrome. In our cohort of classic JME 12 of 126 patients on VPA presented side effects including increased weight in five, obesity in three, and polycystic ovary syndrome in two. Two patients developed pancreatitis during chronic VPA treatment.

Panayiotopoulos et al. (18) successfully reduced VPA to 400 mg/day in 15 patients previously treated with high doses. All patients remained seizure-free. De Toffol et al. (48) treated eleven JME patients with 500 mg/day sustained-release VPA during a mean follow up of 33 months: none of the patients had tonic–clonic seizures, however, some had persistent myoclonic seizures that were considered by the authors as less frequent and less intense. Sundqvist et al. (20) compared 1000 mg vs. 2000 mg VPA in JME during a double-blind, randomized, cross-over study of 16 patients. No significant differences were found in seizure frequency for any seizure type between the two doses. Only 25% of patients were seizure-free throughout the study. In their observation a >5% weight gain was found in 63% of their 16 patients as a common side effect; other side effects reported were gastritis, diarrhea, sedation, tremor, and alopecia. Panagariya et al. (22) showed that 63.1% of 76 patients had good seizure control on 15 mg/kg per day of VPA.

After a 2-year interval of being seizure-free, 58% of patients could be maintained on dosages ranging from 3 to 5 mg/kg per day to 6 to 8 mg/kg per day. Karlovassitou-Koniari et al. (23) in a prospective trial with 14 JME patients, suggested the use of a single-dose extended-release VPA (500 mg per day). Generalized tonic–clonic and absence seizures were controlled in all patients and only one patient had breakthrough myoclonic seizures due to sleep deprivation.

Based on these studies, low dosages of extended-release VPA (400 to 500 mg at hour of sleep) can be safely used to control seizures in JME, after they have been in remission of at least 6 months.

Pregnancy and Juvenile Myoclonic Epilepsy

When planning pregnancy, genetic counseling should be given to all women. Multivitamins with folic acid should be prescribed to all women of childbearing age. If the patient has been completely free from seizures on VPA monotherapy, it can be gradually discontinued or reduced to the lowest plasma level that protects against generalized tonic–clonic seizures. If rare generalized tonic–clonic seizures break through, and VPA has to be used, it should be maintained below 600 mg. Monitoring of pregnancy with ultrasound and alpha-fetoprotein can detect most cases of spina bifida aperta (49–51). VPA has been associated with spina bifida aperta in 1 to 2% (RR 4.9, CI 95%) and with other major birth defects (52–55). We prefer not to use this AED in pregnant women with epilepsy. Lamotrigine is an alternative AED in JME during pregnancy (56). No data is currently available on the use of LEV or TPM in pregnancy.

Decision Point 4:
Associated Clinical Conditions

When obesity or polycystic ovary syndrome occur during VPA therapy, TPM or ZNS can be used, as both can reduce weight. When a history of psychiatric disorders such as depression, agitation or psychosis is present, LTG is preferable. In these cases LEV, TPM, and ZNS should be avoided because they can exacerbate psychiatric conditions.

Decision Point 5: Drug-Resistant Juvenile Myoclonic Epilepsy

In our cohort, JME was truly refractory to AED in 14% (22/161). Gelisse et al. (57) distinguished between "truly resistant group" and the "pseudoresistant" JME. This second group of "pseudoresistant" JME implies poor compliance, risky life style or inadequate choice of drugs; careful attention should be paid to these factors before considering that a patient is refractory. These authors also evaluated clinical factors such as seizure type (namely, the combination of myoclonic, absence, and tonic–clonic seizures) and the coexistence of psychiatric problems that are found in patients with refractory JME.

When seizures persist in JME, add-on therapy to VPA is usually considered first. When this fails, another AED is used as monotherapy. In our cohort, 24 of 161 patients were on VPA polytherapy and 10 (42%) were seizure-free. AEDs used as "add on" to VPA included LTG (five patients), CBZ (one patient), CZP (one patient), lorazepam (one patient), PHT (one patient), and TPM (one patient).

Eighteen patients were on monotherapy with drugs other than VPA. Eleven (61%) were seizure-free. Carbamazepine (three patients), LEV (two patients), LTG (two patients), PB (two patients), PRM (one patient), and TPM (one patient) were also effective as monotherapy.

In 1960, Rabe (58) first reported the effects of methsuximide (MSM) on the myoclonus of four patients with JME. Two were seizure-free and the other two had reduction of 75% in frequency of myoclonus. Hurst (59) used methsuximide (MSM) as an alternative therapy for JME in five female patients. All were seizure-free. One was seizure free for 7 years and had breakthrough seizures during an attempt to discontinue this drug.

Anecdotal reports on the use of other AEDs in JME have been reported. In 1957, Janz (11) recommended PB for the treatment of myoclonic seizures and reported complete control in 24/36 patients. Frequencies of myoclonic seizures were reduced in nine patients. Phenobarbital controlled grand mal in 15/21 patients and reduced incidence in 3. In these earlier years, it was noted that PB and PRM were much more efficient than PHT in the treatment of JME. Although most of their patients were treated with combinations of PB plus PHT at fixed doses, Janz and Christian (11) noted in 1957 that a "predominantly barbituric" regimen controlled 86% of JME patients. Because later series on the treatment of myoclonic epilepsies did not show true benefit from PB because of its secondary effects on cognition and awareness, it is not currently considered a treatment choice for JME.

LEV can be used as monotherapy or in combination with VPA. Cohen (60) reported the use of LEV as monotherapy for primary generalized epilepsy in three patients. One had JME, which was successfully controlled with VPA which had to be stopped because of considerable weight gain. On LEV monotherapy, the patient remained seizure-free for over 6 months. Krauss et al. (61) in a series of ten patients with JME, reported that all tolerated LEV monotherapy, but only two became seizure-free. Antimyoclonic efficacy has also been reported in postanoxic myoclonus and in PME (62) with use of this AED.

Thus, AEDs that can be recommended in uncontrolled JME patients include VPA plus LTG, TPM, LEV, or ZNS, MSM, or FBM. Some of these AEDs can be used as monotherapy.

Antiepileptic Drugs that Aggravate Juvenile Myoclonic Epilepsy

CBZ, OXC, PHT, TGB, VGB, and gabapentin (GBP) can aggravate seizures in JME. In our cohort, CBZ and/or PHT increased seizure frequency in 48% of the patients previously treated with these AEDs.

Genton et al. (12) in 2000, reported that among 40 JME patients treated with CBZ or PHT alone or in combination, 58% (23/40) clearly experienced aggravation, whereas 15% (6/40) improved and 27% (11/40) had no change in seizure frequency. In their series, one patient had absence and myoclonic *status* due to VGB and CBZ.

CBZ and OXC can aggravate myoclonias, increase or precipitate absences, and even cause both myoclonic and absence *status epilepticus* in patients with myoclonic epilepsy. Some authors had proposed their use to control generalized tonic–clonic seizures in myoclonic epilepsies. Due to the risk of seizure exacerbation, it is not advisable to include these drugs as treatment options for JME (12,63–65).

Kivity et al. (66) reported that PHT aggravates seizures in 38%–80% of JME patients.

TGB can also worsen primary generalized epilepsies. It may provoke absences and nonconvulsive *status epilepticus* in idiopathic generalized epilepsy (IGE), including one patient with JME (7).

Gabapentin was reported by Asconape et al. (67) to induce multifocal myoclonus and exacerbation of preexistent myoclonus in ten patients. In all cases, myoclonus was subtle, did not interfere with daily activities, and stopped with discontinuation of this drug.

Case reports have suggested induction of myoclonic status in patients with simple and complex partial seizures who receive vigabatrin (68–70).

Quality of Life in Juvenile Myoclonic Epilepsy

In clinical studies, reduction in seizure frequency is the primary measure of efficacy of an AED. In clinical practice, however, seizure severity and psychological well being are also relevant to the assessment of overall therapeutic benefit (71). A survey of the follow-up and treatment update of JME patients was conducted by Medina et al. (13). Fifty-five patients (35 females and 20 males), responded to a questionnaire, which predominantly concerned quality of life issues. Forty-three patients were taking VPA, seven PHT, five CZP, five CBZ, three PRM, two PB, one ESM, and seven were without treatment. Quality of life was rated very good in 33 patients (60%), good in 12 patients (22%), fair in 7 patients (12%), and bad in 2 patients (4%). Two other patients (2%) did not answer the questionnaire. Patients who considered their quality of life fair or bad, identified problems in work or in school.

REFERENCES

1. Genton P, Dravet C. Treatment of epilepsies with my-oclonias. In: Shorvon S, Dreifuss F, Fish D, Thomas D. eds. *The treatment of epilepsy,* London: Blackwell Science, 1996:247–257.
2. Wallace SJ. Myoclonus and epilepsy in childhood: a review of treatment with valproate, ethosuximide, lamotrigine and zonisamide. *Epilepsy Res* 1998;29:147–154.
3. Wheless JW, Sankar R. Treatment strategies for myoclonic seizures and epilepsy syndromes with myoclonic seizures. *Epilepsia* 2003;44[Suppl 11]:27–37.
4. Tassinari CA, Lyagoubi S, Santos V, et al. Etude des décharges de pointes ondes chez l home II: Les aspects cliniques et électroencéphalographiques des absences myocloniques. *Rev Neurol* 1969;121:379–383.
5. Bureau M, Tassinari CA. The syndrome of myoclonic absence. In: Roger J, Bureau M, Dravet C. Genton P, Tassinari CA, Wolf P. eds. *Epileptic syndromes in infancy, childhood and adolescence.* 3rd ed. London: John Libbey, 2002:305–312.
6. Chadwick, D. Gabapentin and felbamate. In: Duncan JS, Panayiotopoulos CP. eds. *Typical absences and related epileptic syndromes.* London:Churchill Livingstone, 1995:213–220.
7. Knake S, Hammer HM, Schomburg U, et al. Tiagabine-induced absence status in idiopathic generalized epilepsy. *Seizure* 1999;8:314–317.
8. Covanis A, Skiadas K, Loli N, et al. Eyelid Myoclonia with Absence. *Epilepsia* 1994;35[Suppl 7]:13.
9. Giannakodimos S, Panayiotopoulos CP. Eyelid Myoclonia with Absences in Adults: A Clinical and Video-EEG Study. *Epilepsia* 1996;37:36–44.
10. Okino S. Familial benign myoclonus epilepsy of adult onset: A previously unrecognized myoclonic disorder. *J Neurol Sci* 1997;145:113–118.
11. Janz D, Christian W. Impulsiv Petit-Mal. *Deut Z Nervenheilk* 1957;176:346–386.
12. Genton P, Gelisse P, Thomas P, et al. Do carbamazepine and phenytoin aggravate juvenile myoclonic epilepsy? *Neurology* 2000;55:1106–1109.
13. Martínez-Juárez IE, Alonso ME, Medina MT. Long term outcome in subsyndromes of Juvenile Myoclonic Epilepsy. *Neurology* 2004,67[Suppl 5]:A248.
14. Jeavons PM, Clark JE, Maheshwari MC. Treatment of generalized epilepsies of childhood and adolescence with sodium valproate (Epilium). *Develop Med Child Neurol* 1977;19:9–25.
15. Jeavons PM. Monotherapy with sodium valproate. In: Dam M, Gram L, Pedersen B, Orum H. eds. *Valproate in the treatment of seizures.* Hvidore, Denmark: Danish Epilepsy Society, 1981:43–50.
16. Delgado-Escueta AV, Enrile-Bacsal F. Juvenile myoclonic epilepsy of Janz. *Neurology* 1984;34:285–294.
17. Clement MJ, Wallace SJ. Juvenile myoclonic epilepsy. *Arch Dis Childhood* 1988;63:1049–1053.
18. Panayiotopoulos CP, Obeid T, Tahan AR. Juvenile myoclonic epilepsy: A 5-year prospective study. *Epilepsia* 1994;35:285–296.
19. Penry JK, Dean JC, Riela AR. *Juvenile myoclonic epilepsy:* Long-term response to therapy. *Epilepsia* 1994;35(2):302–306.
20. Sundqvist A, Tomson T, Lundkvist B. Valproate as monotherapy for juvenile myoclonic epilepsy: dose-effect study. *Ther Drug Monitor* 1998;20:149–157.
21. Calleja S, Salas-Puig J, Ribacoba R, Lahoz CH. Evolution of juvenile myoclonic epilepsy treated from the outset with sodium valproate. *Seizure* 2001;10:424–427.
22. Panagariya A, Sureka RK, Sardana V. Juvenile Myoclonic Epilepsy—An experience from north western India. *Acta Neurol Scand* 2001;104:12–16.
23. Karlovassitou-Koniari A, Alexiou D, Angelopoulos P, et al. Low dose sodium valproate in the treatment of juvenile myoclonic epilepsy. *J Neurol* 2002;249:396–399.
24. Thibault M, Blume WT, Saint-Hilaire JM, et al. Divalproex extended-release versus the original divalproex tablet: Results of a randomized, crossover study of well-controlled epileptic patients with primary generalized seizures. *Epilepsy Res* 2002;50:243–249.
25. Biton V. Preliminary open-label experience with topiramate in primary generalized seizures. *Epilepsia* 1997;38[Suppl 1]:S42–S44.
26. Biton V, Montouris GD, Ritter F, et al. Topiramate YTC Study Group. A randomized, placebo-controlled study of topiramate in primary generalized tonic-clonic seizures. *Neurology* 1999;52:1330–1337.
27. Kellet MW, Smith DF, Stockton PA, et al. Topiramate in clinical practice: first year's postlicensing experience in a specialist's epilepsy clinic. *J Neurol Neurosurg Psych* 1999;66:759–763.
28. Prasad A, Zuzniecky RI, Knowlton RC, et al. Evolving antiepileptic drug treatment in juvenile myoclonic epilepsy. *Arch Neurol* 2003;60:1100–1105.
29. Biraben A, Allain H, Scarabin JM, et al. Exacerbation of juvenile myoclonic epilepsy with lamotrigine. *Neurology* 2000;55:17508.
30. Carrazana EJ, Wheeler SD. Exacerbation of juvenile myoclonic epilepsy with lamotrigine. *Neurology* 2001;56:1424 [letter to the editor].
31. Trinka E, Dilitz E, Unterberger I, Luef G, et al. Non convulsive status epilepticus after replacement of valproate with lamotrigine. *J Neurol* 2002;249:1417–1422.
32. Timmings PL, Richens A. Lamotrigine in primary generalized epilepsy. *Lancet* 1992;339:1300–1301.
33. Buchanan N. Lamotrigine: clinical experience in 93 patients with epilepsy. *Acta Neurol Scand* 1995;92:28–32.
34. Buchanan N. The use of lamotrigine in juvenile myoclonic epilepsy. *Seizure* 1996;5:149–151.
35. Beran RG, Berkovic SF, Dunagan FM, et al. Double-blind, placebo-controlled, crossover study of lamotrigine in treatment-resistant generalized epilepsy. *Epilepsia* 1998;39:1329–1333.
36. Gericke CA, Picard F, de Saint-Martin A, et al. Efficacy of lamotrigine in idiopathic generalized epilepsy syndromes: A video-EEG-controlled, open study. *Epileptic Disord* 1999;1:159–165.
37. Barron TF, Hunt SL, Timothy CRNP, et al. Lamotrigine Monotherapy in Children. *Pediatr Neurol* 2000;23:160–163.
38. Greenhill L, Betts T, Smith K. Effect of levetiracetam for treatment of drug-resistant generalized epilepsy. *Epilepsia* 2001:42 [Suppl 7]:179 [Abstr.].

39. Mullin P, Stern JM, Delgado-Escueta AV, Eliashiv D. Effectiveness of open-label zonisamide in juvenile myoclonic epilepsy. *Epilepsia* 2001;42[Suppl 7]:184.

40. Chadwick DW, Nicolson A, Smith DF. The relationship between treatment with valproate, lamotrigine, and topiramate and the prognosis of the idiopathic generalized epilepsies. *Epilepsia* 2001;42[Suppl 7]:177 [Abstr.].

41. Nicolson A, Appleton RE, Chadwick DW, et al. The relationship between treatment with valproate, lamotrigine, and topiramate and the prognosis of the idiopathic generalized epilepsies. *J Neurol Neurosurg Psych* 2004;75:75–79.

42. Trinka E, Unterrainer J, Unterberger I, et al. Juvenile myoclonic epilepsy: medical treatment response and prognostic factors for complete seizure remission. *Epilepsia* 2001;42[Suppl 7]:158 [Abstr.].

43. Canadian Clobazam Cooperative Group. Clobazam in treatment of refractory epilepsy: The Canadian experience. A retrospective study. *Epilepsia* 1991;407–416.

44. Mehndiratta MM, Krishnamurthy M, Rajesh KN, et al. Clobazam monotherapy in drug naive adult patients with epilepsy. *Seizure* 2003;12:226–228.

45. Obeid T, Panayiotopoulos CP. Clonazepam in juvenile myoclonic epilepsy. *Epilepsia* 1989;30:603–606.

46. Herzog AG, Klein P, Ransil BJ. Three patterns of catamenial epilepsy. *Epilepsia* 1997;38:1082–1088.

47. Herzog AG. Progesterone therapy in women with epilepsy: A 3 year follow-up. *Neurology* 52:9;1917–1918.

48. De Toffol B, Autret A. Treatment of juvenile myoclonic epilepsy with low-dose sodium valproate. *Rev Neurol (Paris)* 1996;152:708–710.

49. Brock DJ, Sutcliffe RG. Alpha-fetoprotein in the antenatal diagnosis of anencephaly and spina bifida. *Lancet* 1972;29:197–199.

50. Bradai R, Robert E. Prenatal ultrasonographic diagnosis in the epileptic mother on valproic acid. Retrospective study of 161 cases in central eastern France register of congenital malformations. *J Gynecol Obstet Biol Reprod* 1998;27:413–419.

51. Sebire NJ, Spencer K, Noble PL, et al. Maternal serum alpha-fetoprotein in fetal neural tube and abdominal wall defects at 10 to 14 weeks of gestation. *Br J Obstet Gynecol* 1997;104:849–851.

52. Chitayat D, Farrell K, Anderson L, et al. Congenital abnormalities in two sibs exposed to valproic acid in utero. *Am J Med Genet* 1988;31:369–373.

53. Nau H, Hauck RS, Ehlers K. Valproic acid-induced neural tube defects in mouse and human: Aspects of chirality, alternative drug development, pharmacokinetics and possible mechanisms. *Pharmacol Toxicol* 1991;69:310–321.

54. Samren EB, van Duijn CM, Koch S, et al. Maternal use of antiepileptic drugs and the risk of major congenital malformations: A joint European prospective study of human teratogenesis associated with maternal epilepsy. *Epilepsia* 1997;38:957–958.

55. Samren EG, van Duijn CM, Christiaens GC, et al. Antiepileptic drug regimens and major congenital abnormalities in the offspring. *Ann Neurol* 1999;46:739–746.

56. Tennis P, Eldridge RR. International Lamotrigine Pregnancy Registry Scientific Advisory Committee. *Epilepsia* 2002;43:1161–1167.

57. Gelisse P, Genton P, Thomas P, et al. Clinical factors of drug resistance in juvenile myoclonic epilepsy. *J Neurol Neurosurg Psych* 2001;70:240–243.

58. Rabe F. Celontin (Petinutin)—Ein Beitrag zur differenzierten Epilepsiebehandlung. *Nervenarzi* 1960;7:306–312.

59. Hurst DL. Methsuximide therapy of juvenile myoclonic epilepsy. *Seizure* 1996;5:47–50.

60. Cohen J. Levetiracetam monotherapy for primary generalized epilepsy. *Seizure* 2003;12:150–153.

61. Krauss GL, Abou-Khalil B, Sheth SG, et al. Efficacy of levetiracetam for treatment of drug-resistant generalized epilepsies. *Epilepsia* 2001;42[Suppl. 7]:184.

62. Genton P, Gélisse PH. Antimyoclonic effect of levetiracetam. *Epil Dis* 2000;2:209–212.

63. Mc Lean MJ, Schmutz M, Wamil AW, et al. Oxcarbazepine: mechanisms of action. *Epilepsia* 1994;35 [Suppl 3]:5–9.

64. Knott C, Panayiotopoulos CP. Carbamazepine in the treatment of generalized tonic clonic seizures in juvenile myoclonic epilepsy. *J Neurol Neurosurg Psych* 1994;57:503 [Letter].

65. Sozuer DT, Atakli D, Atay T, et al. Evaluation of various antiepileptic drugs in juvenile myoclonic epilepsy. *Epilepsia* 1996;37[Suppl 4]:S77 [Abstr.].

66. Kivity S, Rechtman E. Juvenile myoclonic epilepsy: serious consequences due to pitfalls in diagnosis and management. *Epilepsia* 1995;36[Suppl 3]:S66 [Abstr.].

67. Asconape J, Diedrich A, DellaBadia J. Myoclonus associated with the use of gabapentin. *Epilepsia* 2000;41:479–481.

68. Marciani MG, Maschio M, Spanedda F, et al. Development of myoclonus in patients with partial epilepsy during treatment with vigabatrin: an electroencephalographic study. *Acta Neurol Scand* 1995;91:1–5.

69. Neufeld NY, Vishnevska S. Vigabatrin and multifocal myoclonus in adults with partial seizures. *Clin Neuropharmacol* 1995;18:280–283.

70. Garcia-Pastor A, Garcia-Zarza E, Peraita-Adrados R. Acute encephalopathy and myoclonic status induced by vigabatrin monotherapy. *Neurologia* 2000;15:370–374.

71. Devinsky O, Penry JK. Quality of life in epilepsy: Clinician's view. *Epilepsia* 1993;34[Suppl 4]:4–7.

Subject Index

Page numbers followed by *f* indicate a figure; *t* following a page number indicates tabular material